Music and Empathy

T0384824

In recent years, empathy has received considerable research attention as a means of understanding a range of psychological phenomena, and it is fast drawing attention within the fields of music psychology and music education. This volume seeks to promote and stimulate further research in music and empathy, with contributions from many of the leading scholars in the fields of music psychology, neuroscience, music philosophy and education. It exposes current developmental, cognitive, social and philosophical perspectives on research in music and empathy, and considers the notion in relation to our engagement with different types of music and media. Following a Prologue, the volume presents twelve chapters organised into two main areas of enquiry. The first section, entitled 'Empathy and Musical Engagement', explores empathy in music education and therapy settings, and provides social, cognitive and philosophical perspectives about empathy in relation to our interaction with music. The second section, entitled 'Empathy in Performing Together', provides insights into the role of empathy across non-Western, classical, jazz and popular performance domains. This book will be of interest to music educators, musicologists, performers and practitioners, as well as scholars from other disciplines with an interest in empathy research.

Elaine King is Senior Lecturer in Music at the University of Hull. She co-edited *Music and Gesture* (Ashgate 2006), *New Perspectives on Music and Gesture* (Ashgate 2011) and *Music and Familiarity* (Ashgate 2013), and has published book chapters and articles on aspects of ensemble rehearsal and performance. She is a member of the Royal Musical Association (Council, 2009–12) and Society for Education, Music and Psychology Research (Conference Secretary, 2006–12) as well as Associate Editor of *Psychology of Music*. She is an active cellist, pianist and conductor.

Caroline Waddington received her Master of Music in Solo Performance from the Royal Northern College of Music and her PhD in Music from the University of Hull, for which she carried out research on peak performance and empathy in ensemble playing. She enjoys a busy portfolio career in music performance, research and education. Caroline also has a strong commitment to arts and health work and delivers various projects in hospitals, hospices and special schools around the UK.

SEMPRE Studies in The Psychology of Music
Series Editors:
Graham Welch, University of London, UK, Adam Ockelford, Roehampton
University, UK and Ian Cross, University of Cambridge, UK

The theme for the series is the psychology of music, broadly defined. Topics include (i) musical development at different ages, (ii) exceptional musical development in the context of special educational needs, (iii) musical cognition and context, (iv) culture, mind and music, (v) micro to macro perspectives on the impact of music on the individual (from neurological studies through to social psychology), (vi) the development of advanced performance skills and (vii) affective perspectives on musical learning. The series presents the implications of research findings for a wide readership, including user-groups (music teachers, policy makers, parents) as well as the international academic and research communities. This expansive embrace, in terms of both subject matter and intended audience (drawing on basic and applied research from across the globe), is the distinguishing feature of the series, and it serves SEMPRE's distinctive mission, which is to promote and ensure coherent and symbiotic links between education, music and psychology research.

Recent titles in the series:

Listening in Action
Rebecca M. Rinsema

Embodiment of Musical Creativity
Zvonimir Nagy

Communities of Musical Practice
Ailbhe Kenny

Music, Technology and Education
Edited by Andrew King and Evangelos Himonides

Creative Teaching for Creative Learning in Higher Music Education
Edited by Elizabeth Haddon and Pamela Burnard

Collaborative Creative Thought and Practice in Music
Edited by Margaret S. Barrett

The Tangible in Music
Marko Aho

Music and Empathy

Edited by Elaine King and
Caroline Waddington

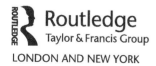
Routledge
Taylor & Francis Group
LONDON AND NEW YORK

First published 2017 by Routledge

2 Park Square, Milton Park, Abingdon, Oxfordshire OX14 4RN

711 Third Avenue, New York, NY 10017

Routledge is an imprint of the Taylor & Francis Group, an informa business

First issued in paperback 2018

British Library Cataloguing-in-Publication Data
A catalogue record for this book is available from the British Library

Library of Congress Cataloging-in-Publication Data
Names: King, Elaine, 1974– | Waddington, Caroline.
Title: Music and empathy / edited by Elaine King and Caroline Waddington.
Description: Abingdon, Oxon; New York: Routledge, 2017. | Includes bibliographical references and index.
Identifiers: LCCN 2016038682 | ISBN 9781472445803 (hardback) | ISBN 9781315596587 (ebook)
Subjects: LCSH: Music—Psychological aspects. | Empathy.
Classification: LCC ML3838 .M948 2017 | DDC 781.1/1—dc23
LC record available at https://lccn.loc.gov/2016038682

ISBN: 978-1-4724-4580-3 (hbk)
ISBN: 978-1-138-58682-6 (pbk)

Typeset in Times New Roman
by codeMantra

Contents

Figures

Tables

Music examples

Notes on contributors

Claudio Babiloni is Associate Professor in the Department of Physiology and Pharmacology at the University of Rome, *La Sapienza* (Rome, Italy) and at the Institute for Research and Medical Care, IRCCS San Raffaele Pisana (Rome, Italy). He has a PhD in Biomedical Sciences and is an experienced neurophysiologist with a special interest in the study of biological and neuroimaging underpinnings of cognitive–motor functions in humans. He has published extensively on neurophysiology and clinical neurophysiology, many of his papers on quantitative electroencephalography (EEG).

Ivo Bruni is a biomedical engineer, and a past and honorary president of EB-NEURO S.p.A.

Claudio Del Percio received a PhD in Neurophysiology at the University of Rome *La Sapienza* (Rome, Italy). He is affiliated to the Department of Integrated Imaging, IRCCS SDN (Naples, Italy). He is an experienced neurophysiologist with a special interest in the study of quantitative electroencephalography (EEG) and he has published widely on neurophysiology and clinical neurophysiology.

Peter Elsdon is Senior Lecturer in Music at the University of Hull. His book on Keith Jarrett's *The Köln Concert* was published by Oxford University Press in 2013. He has also published work on Jarrett, John Coltrane and Icelandic rock band Sigur Rós. With Jenny Doctor and Björn Heile, he is co-editor of the forthcoming volume *Watching Jazz: Encountering Jazz Performance on Film and Television* (OUP).

Anthony Gritten is Head of Undergraduate Programmes at the Royal Academy of Music, London. His publications include two co-edited volumes on *Music and Gesture* (Ashgate, 2006, 2011) and essays in visual artists' catalogues, on the thought of Lyotard, Nancy and Bakhtin, and on the music of Stravinsky, Cage and Delius. His articles in *Performance Studies* have considered issues including distraction, problem solving, ethics, ergonomics and technology. He is a Fellow of the Royal College of Organists, and has performed across the UK, France and Canada. Projects have included premieres of pieces by Daniel Roth, including his magnum opus, *Livre d'Orgue pour le Magnificat*, and anniversary cycles of the complete works of Tunder, Buxtehude, Homilius and Mendelssohn.

Elaine King is Senior Lecturer in Music at the University of Hull. She co-edited *Music and Gesture* (Ashgate, 2006), *New Perspectives on Music and Gesture* (Ashgate, 2011) and *Music and Familiarity* (Ashgate, 2013), and has published book chapters and articles on aspects of ensemble rehearsal and performance in various journals, including *Psychology of Music* and *Musicae Scientiae*. She is a member of the Royal Musical Association (Council, 2009–12) and Society for Education, Music and Psychology Research (Conference Secretary, 2006–12) as well as Associate Editor of *Psychology of Music*. She is an active cellist, pianist and conductor.

Felicity Laurence has an international background as music educationist, composer and researcher in intercultural musical work, most recently conducted in Palestine and Israel. She has researched and published in the area of empathy and musicking within various disciplinary fields including that of music education, music and conflict resolution and applied ethnomusicology. Her recent publications include edited volumes entitled *Masterclass in Music Education* (Bloomsbury, 2013) and *Music and Solidarity* (Rutgers University, 2011), and chapters in *The Oxford Handbook of Music Education* (OUP, 2012), *Sociology and Music Education* (Ashgate, 2010) and *Music and Conflict Transformation* (Tauris, 2008).

Andrei C. Miu is Director of the Cognitive Neuroscience Laboratory and Professor at the Department of Psychology, Babeş-Bolyai University from Cluj-Napoca, Romania. His research has focused on human emotions, including the influence of emotions on cognitive processes, physiological correlates of emotions and genetic influences on emotions. As a result of his taste for opera music and his scientific interest in emotions, he started studying music-induced emotions. His recent work on the psychophysiology and genetics of music-induced emotions was supported by an 'Arnold Bentley Award' and a 'Reg and Molly Buck Award' from the Society for Education, Music and Psychology Research (SEMPRE). He is on the editorial boards of several international journals, including *Emotion* and *Translational Neuroscience*.

Istvan Molnar-Szakacs received a Bachelor of Science with Honours from Dalhousie University, Canada in Neuroscience and Biology in 2000. He earned his doctorate in Neuroscience from UCLA in 2005, studying the neural basis of non-verbal social communication. He is also a graduate of the FPR-UCLA Center for Culture, Brain and Development's pre-doctoral training program. He spent a year as a post-doctoral fellow at the Swiss Federal Institute of Technology (EPFL) in Lausanne, Switzerland. In 2006, he joined UCLA's Semel Institute for Neuroscience and Human Behavior as a Research Neuroscientist and co-ordinator of the Tenenbaum Center for the Biology of Creativity, staying until 2010. Istvan is currently living and writing in Canada.

Adam Ockelford is Professor of Music at the University of Roehampton, London. He studied oboe, piano, harpsichord and composition at the Royal Academy of Music from 1977–81 where he developed a lifelong fascination for music, as a composer, performer, teacher and researcher. While attending the Academy, he started working with children with special needs – a number of whom, he noticed, had special musical abilities too – and he became interested in how we all intuitively make sense of music without the need for formal education. He pursued this line of enquiry, and gained a PhD in music at Goldsmith's College, London in 1993 in which he set out his 'zygonic' theory of musical understanding. This theory has proved a valuable tool in music theory and analysis, in investigating musical development, and exploring interaction in music therapy and education. He is Secretary of the Society for Education, Music and Psychology Research (SEMPRE); Chair of Soundabout, an Oxfordshire-based charity that supports music provision for children and young people with complex needs; and founder of The AMBER Trust, a charity that supports visually impaired children in their pursuit of music.

Rowan Oliver is Lecturer in Popular Music at the University of Hull. His musicological research deals primarily with groove and technology in African–American and African diasporic popular music, and he is an associate member of the Center for Black Music Research. As a professional musician he has worked internationally with a number of artists, including seven years as the drummer with *Goldfrapp*. Rowan continues to record, perform, produce, and remix in a range of genres alongside his academic career. He is book reviews editor for the *Journal of Music, Technology and Education*.

Daniela Perani, MD, neurologist, and radiologist, is Professor of Neuroscience at the University *Vita-Salute San Raffaele* (Milan, Italy). She is the coordinator of several national and international research projects in neurology and neuroscience. Her research deals with *in vivo* molecular and functional imaging applied to neurology and neuroscience research fields, in particular in neurodegenerative dementias, language, memory systems, and music perception. She has authored more than 200 full papers (HI 80) and several books and book chapters.

Tal-Chen Rabinowitch is a postdoctoral fellow at the Institute for Learning and Brain Sciences at the University of Washington. Her research examines the connections between music, synchrony and emotional and social interaction in toddlers and young children. She obtained her PhD at the Centre for Music and Science, University of Cambridge, where she investigated the relationship between music and empathy.

Matthew Rahaim is Associate Professor of Ethnomusicology at the University of Minnesota. He is author of *Musicking Bodies: Gesture and Voice in Hindustani Music* (Wesleyan University Press, 2012) and his articles have appeared in the *Journal of Asian Studies, World of Music, Gesture, Asian Music* and *New Perspectives on Music and Gesture* (Ashgate, 2011). He has taught at the University of California, Berkeley; Stanford University; and St. Olaf College. Rahaim also is an avid performer of Hindustani vocal music, both in India and in North America.

Evgenia Roussou is currently a doctoral student specialising in the study of piano accompaniment at the University of Hull. She holds a Bachelor of Music with Honours degree from the same institution and a Masters degree in performance with specialisation in piano accompaniment from the University of Leeds. Her doctoral research explores the techniques, skills and roles (both socio-emotional and functional) of experienced piano accompanists in the Western solo–accompaniment art duo context. Her research interests include all facets of performance studies, psychology of music, piano pedagogy, and aural training. She is an active piano accompanist involved in a variety of concerts and performances.

Jonna K. Vuoskoski currently holds postdoctoral fellowships at the University of Oxford, UK, and at the University of Jyväskylä, Finland. She received her doctorate in 2012 from the University of Jyväskylä, where she carried out research on the role of empathy and personality in music-induced emotions. Her research findings have been published in the leading journals of the field, including *Music Perception, Psychology of Music, Musicae Scientiae, Psychology of Aesthetics, Creativity, and the Arts*, and *Cortex*. Her current research interests include music and empathy, music and emotion, and cross-modal interactions in music perception.

Caroline Waddington received her Master of Music in Solo Performance from the Royal Northern College of Music and her PhD in Music from the University of Hull, where she carried out research on peak performance and co-performer empathy in expert ensemble playing. She enjoys a busy portfolio career as a freelance musician, teacher and researcher. Caroline is a founding member of the Phoenix Clarinet Quartet, with whom she won the international competition *Clarinetissim* (Spain, 2012), and the VISTA Trio, with whom she performs regularly across the UK. She has a strong commitment to education and outreach work, delivering workshops, residencies and interactive performances in various community settings on behalf of *Live Music Now* and *Music in Hospitals*.

Clemens Wöllner is Professor of Systematic Musicology at the University of Hamburg, Germany. He received an MA in Psychology of Music at the University of Sheffield and a PhD on the perception of expressiveness in conducting from Martin Luther University Halle Wittenberg. His research focuses on psychological approaches to music performance, musical gestures, multimodal perception, expertise and skill acquisition. He serves on the editorial boards of *Psychology of Music, Musicae Scientiae* and *Music Performance Research*.

Series editors' preface

The enormous growth of research that has been evidenced over the past three decades continues into the many different phenomena that are embraced under the psychology of music 'umbrella'. Growth is evidenced in new journals, books, media interest, an expansion of professional associations (regionally and nationally, such as in Southern Europe, Latin America, Asia), and with increasing and diverse opportunities for formal study, including within non-English-speaking countries. Such growth of interest is not only from psychologists and musicians, but also from colleagues working in the clinical sciences, neurosciences, therapies, in the lifelong health and well-being communities, philosophy, musicology, social psychology, ethnomusicology and education across the lifespan. As part of this global community, the Society for Education, Music and Psychology Research (SEMPRE) celebrated its 40th Anniversary in 2012 and continues to be one of the world's leading and longstanding professional associations in the field. SEMPRE is the only international society that embraces formally an interest in the psychology of music, research and education, seeking to promote knowledge at the interface between the twin social sciences of psychology and education with one of the world's most pervasive art forms, music. SEMPRE was founded in 1972 and has published the journals *Psychology of Music* since 1973 and *Research Studies in Music Education* since 2008, both now produced in partnership with SAGE (see www.sempre.org.uk), and we continue to seek new ways to reach out globally, both in print and online. This includes the launch of a new online journal *Music and Science* in 2017. We recognise that there is an ongoing need to promote the latest research findings to the widest possible audience. Through more extended publication formats, especially books, we believe that we are more likely to fulfil a key component of our mission, which is to have a distinctive and positive impact on individual and collective understanding, as well as on policy and practice internationally, both within and across our disciplinary boundaries. Hence, we welcome the strong collaborative partnership between SEMPRE and Routledge (formerly Ashgate Publishing).

The *SEMPRE Studies in The Psychology of Music* series has been designed to address this international need since its inception in 2007. The theme for the series is the psychology of music, broadly defined. Topics include (amongst others): musical development and learning at different ages; musical cognition and context; culture, mind and music; creativity, composition, and collaboration; micro to macro perspectives on the impact of music on the individual (from neurological studies through to social psychology); the development of advanced performance skills; musical behaviour and development in the context of special educational needs; and affective perspectives on musical learning. The series seeks to present the implications of research findings for a wide readership, including user-groups (music teachers, policy makers, parents and carers, music professionals working in a range of formal, non-formal and informal settings), as well as the international academic teaching and research communities and their students. A key distinguishing feature of the series is its broad focus that draws on basic and applied research from across the globe under the umbrella of SEMPRE's distinctive mission, which is to promote and ensure coherent and symbiotic links between education, music and psychology research.

We are very pleased to welcome this new text in the SEMPRE series, edited by Elaine King and Caroline Waddington, both from the University of Hull. *Music and Empathy* brings together an excellent international combination of relatively new and established authors who offer diverse yet complimentary insights into how we might make sense of the contested notion of empathy in the context of musical experience. The twelve chapters, organised into two groups, draw on current philosophical, developmental, cognitive, social, and educational perspectives on research about music and empathy. The opening cluster of chapters focuses on how to make sense of empathy in our individual engagement with music, whereas the second cluster focuses more on the nature of empathy when performing together, when we make music/experience music with others. This is an excellent and enriching addition to the SEMPRE series, not least because it seeks to get at the heart of why we are so emotionally engaged with music.

Graham Welch
UCL Institute of Education, London, UK

Adam Ockelford
Roehampton University, UK

Ian Cross
University of Cambridge, UK

Acknowledgements

We wish to thank the authors for their contributions to this volume. In addition, we should like to thank Emma Gallon, Heidi Bishop, Annie Vaughan, Rebecca Dunn and Laura Macy at Routledge for their support and guidance in enabling this volume to come together as well as the members of the production team for their assistance in the delivery of the book. We are grateful to the SEMPRE Series Editors for their support and enthusiasm in this project too.

Introduction

Elaine King and Caroline Waddington

In recent years, empathy has received considerable attention by researchers as a means of understanding a range of psychological and mental phenomena, including communication, social interaction, consciousness and emotion. The history of empathy research is both varied and colourful, reflected in the number of conflicting definitions and conceptualisations of the term across numerous scientific and non-scientific fields. The genesis of the term 'empathy' is inextricably linked to the earlier concept of 'sympathy' that had its roots in eighteenth-century philosophy (Hume, 1739/1978; Smith, 1759/1976). These early conceptualisations of sympathy suggested a kind of fellow feeling, associated with the word's etymological roots in Greek (*sym* + *pathos*). 'Empathy' emerged in the nineteenth century in German aesthetics: *Einfühlung* ('feeling into') originally described the tendency of observers to project themselves and their feelings into a work of beauty (Vischer, 1873/1994) in order to increase their understanding or deepen their appreciation of the work. It was Theodor Lipps (1903) who first transformed empathy from a concept of philosophical aesthetics into a more psychological context as he used the term to describe the process by which we come to know others' mental states. According to Lipps, empathy is a process of inner imitation in which a person imitates the movements or expressions of an object or individual. When observing another's emotional state, the observer is prompted to imitate internally the other's emotional cues and, as a result, shares the emotional state even if experiencing a weaker version of it. It was this more psychological concept of *Einfühlung* that Edward Titchener (1909) translated into English as empathy (for a more comprehensive account of empathy, see Laurence, this volume).

Music and empathy research

Over the last ten years, a large body of research has examined emotional expression and emotional responses to music (see Juslin, 2001). Studies have suggested that listeners value music partly for its ability to evoke emotions; however, it is still unclear which emotions listeners experience when they listen to music or how these emotions are triggered. Researchers have also sought to understand the underlying mechanisms of musical emotions in more detail (Juslin & Västfjäll, 2008). Deniz Peters (2015) has considered how listening to music can allow us to experience emotions that are not our own. He argues that empathy is with a 'musical other' that comes into existence through the attribution of the emotional ownership to an imagined agent that is not the listener. Meanwhile, Stephen Davies (2011) argues that a listener's response to emotion in music is a mirroring response brought about by emotional contagion, while Clemens Wöllner (2012) claims that perceptions of emotional expression in music can be related to cognitive and affective empathy.

Alongside research on music and emotions, the concept of empathy has been closely related to music in terms of developmental issues as well as listening and performing experiences. The development of empathy in children has been linked particularly to music education. Mirja Kalliopuska and Inkeri Ruókonen (1986) used a self–other perspective-taking definition for empathy so as to investigate the role of music education in the development of empathy in children, while M. Hietolahti-Ansten and Kalliopuska (1991) examined the influence of instrumental study on children's development of empathy. Tal-Chen Rabinowitch, Ian Cross and Pamela Burnard (2012) extended this work by investigating the relationship between Musical Group Interaction (MGI) and the development of emotional empathy in children.

Music is a social activity in which composers, performers and listeners can interact in a variety of different ways (North & Hargreaves, 2008). It is possible that empathy facilitates these interactions and may be central to our understanding of group dynamics within performing ensembles. In his study of the working process of musicians in a jazz sextet, Frederick Seddon (2005) put forward two new concepts relating to co-performer empathy: 'empathetic attunement' and 'empathetic creativity'. He defined the former as the process in which members of an ensemble agree on interpretation and expressive ideas, and the latter as the corresponding product of novel expressive variations (see also Seddon & Biasutti, 2009). Interestingly, Sharon Myers and Catherine White (2011) carried out a study examining the parallels between empathy in musicians' performing experiences and the role of empathy in the therapeutic process. In the context of musical performance they found that empathy was essential for musicians to be able to work together at the highest level.

Istvan Molnar-Szakacs and Katie Overy (2006) have proposed the Shared Affective Motion Experience (SAME) model, which suggests that 'musical sound is perceived not only in terms of the auditory signal, but also in terms of the intentional, hierarchically organised sequences of motor acts behind the signal' (Overy & Molnar-Szakacs, 2009, p. 492). The researchers propose that music can provide an auditory representation of the presence of another person or social group. In the context of group musical performance, the SAME model suggests that there is the potential for synchronised, affective experience and communication. A study by Sebastian Kirschener and Michael Tomasello (2010) has provided further evidence for the SAME model, and suggests that shared experiences of musical interaction may result in the development of greater empathic concern, or prosocial behaviour.

Despite the growing body of research about music and empathy, there is no existing book or journal that focuses specifically on the subject or attempts to draw together the emerging strands. This volume exposes current philosophical, developmental, cognitive, social and educational perspectives on research about music and empathy through considering the notion in relation to our development and engagement with different types of music and media. It includes contributions from new and established scholars who have produced research to date on music and empathy, as well as material from those with leading reputations for endeavour that promises to enrich our understanding of the subject.

With regard to definitions and use of terminology in this volume, it should be noted that authors provide complementary and sometimes competing understandings of central terms and concepts, including 'empathy'. There are two adjectives of the noun 'empathy', namely 'empathic' and 'empathetic', which may be used in different discourses, normally depending on authors' or speakers' preferences. Both can be used interchangeably and are effectively synonymous. While the former may pre-date the latter in usage (see Oxford English Dictionary online), empathetic resonates with adjectival versions of sympathy (that is, sympathetic), so is sometimes preferred. In this volume, we have encouraged authors to adopt the term 'empathic' wherever possible for consistency, although some have chosen to use 'empathetic' for specific reasons and when citing the works of others who have adopted this version of the adjective.

Overview of *Music and Empathy*

Following a Prologue, the twelve chapters of this volume are organised into two main areas of enquiry. Part I ('Empathy and musical engagement', Chapters 1–6) focuses on empathy from a range of perspectives concerned with the ways in which individuals develop responses to and experiences about music. Part II ('Empathy in performing together', Chapters 7–12) considers empathy in collaborative performance contexts, embracing philosophical, socio-cultural, neuroscientific and other arguments through theoretical and empirical research.

In the Prologue ('Revisiting the Problem of Empathy'), Felicity Laurence dissects the concept of empathy, arguing that the term 'empathy' can and does take a number of meanings that are, upon examination, unrelated, although at times conflated. From the initial discussion of ways in which empathy is conceived both in lay and scholarly contexts, the account then looks at specific sources of and conundrums in this conceptual eclecticism, bringing into view several challenges to areas of current consensus. The discussion then moves to a consideration of the work of Edith Stein, and her efforts a century ago to disentangle some of the already apparent confusions that had arisen around what was still a young concept in Western thought. The Prologue concludes with reflections on the conceptual distinction between the notion of a specific 'musical empathy' – the topic of many of the chapters that follow – and the separate idea of music's potential to promote a 'general' empathy. In addressing the underlying and persistent dilemmas of empathy as a central concept, and in trying to tease out conceptual resonances and dissonances in the ways described, Laurence's Prologue sets the scene for the entire volume and provides an initial sense of the interconnectedness of the ideas contained therein.

In Chapter 1 ('Towards a developmental model of musical empathy using insights from children who are on the autism spectrum or who have learning difficulties'), Adam Ockelford offers insight into the ways in which music can be used to promote development within a specific therapeutic learning environment. He explores how music can function not only as a proxy language for some children on the autism spectrum, but also provide them with a vehicle for understanding how others think and feel, and a grasp of why they act in certain ways. He argues that comprehension can arise non-verbally since music can convey intentionality and influence in interactions (Ockelford, 2013a); moreover, music can evoke emotion directly (through the content and structure of its constituent sounds) or indirectly, through learnt symbolic meanings. The chapter reports on research that shows how children on the autism spectrum are able to use both these channels to express their own feelings with the aim of communicating these to others, as well as understanding how others think and feel (Ockelford, 2013b).

In Chapter 2 ('Synchronisation – a musical substrate for positive social interaction and empathy'), Rabinowitch explores the nature of musical interaction in a structured music–educational setting, specifically through analysis of the cognitive, social and physiological aspects of 'Musical Group Interaction' (MGI) via consideration of both group and individual relationships. While previous research has demonstrated that repeated participation of school children in structured sessions of MGI can contribute to an increased capacity for empathy, presumably through mechanisms of skill transfer, this chapter provides new insights about the foundations of synchronisation in MGI as a substrate for positive social interaction and empathy. MGI is described as a considerably complex environment demanding from its participants high levels of cognitive, social, and emotional engagement and influenced by their individual capabilities, personality traits and attitudes. Synchronisation, a fundamental building block of group music-making and MGI, is shown to be vital for prosocial behaviour.

Chapter 3 ('Music: the language of empathy') focuses more closely on the ways in which individuals develop empathic neurological connections through music. Molnar-Szakacs argues that music can unite us as well as promote a sense of spirituality, mutual understanding and cooperation. He suggests that music allows us to get inside each other's minds and to feel a sense of shared humanity – to have empathy for one another. This chapter reports on studies of the brain that have found a large network of structures including the human mirror neuron system and the limbic system to be recruited during emotional empathy. The 'Shared Affective Motion Experience' (SAME) model of emotional music perception is discussed (Molnar-Szakacs, Green, & Overy, 2012; Molnar-Szakacs & Overy, 2006; Overy & Molnar-Szakacs, 2009) and used to describe how music may be able to exert profound effects on our desire to connect socially as well as to guide research in therapeutic settings.

In pursuing research on the development of emotional responses to music, Chapter 4 ('The social side of music listening: empathy and contagion in music-induced emotions') introduces and examines different theories about musical emotion induction via empathy. Andrei Miu and Jonna Vuoskoski indicate that music may induce emotional responses through multiple different mechanisms (for example, Juslin & Västfjäll, 2008), while empathy and its subcomponent emotional contagion may offer a persuasive explanation for how music could be able to induce emotional responses in the absence of extramusical or autobiographical associations. It is reported that during the last decade, several researchers have suggested that some form of empathy may be involved in the emotional responses induced by music (for example, Juslin & Västfjäll, 2008; Livingstone & Thompson, 2009; Scherer & Zentner, 2001); however, empirical investigations on the matter have only recently started to emerge. This chapter highlights the emergence of music from the theory of mind (Livingstone & Thompson, 2009) and emotional contagion as a mechanism of emotion induction (Juslin & Västfjäll, 2008). In addition, it summarises recent empirical findings regarding the role of trait empathy in the susceptibility of music-induced emotions (Vuoskoski & Eerola, 2012), the contribution of dispositional empathy to emotion-related music preferences (Garrido & Schubert, 2011; Vuoskoski *et al.*, 2012), and the effect of empathy-related instructions on music-induced emotions (Miu & Balteş, 2012).

In Chapter 5 ('Audience responses in the light of perception–action theories of empathy'), Wöllner reviews theories of cognitive and affective empathy and focuses particularly on perceived actions. He claims that music performance is based on bodily actions, so observing other individuals' acting may resonate in the perceiver's motion system and subsequently cause bodily responses. Indeed, numerous studies have shown that seeing the musicians' body movements has a strong impact on the experience of music. While recent research has attempted to attribute this impact to processes that play a role in empathic responses when observing other individuals, Wöllner raises key questions about how audience members grasp the performer's expressive intentions, what role body concepts play in these processes, and how empathy may enable and modulate the understanding of what is conveyed in a performance. In this chapter, the findings for performing arts in the domains of music and dance are discussed, and explanations for individual differences in aesthetic responsiveness are proposed.

Within the area of jazz performance, Peter Elsdon further considers audience perspectives about empathy in Chapter 6 ('Viewing empathy in jazz performance'). He explores empathy through the metaphor of conversation (Berliner, 1994; Monson, 1996) in the sense that different voices are heard, understood, responded to, and so on, in a democratic manner. Empathy is understood as appropriate action, following what is often called the 'simulation model'. Empathic performance, in other words, is considered to be that in which musical gestures complement each other, and seem stylistically appropriate. Elsdon builds on this understanding by considering empathy as a quality that is emergent from performances and representations of performances. His approach uses audio–visual texts of jazz performance to examine representations of music-making, and to analyse how these representations frame ideas about musicality, interaction and appropriate action. He suggests that in the context of viewing music-making on film, a sense of empathy among jazz performers can be created as

much by the framing devices employed, as by musical gestures which are stylistically appropriate. To this end, empathy is considered to be an idea that we
construct in the course of viewing a performance, mediated by the representational devices at work.

Research on empathy and performance continues in Part II of the volume as
our interactions with music through performing together are scrutinised across
different contexts. In Chapter 7 ('Otherwise than participation: unity and alterity
in musical encounters'), Matthew Rahaim explores the concept of empathy via
discussion of rapport, ethics and musical 'otherness' in his research with Hindustani musicians. Rahaim is concerned with the ways in which encounters with
musical strangers produce the appearance of radical human alterity. Even though
it is pointed out that model cases for such studies are usually those reflecting
savage or inhuman interactions, Rahaim claims that, in fact, certain kinds of
encounters with musical 'otherness' can produce a special kind of rapport, ethics
and empathy not possible between those who take their sameness for granted.
Drawing on the philosophy of Emmanuel Levinas and the author's original ethnographic work in India, case studies of such encounters are discussed and, in
each case, Rahaim offers a phenomenological account of the various kinds of
empathy that come into play as well as the kinds of ethical demands made on
those involved.

In Chapter 8 ('In dub conference: empathy, groove and technology in Jamaican
popular music'), Rowan Oliver examines the rhythmic interrelationships that exist between instrumentalists when grooving. He argues that groove relationships
rely upon a multi-layered empathic understanding between musicians, both in
terms of the way that they play together and also how their collective sound
fits within – or outside – stylistic conventions. Building on the work of Mark
Doffman (2008) and Anne Danielson (2006) as well as by taking Christopher
Small's (1998) ideas around musicking into account, the chapter discusses some
empathic aspects of the ways that groove is constructed in Jamaican reggae,
focusing initially on the stylistically specific relationship between the drums
and the bass (as well as other instruments in the ensemble) before broadening
the scope to include the contribution of the producer, both when mixing a band
recording session and, crucially, when creating a dub version of a pre-existing
track (or 'riddim'). The significance of timbre as a defining factor in groove is
also noted as an idea that links with Jamaican sonic priorities (Goodman, 2010;
Henriques, 2011) and Olly Wilson's (1992) seminal ideas around the 'heterogeneous sound ideal' in Afro-diasporic musicking. Given the central role which studio
production plays in defining the sound of a particular recording, Oliver suggests
that the Jamaican producer can be seen as a vital participant in the distinctive
construction of reggae groove, a participant whose empathic relationships with
musicians and stylistic convention are akin to those found among instrumentalists, but which additionally incorporate a significant technological dimension.

Claudio Babiloni, Claudio Del Percio, Ivo Bruni and Daniela Perani look more
closely at emotional and cognitive empathy in the development of empathic relationships among performing musicians. In Chapter 9 ('Empathy of the musical

brain in musicians playing in ensemble'), theories about the neural basis for empathy are discussed and then investigated further in two experiments. The first
experiment tests an important new method for measuring ensemble musicians'
electroencephalogram (EEG) rhythms simultaneously. In the second experiment
the EEG measurements and empathy quotient test scores of different quartets are
compared among ensemble players when performing, observing their playing,
undertaking a control task, and resting. It was found that the higher the empathy
quotient test score, the higher the alpha rhythms in particular brain regions during the observation condition only, suggesting that alpha rhythms reflect emotional empathy in musicians when observing their own performance.

Moving into the domain of Western art performance, ensemble playing has
become a key area of research in music psychology and education, since almost
all musicians perform, rehearse or create music with others. Recent studies
have explored chamber musicians' optimal experiences of performing together,
whereby players have spoken of achieving a collective state of mind, described
variously as 'in the groove' (Berliner, 1994), a 'group flow state' (Sawyer, 2006),
and 'empathetic attunement' (Seddon, 2005). This collective state of mind seems
to be the key difference between solo and ensemble optimal experiences of performance and seems to be linked to empathy. Elsewhere, it has been suggested
that empathy is key for ensembles to function at the highest level (Keller, 2014;
Myers & White, 2011). In Chapter 10 ('When it clicks: co-performer empathy in
ensemble playing'), Caroline Waddington considers the nature and importance
of co-performer empathy among established professional chamber ensembles.
Through a thematic analysis of focus group interviews with these ensembles, as
well as two observational case studies, she examines the process of co-performer
empathy and its relationship to creativity in expert ensemble performance.

Following on from this, in Chapter 11 ('Developing trust in others; or, how to
empathise like a performer') Anthony Gritten takes an in-depth look at the role
and importance of trust in ensemble playing, and its relationship to empathy.
Gritten argues that trust is the basis for empathy's emergence, integral to ensemble musicians' communication and interaction, and posits that empathy can
only be understood fully as a function of trust and trustworthiness. The chapter
culminates with a brief comparison of trust and empathy, noting two aspects that
empathy alone is unable to explain and aims to synthesise the two concepts in the
direction of a full explanation of interaction's social value.

The final contribution of this volume looks specifically at the unique socio–
musical dynamic of duo partnerships through consideration of empathy in the
Western solo–accompaniment ensemble context. In Chapter 12 ('The empathic
nature of a piano accompanist'), Elaine King and Evgenia Roussou review existing studies on empathy with ensemble performers as well as relevant historical
and pedagogical perspectives on piano accompanists. Thematic analysis of data
retrieved from an interview study with professional soloists and piano accompanists about their understandings of empathy in duo partnerships indicates that
accompanists are perceived to offer higher levels of moral and musical support
and reassurance in ensemble playing than other co-performers. The findings

suggest that the empathic nature of the piano accompanist is potentially more one-sided or uneven than in other Western art chamber ensembles. Furthermore, the different functions of empathy and influences upon performers' experiences of empathy in this context indicate that it may be regarded as a divergent, rather than emergent, phenomenon.

As a whole, this book is securely bound together by its overall theme of empathy, yet clear overlaps and links exist across the two sections and between chapters. Emerging themes include consideration of empathy through 'musicking' (all chapters); emotional contagion (Chapters 3–5, 9); bodily interaction (Chapters 5–8, 10); socio-emotional interaction (Chapters 1–2, 6–8, 10–12); and musical interaction (Chapters 1–2, 7–12). The diversity of perspective and methodology evident across the volume reflects the cross-disciplinarity of contemporary thinking about the subject as there is representation from scholars working in the fields of music psychology and music education as well as related disciplines, including neuroscience and philosophy. It is hoped that the book will inspire further research on empathy and music as well as provide fruitful discussion among researchers, music practitioners, students and professionals about the ways in which we think, feel and respond empathically to one another in our everyday musical lives.

References

Berliner, P. (1994). *Thinking in jazz: The infinite art of improvisation*. Chicago, IL: University of Chicago Press.

Danielson, A. (2006). *Presence and pleasure: The funk grooves of James Brown and Parliament*. Middletown, CT: Wesleyan University Press.

Davies, S. (2011). Infectious music: Music-listener emotional contagion. In A. Coplan & P. Goldie (Eds.), *Empathy: Philosophical and psychological perspectives* (pp. 134–48). Oxford: Oxford University Press.

Doffman, M. (2008). *Feeling the groove: Shared time and its meanings for three jazz trios* (Unpublished doctoral dissertation). The Open University, UK.

Garrido, S., & Schubert, E. (2011). Individual differences in the enjoyment of negative emotion in music: A literature review and experiment. *Music Perception, 28*(3), 279–96.

Goodman, S. (2010). *Sonic warfare: Sound, affect and the ecology of fear*. Cambridge, MA: Massachusetts Institute Technology Press.

Henriques, J. (2011). *Sonic bodies: Reggae sound systems, performance techniques, and ways of knowing*. London: Continuum Press.

Hietolahti-Ansten, M., & Kalliopuska, M. (1991). Self-esteem and empathy among children actively involved in music. *Perceptual and Motor Skills, 71*(3), 1364–66.

Hume, D. (1739/1978). *A treatise of human nature*. P. H. Nidditch (Ed.). Oxford: Oxford University Press.

Juslin, P. N. (2001). Communicating emotion in music performance: A review and a theoretical framework. In P. N. Juslin & J. A. Sloboda (Eds.), *Music and emotion: Theory and research* (pp. 309–337). Oxford: Oxford University Press.

Juslin, P. N., & Västfjäll, D. (2008). Emotional response to music: The need to consider underlying mechanisms. *Behavioral and Brain Sciences, 31*(5), 559–75.

Kalliopuska, M., & Ruókonen, I. (1986). Effects of music education on development of holistic empathy. *Perceptual and Motor Skills, 62*(1), 187–91.

Keller, P. E. (2014). Ensemble performance: Interpersonal alignment of musical expression. In D. Fabian, R. Timmers & E. Schubert (Eds.), *Expressiveness in music performance: Empirical approaches across styles and cultures* (pp. 260–82). Oxford: Oxford University Press.

Kirschener, S., & Tomasello, M. (2010). Joint music making promotes prosocial behavior in 4-year-old children. *Evolution and Human Behavior, 31*(5), 354–64.

Lipps, T. (1903). *Aesthetik: Psychologie des schonen und der kunst, erster teil.* Hamburg: Leopold Voss Verlag.

Livingstone, S., & Thompson, W. F. (2009). The emergence of music from the theory of mind. *Musica Scientiae, 2009/10,* 83–115.

Miu A. C., & Balteş, F. R. (2012). Empathy manipulation impacts music-induced emotions: A psychophysiological study opera. *PLoS ONE, 7*(1). DOI: 10.1371/journal.pone. 0030618.

Molnar-Szakacs, I., & Overy, K. (2006). Music and mirror neurons: From motion to 'e'motion. *Social Cognitive and Affective Neuroscience, 1*(3), 235–41.

Molnar-Szakacs, I., Green, V., & Overy, K. (2012). Shared Affective Motion Experience (SAME) and Creative, interactive music therapy. In D. Hargreaves, R. MacDonald & D. Miell (Eds.), *Musical imaginations: Multidisciplinary perspectives on creativity, performance and perception* (pp. 313–31). Oxford: Oxford University Press.

Monson, I. (1996). *Saying something: Jazz improvisation and interaction.* Chicago, IL: University of Chicago Press.

Myers, S. A., & White, C. M. (2011). 'Listening with the third ear': An exploration of empathy in musical performance. *Journal of Humanistic Psychology [published online].*

North, A. C., & Hargreaves, D. J. (2008). *The social and applied psychology of music.* Oxford: Oxford University Press.

Ockelford, A. (2013a). *Applied musicology: Using zygonic theory to inform music education, therapy). Music, language and autism: Exceptional strategies for exceptional minds.* London: Jessica Kingsley.

Ockelford, A. (2013b). *Music, language and autism.* London: Jessica Kingsley Publishers.

Overy, K., & Molnar-Szakacs, I. (2009). Being together in time: Musical experience and the mirror neuron system. *Music Percept, 26*(5), 489–504.

Peters, D. (2015). Musical empathy, emotional co-constitution, and the 'musical other'. *Empirical Musicology Review, 10*(1), 2–15.

Rabinowitch, T. C., Cross, I., & Burnard, P. (2012). Long-term musical group interaction has a positive influence on empathy in children. *Psychology of Music, 41*(4), 484–98.

Roussou, E. (2013). An exploration of the pianist's multiple roles within the duo chamber ensemble. In. A. Williamon & W. Goebl (Eds.), *Proceedings of the International Symposium of Performance Science 2013.* Brussels: AEC.

Sawyer, K. (2006). *Explaining creativity: The science of human innovation.* Oxford: Oxford University Press.

Scherer, K., & Zentner, M. (2001). Emotional effects of music: production rules. In P. Juslin & J. Sloboda (Eds.), *Music and emotion: Theory and research* (pp. 361–92). Oxford: Oxford University Press.

Seddon, F. A. (2005). Modes of communication during jazz improvisation. *British Journal of Music Education, 22*(1), 47–61.

Seddon, F. A., & Biasutti, M. (2009). A comparison of modes of communication between a string quartet and a jazz sextet. *Psychology of Music, 37*(4), 395–415.

Small, C. (1998). *Musicking: The meanings of performing and listening.* Hanover, NE: Wesleyan University Press.

Smith, A. (1759/1976). *The theory of moral sentiments.* D. D. Raphael & A. L. Macfie (Eds.). Oxford: Clarendon.

Titchener, E. (1909). *Lectures on the experimental psychology of the thought process.* New York: Macmillan.

Vischer, R. (1873/1994). 'Uber das optische formgefuhl'. In H. Mallgrave & E. Ikonomou (Eds. and Trans.), *Empathy, form and space: Problems in German aesthetics, 1873–1893* (pp. 89–124). Santa Monica, CA: Getty Centre for the History of Art and the Humanities.

Vuoskoski, J. K., & Eerola, T. (2012). Can sad music really make you sad? Indirect measures of affective states induced by music and autobiographical memories. *Psychology of Aesthetics, Creativity, and the Arts, 6*(3), 204–13.

Vuoskoski, J. K., Thompson, B., McIlwain, D., & Eerola, T. (2012). Who enjoys listening to sad music and why? *Music Perception, 29*(3), 311–17.

Wilson, O. (1992). The heterogeneous sound ideal in African–American Music. In J. Wright (Ed.), *New perspectives on music* (pp. 326–37). Sterling Heights, MI: Harmonie Park Press.

Wöllner, C. (2012). Is empathy related to the perception of emotional expression in music? A multimodal time-series analysis. *Psychology of Aesthetics, Creativity, and the Arts, 6*(3), 214–23.

Prologue

Revisiting the problem of empathy

Felicity Laurence

The enduring problem of empathy

Long ago, William Blake captured the sense of human intersubjective resonance in his poem *On Another's Sorrow*:

> Can I see another's woe,
> And not be in sorrow too?
> Can I see another's grief,
> And not seek for kind relief?
>
> Can I see a falling tear,
> And not feel my sorrow's share?

(Blake, 1789; from verses 1 and 2)

In essence, Blake is invoking Adam Smith's 'fellow-feeling', a fundamental tenet in what in African thought is called *Ubuntu* – the concept that we are not just human, but human-and-fellow-human, which in turn allows and even obliges us to take on another's feeling and be moved to try to alleviate another's pain where we recognise that pain. It is this kind of notion that has come to be associated with the more recent concept of empathy, an expression now so generously used in current discourse that we might be forgiven for assuming an uncomplicated consensus in its construal.

But the question of what we might construe as empathy is in fact a conundrum. This Prologue considers some of its sharper 'edges' in probing a little the concept that we, in our disparate ways, are bringing here into the musical realm. To this end, I sketch first an overview of how empathy is currently understood, and aspects of ambiguity besetting the concept from its inception; to further tease out these latter, I then draw in particular upon one of the early philosophical investigations into what had already been signalled as a 'problem' by the early twentieth century – namely, the account of Edith Stein. I conclude with several thoughts about some things we might keep in mind as we proceed in our collective exploration of this somewhat fragile concept within various music-centred contexts.

While the 'age of empathy' proclaimed by Frans de Waal, and Jeremy Rifkin's 'empathic civilisation' may seem hardly supportable in view of the world's current multiple trauma,[1] the idea of empathy is nonetheless extraordinarily ubiquitous in Western thought, with the current upsurge of interest fuelled by the discovery in the 1990s of 'mirror neurons' (decreed widely and with a certain impunity as 'empathy neurons', although their role in elucidating whatever is meant by 'empathy' is unstraightforward and the site of ongoing scrutiny).[2]

Empathy frequently connotes some kind of universal panacea (our pundits quick to assume its relevance, potency and effectiveness),[3] accepted uncritically as a 'good thing' of which the more we 'have' the better.[4] Indeed, in the light of its current catch-all manifestation, we might recall and extend moral theorist Martin Hoffman's earlier suggestion of the possibility of 'promiscuous' empathy – a state on which the concept might be argued to be verging.[5]

However, despite its irrepressibility in lay discourse and a rich seam of scholarly investigations from various disciplines,[6] and as variously noted by my co-authors in this volume, the concept of empathy remains beset by a lack of conceptual lucidity that has been a problem since the concept was first introduced, initially in the German as *Einfühlung* in 1873, and just over a hundred years ago in its English form, 'empathy'. Despite a consensus about the underpinning concern with the connection of one consciousness with another, it remains the case that what is designated as empathy very often differs not only from one person to the next, but also even within one individual's explanations – sometimes within one paragraph or even a single sentence.[7]

Empathy is variously, and *differently*, given as: something you 'have' (or don't have);[8] something you 'feel'; something you 'do'; and our lexicon these days also encompasses such notions as: a 'global empathic consciousness'; 'empathic resonance'; the 'empathic brain'; empathy as a 'political act'; (and now, even 'empathic solutions'). Empathy itself appears as synonymous with: mimicry; attunement; compassion; sympathy (and indeed even with kindness and helpfulness);[9] moments of connection; feelings of mutual understanding.

In broader conceptions, empathy is given as an imaginative, cognitive, affective and communicative *process*; with 'levels' and 'kinds' of empathy, 'complex' versus 'primitive' empathy – the latter conceived in turn as emotional contagion, or, as explained by Goldie, 'a kind of "resonance" which is more or less non-conscious' for which evidence is now sought from the afore-mentioned mirror neurons (Goldie, 2011, p. 304). From anthropological inquiry, leaning in turn upon Stueber's distinction of a 'basic' from 'reenactive' empathy, comes the assertion that empathy is culturally dependent for its manifestation and expression. As Hollan puts it:

> 'basic', evolved capacities to attend and to attune to others [are then] culturally elaborated and expressed or suppressed in specific social and moral contexts.
>
> (Hollan, 2012, p. 71)

thus echoing de Waal's suggestion of emotional contagion as the 'first step on the road to full-blown empathy' (de Waal, 2010, p. 74).

Within this 'colourful' (as Elaine King and Caroline Waddington phrase it above) semantic display, we can discern three main recurrent 'takes' on empathy, namely: 1) 'standing in another's shoes' in order to take the other's role or perspective; 2) the sharing of another's feeling (here I am subsuming the notion also of directly 'feeling the other's feeling'); and 3) a concomitant, inherent caring, prosocial or altruistic response to both: three ideas that are not the same conceptually, may have quite different neurological bases, and may or *may not* be correlated with, or lead to, another.

This kaleidoscope of meaning is fraught with quandary. Seeing things from another's viewpoint does not in fact equate to sharing what that person is *feeling*, nor even to being *interested* in trying to understand what that person is feeling. Nor does it necessarily mean that, having understood how someone else is seeing the world, one might be thereby *enabled* ipso facto to share – let alone to *feel* – exactly what that person is feeling; and nor does either sharing of feeling or perspective-taking necessarily incorporate, result in, or indeed require in the first place the desire – whether this precedes or follows – to alleviate suffering or to help.

Understanding what another person is thinking is certainly not *necessarily* accompanied by any beneficent intent, as apparent in military contexts where 'getting inside' the enemy's way of thinking has ever been a vital element of warfare. Even without directly malevolent intent, it is perfectly possible to imagine someone's thoughts – correctly or not – and simply not to care; it is unproblematic enough to imagine the anxiety and emotional and physical distress of people crossing the sea in flimsy rafts from war zones to hoped-for safety in Europe, but by no means is this understanding inevitably accompanied by sympathy. As Hoffman asks: 'why should perspective-taking serve prosocial rather than egoistic ends?' (Hoffman, 2000, p. 131).

Many of these disparate phenomena are positioned as legitimate elements within composite concepts. One such concept is Mark Davis's multifaceted model, which distinguishes between 'cognitive role taking' and 'affective reactivity to others' (Davis, 1994, p. 9), and between 'process' and 'outcome' (Davis, 1994, p. 10), arguing that role taking, a *process*, is inappropriately compared with (inner) emotional or (exhibited) behavioural responses that are *outcomes* which may *result from* such a process.[10] The four pivotal constituents of his framework: Antecedents (traits and situations), Processes, Intrapersonal Outcomes, and Interpersonal Outcomes, form a 'multidimensional' complex of related constructs, not all of which need to be involved in every instance of empathising; indeed, empathy itself lies only within the areas of 'processes' and 'intrapersonal outcomes' (Davis, 1994).

Davis's framework underpins his 'Interpersonal Reactivity Index' (IRI) (1983)[11] which over the ensuing decades has become a main point of reference for analysis within psychological research, correlations being sought between perceived neural and other events and people's self-report (itself not unproblematic) according to Davis's questionnaire. This of course poses the problem that findings are then inherently committed to Davis's specific concept of empathy – even though this is by no means universally approved (and disparaged as a 'conglom-eration' (Schertz, 2004) – and indeed upon the quantitative basis of his apportion-ing of its four constituent elements. Were empirical work drawing upon Davis's IRI to be reanalysed according to another theoretical framework, we might have an essentially different set of understandings.[12]

Davis's work draws in part from Martin Hoffman's theory of prosocial moral development (in Western society), which posits empathy as its linchpin. Hoffman's account carries a particular relevance to our current discussion, where the moral valence of music ripples constantly under, and sometimes on, the surface. Hoffman's own definition of empathy as 'an affective response more appropriate to another's situation than one's own' (Hoffman, 2000, p. 4) applies, however, only to the empathic response to another's suffering, with a hard-wired 'empathic distress' which can ultimately become 'embedded' into moral principle and structures. However, his five 'modes of empathic arousal', linked in turn with five stages of empathic development (the first three prever-bal and involuntary, including mimicry, the fourth and fifth requiring higher order cognitive function, with role taking at the top), resonate variously in en-suing accounts in subsequent chapters, in other forms. Interestingly, Hoffman argues that *all* modes of empathic arousal *remain in force* once established, the more advanced building on the earlier levels, continuing to influence a per-son's empathic responding into adulthood, invoked according to the specific situation.

I turn now to the thorniest of questions: can we in fact ever feel another per-son's feeling? Recurrent neural processes may be discerned, as indeed discussed in subsequent chapters, but we can never *know* what the experience of the intri-cate inner state of another person actually *feels like* to *them*. We can *try* to un-derstand this, we can infer from our own similar experience, we can project our own responses, and we may certainly feel our own resulting feelings in response to what we witness of another's expression of emotion or thoughts, and to what we *think* we understand of these (and here the question of 'empathic accuracy' arises – a huge topic in itself in which various authors have conducted extensive investigations).[13] But what *I* feel and experience inwardly is surely a function of my entire history, and of my entire physical and mental 'makeup' – conditioned by myriad previous experiences, traits of my personality, my current states of awareness and emotional being. You – surely – cannot feel *my* pain, the precise and specific shade of that or any other feeling I experience, although you can *try* to imagine it, feel another feeling that is close, or feel a congruent feeling that is your own.

Peter Goldie teases out further niceties of meaning here, coming to a robust rejection of the notion that we can (or even should try to) imagine being the other at all, which he somewhat startlingly pronounces to be 'anti-empathy', and he himself thoroughly against it (Goldie, 2011, p. 302). Distinguishing two kinds of perspective-taking,[14] Goldie allows '*in-his-shoes perspective-shifting*' (Goldie, 2011, p. 302, original italics):

[that is] consciously and intentionally shifting your perspective in order to imagine what thoughts, feelings, decisions, and so on *you* would arrive at if you were in the other's circumstances.

(Goldie, 2011, p. 303, original italics)

But he rejects what he describes as '*empathetic perspective-shifting*':

consciously and intentionally shifting your perspective in order to imagine *being* the other person, and thereby sharing in *his* or *her* thoughts, feelings, decisions, and other aspects of their psychology.

(Goldie, 2011, p. 303, original italics)[15]

Goldie argues that these two ways of shifting perspective are utterly different, the latter deeply problematic, being 'conceptually unable to operate with the appropriately *full-blooded notion of first-personal agency* that is involved in deliberation' (Goldie, 2011, p. 303, original italics). Goldie insists that only *I* can take my own stance towards my own thoughts, feelings and intentions:

Thoughts are thought, feelings felt, decisions and choices made, *by particular agents*, and the identity of the agent in this full-blooded sense can make a difference to what is thought, felt, decided on, or chosen. It is not as though all thoughts, feelings, decisions, and choices can be 'processed' by *any* agent, impersonally, just so long as that agent is minimally rational.

(Goldie, 2011, p. 315, original italics)

Goldie becomes more emphatic still: where the would-be empathiser attempts to think the thoughts of the other, she in fact '*usurps* the other's agency, replacing it with her own' (Goldie, 2011, p. 316, original italics). Goldie declares that if in empathising we were to attempt to take aboard the other's character, we 'would still be left with [our] own full-blooded agency, which would continue to play its covert, non-speaking part in the deliberation – a particularly virulent form of contamination' (Goldie, 2011, p. 316).[16]

In this view, empathy is not at all always a 'good thing', a point arising with comparable insistence from a quite other disciplinary milieu, and from beyond the Western arena in which the concept flourishes so densely at the moment. Here are Hollan and Throop reporting from the anthropological field:

One thing that is clear … is that first-person-like knowledge of others in the context of everyday social practice is rarely, if ever, considered an unambiguously good thing. … people all over the world seem just as concerned with concealing their first-person subjective experience from others as in revealing it.

(Hollan & Throop, 2008, p. 389)

Echoing Goldie's vehement call to us to be careful, Hollan and Throop also pose fundamental questions about not only the possibility, but the desirability of such 'empathic' knowledge, often considered potentially more harmful than helpful by those whose cultures they and their colleagues explore. Touching upon a further layer of conundrum – the notion of 'self' and its integrity – they state:

> Everywhere, we find complex concepts of personhood that convey what is appropriate to know about people and what not, that sketch out how porous or impermeable the boundaries of the self should be ideally, that hint at the damage done when psychic integrity (however defined) is breached.
>
> (Hollan & Throop, 2008, p. 389)

These counterpointings to the current narrative of a benign empathy at the core of being both human and humane shift that ground a little; it jars to encounter Goldie's empathy as potential 'contamination', and as in fact a site of fear and potential injury as soon as we step outside the Western setting – thoughts to hold in mind as we proceed to explore here our field of empathy and musical experience.

I return now to our Western setting to examine a little more closely a specific instance of conceptual variegation, and its role in the history and ongoing existential tussles enveloping our core topic.

Sympathy and empathy: origins

> In empathy I try to feel your pain. In sympathy I know you are in pain, and I sympathize with you, but I feel my sympathy and my pain, not your anguish and your pain.
>
> (Wispé, 1968, para. 2)

The conflation – the '*Ur*' conflation perhaps – of empathy with sympathy is particularly tenacious, the terms popping up synonymously from one sentence to another in tract after tract, sometimes with provisos, often unremarked. Despite Wispé's painstaking attempt at elucidation more than four decades ago, and the many others that have ensued, this particular slippage seems still to defy efforts to resolve it.[17]

One primary origin of this state of affairs lies in the new understanding of 'sympathy' articulated in the context of the Scottish Enlightenment. Shades of what we might mean by 'empathy' in David Hume's account in 1738–39 of 'sympathy' as the understanding of one person's inner states by another are clear enough, and echoed in his younger colleague Adam Smith's further (1759/1790) contributions to this inquiry, which share Hume's notion of 'fellow-feeling' and its integral salience to moral judgement. In this construal, sympathy was now given as pertaining to the understanding of *any* feeling experienced by another, and not just the suffering to which the concept had hitherto been limited (as in Blake's appeal above, and which of course we reencounter in current discourses of both sympathy and empathy).[18] Smith distinguishes pity and compassion from sympathy:

> Pity and compassion are words appropriated to signify our fellow-feeling with the sorrow of others. Sympathy, though its meaning was, perhaps, originally the same, may now, however, without much impropriety, be made use of to denote our fellow-feeling with any passion whatever.
>
> (Smith, 1759/1790, I.I.5)

Sympathy is seen as an act of imagination rather than a function of direct perception via the senses or as reducible to 'catching' someone else's emotion (the 'emotional contagion' mentioned above and further discussed below and in subsequent chapters); for Hume, as Terence Penelhum explains, it is a 'psychic mechanism' which 'generates a special sort of emotional involvement with the experiences of others that leads to the sentiments of approval and disapproval' (Penelhum, 1992, p. 153).

While there were also significant differences between their accounts, Geoffrey Sayre-McCord notes that both Hume and Smith argue 'our capacity to imagine ourselves (more or less successfully) in the other's place' (Sayre-McCord, 2015, p. 217). They also switch between requiring the feeling of the other's feeling and not doing so:

> Hume and Smith sometimes have in mind just the process by which we … come to feel as others do, and sometimes have in mind just the product, the fellow-feeling, without regard to how it came about. So they each end up allowing that we might sympathize with another despite not actually feeling as the other person does …
>
> (Sayre-McCord, 2015, p. 212)[19]

Penelhum paraphrases what he calls Hume's 'mechanism of sympathy' (Penelhum, 1992, p. 153), retaining much of Hume's original vocabulary:

> I become aware of the passion of another person through observation of the behavioural signs of it that are familiar in my own case. This gives me the idea of the other's emotion. This becomes enlivened in me to the point where it develops into an impression, that is, a counterpart in me of the very emotion the other is feeling. What communicates the vivacity necessary for this transformation is the 'idea, or rather the impression' of myself. The closer a person is to me and the more recognizably like me he or she is, the more intensively this vivacity is communicated …; but all human beings bear some significant resemblance to one another, so there is in principle no one for whom I cannot feel a passion sympathetically.
>
> (Penelhum, 1991, p. 154)

The new idea of sympathy swiftly became, as Remy Debes puts it, 'eclectic' (Debes, 2015, p. 287),[20] lying in wait, as it were, for the later idea of *Einfühlung*

18   *Felicity Laurence*

to appear on the nineteenth-century Western aesthetic scene, by which point the
notion of 'sympathy' – however manifold its connotations had become – was
deeply rooted in Western thought.

It was not long before the intertwining of the two concepts occurred. In a first
attempt to bring the insights of Robert Vischer's *Einfühlung* to a non-German
but English-speaking audience, the aesthetician Violet Paget informally translated *Einfühlung* as 'sympathy' in 1895, at this point openly equating sympathy's 'feeling with' with *Einfühlung*'s 'feeling into'.[21] (Violet Paget was the real
name of the aesthetician Vernon Lee. She later adopted Titchener's term in her
own work on empathy.) This initial outing into the English language clearly did
not endure, although given the etymological fragility of the neologism that did
survive – Titchener's 'empathy' – some would argue that this was a pity. Titchener's eventual (re)translation of the German term into English in 1909 drew upon
the Aristotelian *empatheia* ('in suffering' or 'in passion'):

> Not only do I see gravity and modesty and pride and courtesy and stateli-
> ness, but I feel or act them in the mind's muscle. That is, I suppose, a simple
> case of empathy, if we may coin that term as a rendering of *Einfühlung.*
>
> (Titchener, cited in Wispé, 1987, p. 21)

a coining which, according to Debes (2015, p. 286) hardly reflects even
Titchener's own usage of it, let alone what we, variously, mean now. Trans-
porting concepts from one language to another that doesn't have them was, and
remains, sticky; nuances are readily 'lost in translation'. From a further disciplinary vantage point, the biologist Colwyn Trevarthen, who places sympathetic
communication at the core of his notion of infant intersubjectivity, contends
that 'sympathy' – the 'feeling with' – best describes the resonant bonds one
consciousness may experience with another. He is clear: 'It is unfortunate, I believe, that "empathy" has become the preferred word in English' (Trevarthen,
2010, p. 1).[22]

Thus, although Titchener's somewhat capricious translation brought the 'new'
concept into the English-speaking world, it arguably did little to assist its trajectory, as distinct from sympathy, from that point.[23] Debes records complaints
about the 'ever-expanding taxonomy of meanings for "empathy"' (Debes, 2015,
p. 297) emerging already in the 1930s, and the Gestalt researcher Adam Luchins's
avowal in 1957 'that "empathy" had become so thin', as to require semantic spec-
ification before the term might meaningfully be employed (ibid.).

It may well be that a notion of 'sympathy' (especially given a tradition of meta-
phors involving that concept, including 'sympathetic resonance' in music) seems
better suited to explaining at least some of whatever it is that we are finding,
exploring, testing, bringing into being as we look at questions of empathy and
musical experience. While Rae Greiner notes that 'the moral and social theories of Smith and Hume [concerning sympathy] are thick with references to the
mental activities, perceptual and imaginative acuities, and ethical conundrums
that in the parlance of our own day, can seem to belong exclusively to empathy'

(Greiner, 2012), Debes wonders about the sense in trying now – a hundred years on – to insist upon the distinction between them; as he puts it, to 'establish an objective, nonstipulated distinction between "empathy" and "sympathy" – a distinction which now seems never really existed anyway' (Debes, 2015, p. 322). And yet, perhaps we might have done better simply to stick to what the German was telling us – *Einfühlung*'s 'feeling into'.

It is to this 'feeling into' that we now return. There are recent attempts to go back to scratch and listen again to the earliest philosophers who were also struggling with the idea of empathy about one hundred years ago, invoking for example Theodor Lipps who explained it via a notion of 'inner imitation' of the other's state;[24] others are returning to the phenomenologist philosopher Edmund Husserl, as with Zahavi's quest to see whether and how the idea of mirror neurons fits with Husserl's writings on intersubjectivity (see endnote 2).

I turn now to Edith Stein's beautifully elaborate scrutiny of empathy, which deals not only with the sympathy–empathy dyad, but further pivotal distinctions, including of perspective-taking, emotional contagion, and the smouldering question of whether it is conceivable that we can feel precisely what another is feeling.

'Zum Problem der Einfühlung'

Although Edith Stein's exploration of empathy continued beyond her initial doctoral exposition, *Zum Problem der Einfühlung* ('On the Problem of Empathy' – supervised by Husserl, and published in 1917), two main factors impeded her progress and the dissemination of her insights. Her gender was the first obstacle: she was only the second woman in Germany to be awarded a doctorate in philosophy and academic positions were hardly available to women, and Husserl himself was pretty unsupportive in helping her along her own academic path.[25] But although she later converted to Catholicism and indeed took orders as a nun, it was her Jewishness which put paid not only to her career altogether in the early 1930s, but also eventually to her life itself: she was murdered in Auschwitz in 1942, her work on empathy having already slipped into obscurity. Though she remains fairly hard to find in English-language discussions (indeed, in the three accounts I have singled out in endnote 6 she is barely mentioned), there are occasional moments when she suddenly appears again, lauded for example as a rare credible theorist of the topic (Schertz, 2004), implicit in Debes's expression of relief that she is 'getting better recognition' (Debes, 2015, p. 295) and indeed in the salutation by my co-contributor Matt Rahaim who hails her in passing as 'philosopher of empathy *par excellence*'.[26] She is better known in the German philosophical context: recent discussion of her thought appears for example in Angelika Krebs' examination of the 'dialogic' nature of love (Krebs, 2015).

However, Stein's work has gradually been re-emerging from its long overshadowing by Husserl's discussions which built upon it, with a growing awareness of her own, unacknowledged, contribution to these from her continued work as his post-doctoral assistant. Initially, this renewed visibility arose mainly as a result of her canonisation in 1998 and its accompanying publicity arising from Jewish perceptions of her 'appropriation' by those considered to have let her down in the first place, and also the ensuing reissuing of her collected writings. Stein's inclusion in the volume *Ten Neglected Classics of Philosophy* (in Kris McDaniel's astute study of her main themes) signals an increasing acknowledgement of her significance.

I like to draw attention to Edith Stein's work because it makes such an elegant attempt to open up the black box of the inner workings of empathy, because it is indeed such a seminal part of the original philosophical inquiries, and because she has been, as McDaniel puts it, so 'unfairly marginalized' (McDaniel, 2016, p. 199). Stein's work not only presciently pinpoints many of our current semantic and conceptual conundrums, but also offers, a century on, illuminative ways of considering these.

I hope that this gossamer-light depiction of Stein's investigation (itself pithy in the extreme and demanding utmost mental agility to keep up with) will recall for the reader some of the profound concerns aired in previous pages, and provide one 'pivot' for the succeeding collective discussion.

As McDaniel notes, Stein is concerned with 'the problem of other minds' (McDaniel, 2016, p. 199). McDaniel paraphrases Stein's central concern thus: 'I know that there are persons other than myself, and I know that these persons have various psychological states and experiences. How do I know these things?' (ibid.). In this sense, and crucially, Stein is exploring empathy (which for her of course was in fact *Einfühlung*, a term which carries, as we have seen, a far more directly descriptive connotation than the term we have ended up with in English) as a *mechanism* of knowledge of the other's inner states, rather than as either an affective or cognitive response to the other.

Edith Stein's 'Einfühlung'

When Stein began her doctoral study of *Einfühlung*, it was already sizzling away in psychological and philosophical circles, as Wispé observes '– intellectually speaking – everywhere' (Wispé, 1987, p. 24).[27]

Stein initially approached her study from the perspective of psychology, but quickly found this premature, and was fairly forthright in explaining that:

> [psychology] possessed neither the required foundations of refined first principles nor the capacity to formulate them on its own.
> (Stein, cited in Herbstrith, 1985, p. 11)

and, reiterating the primacy of philosophical validity:

> Genetic psychology, presupposing the phenomenon of empathy, investigates the process of this realization and must be led back to the phenomenon when its task is completed.
> (Stein, 1917/1989, p. 22)

Here is a first 'prequel'; in much reporting of the subsequent empirical research which proceeded apace despite the persistent theoretical murkiness, we find either a cursory definition of empathy or none at all, so that we are left to infer which particular aspect is being investigated from available clues and the actual test instruments being used.

Using Husserl's methodology of phenomenology, Stein explains its thesis that transcendental, 'pure' consciousness is the only area of *certain* knowledge, and argues that objects appear to consciousness within four so-called 'phenomenal realms', corresponding to interconnected layers of the human being. Of these four realms (the physical, the personal/individual, the mental/intellectual and the sensory), it is only the latter two that are empathisable. So when de Waal writes now that 'we can't feel anything that happens outside ourselves' (de Waal, 2010, p. 65), he is reflecting Stein's notion that what is *physically felt* cannot be replicated by another, though we might be able indirectly to sense what it might be *like* for another to feel the pain; and while we can communicate on an intellectual level, our respective personalities resist (empathic) 'knowing' by another as resiliently as does our physical state. This recalls both Goldie's rejection of our ability to imagine the other person's inner state as if you were she, or he (Goldie, 2015; see above), and also Hollan and Throop's attention to the capacity (and they consider also the willingness) to be *empathised* (Hollan & Throop, 2008, p. 392).[28]

Primordial experience

From these perspectives, Stein investigates 'empathy as a particular act of cognition' (Stein, 1917/1989, p. 397), that is, in turn, a composite act of comprehension, in which the 'primordiality' of our own present experiences is differentiated from precise and direct experience of another's feeling. ('Primordial' is her translator's rendition of the original term *originär*).[29] While we can, via empathic comprehension, come to an experience of our own 'primordial' feeling in response to another's feeling or other aspect of their inner experience, the feeling of the other that we have perceived and 'empathised' is not our own, however strongly we may recognise its congruence to our own experience. In phenomenological terms, the empathised experience 'appears differently' for the person directly experiencing it from how it appears for the empathiser, for whom it is therefore non-primordial. Empathy is thus a kind of inner understanding, different from, but related to, outer perception: 'an act which is primordial as present experience though non-primordial in content' (Stein 1917/1989, p. 10). Others' experiences therefore can be grasped, but they do not have the same quality of 'givenness' or reality for us, though the resulting feeling we may have is indeed our own, and therefore in her conception, 'primordial'.

Stein rejects earlier 'inner imitation' theories' implication of 'complete coincidence' of original with empathised experience (including that of Lipps).[30] In fact, she turns inner imitation somewhat on its head. Where Paget, Titchener and others suppose an internal mimicry *leading to* empathic understanding of the other, Stein claims a reverse process in which empathy *precedes* any mimicry:

> I do not arrive at the phenomenon of foreign experience, but at an experience of my own that arouses in me the foreign gestures witnessed.
>
> (Stein, 1917/1989, p. 23)

Stein allows that internal imitation may be a mechanism of the direct transference of *feeling* from one person to another, leading to an emotional response to the other's expression of feeling, but suggests that this in itself is not empathy. In empathising, we respond to another's experience in a 'con-primordial' way with our own, recapitulating, although not precisely sharing, the other's experience:

> My friend comes to me beaming with joy and tells me he has passed his examination. I comprehend his joy empathically; transferring myself into it, I comprehend the joyfulness of the event and am now primordially joyful over it myself.
>
> (Stein, 1917/1989, p. 13)

Empathy as processual act

Stein refers constantly to the 'act of empathy' – empathising as something we do as well as experience. She also intimates that empathy is a process rather than a discrete event or action, here with first 'grasping' or comprehending her friend's joy, then 'transferring herself into it', grasping directly the joyfulness of the event, and finally feeling her own, primordial, joy. And it is here that we come to Stein's location of sympathy.

Sympathy

Stein positions *Mitgefühl* (sympathy) as *essentially* different from *Einfühlung* (empathy), in that the former is indeed primordial experience, in fact that direct experience described above which ensues from the initial empathic act during which the other's experience is first perceived or grasped. In the example given above, it is her own, resulting joy, which is 'joy-with-him', the fellow-feeling aroused by the empathic act, and which is her own, different joy, possibly even stronger than her friend's joy. In Stein's terms therefore, we can envisage sympathy quite simply as the sharing, or 'taking on' of a feeling, *after* its initial 'grasping' in the first act within the empathic process. Thus, in Stein's account, the two concepts are different in *kind*. Empathy is a *mechanism* of 'receiving' the other's inner state; sympathy, a *feeling* that might (or might not) arise from it.

Stein is also clear that one's capacity to empathise is subject to certain accompanying inbuilt aspects ('my actual lifelong habits of intuiting and thinking'

(Stein, 1917/1989, p. 62)), or extraneous factors – what others respectively designate as extant traits and one's specific situation (as in Mark Davis's 'Antecedents', see above). She reiterates this point in her description of 'negative empathy' (a term she accepts from Lipps), explaining that while sympathy *may* arise from empathising, it also may not. 'Negative empathy', which excludes fellow-feeling, occurs when:

> the tendency of the empathic experience to become a primordial experience of my own cannot be realized because 'something in me' opposes it. This may be either a momentary experience of my own or my kind of personality.
>
> (Stein, 1917/1989, p. 15)

Referring once more to her example above, Stein imagines being informed of her friend's good news at a time of her own grief over a bereavement. This results in a 'phenomenal conflict', where, in one of our phenomenal realms (see above), we go through the empathic process and feel the resulting sympathetic 'joy-with-him', while on another level, the process cannot be completed, resulting (by definition) in her form of negative empathy. Indeed, she suggests that we can move between levels, 'without conflict' – the interesting implication here being that we can function mentally on different levels, and possibly feel different feelings, simultaneously.

Feeling of oneness

Essential to Stein's argument is the distinction between 'I' and the other 'I'. She acknowledges that while one may well experience the relinquishing of the self and the consequent surrendering to and dissolution in the other, this is not a process of empathy but of 'self-forgetfulness'. But the absolute and constant retention of awareness of self as separate from the foreign consciousness and its experiences, is for Stein a core tenet of empathy.[31] However, she does conceive a 'feeling of oneness', which arises neither as a function of the dissolution of interpersonal boundaries, nor as a way of experiencing others, but, possibly, where a number of people are experiencing the same occurrence (or idea, or event) in very similar ways.

> I feel my joy while I empathically comprehend the others' and see it as the same. And, seeing this, it seems that the non-primordial character of the foreign joy has vanished. Indeed, this phantom joy coincides in every respect with my real live joy, and theirs is just as alive to them as mine is to me. Now I intuitively have before me what they feel. It comes to life in my feeling, *and from the 'I' and 'you' arises the 'we' as a subject of a higher level.*
>
> (Stein, 1917/1989, p. 17, my italics)

She continues:

> we empathically enrich our feeling so that 'we' now feel a different joy from
> 'I', 'you' and 'he' in isolation. But 'I', 'you' and 'he' are retained in 'we'.
>
> (Stein, 1917/1989, p. 18)

Thus, empathy both precedes and makes possible this feeling of oneness, the resulting enrichment of individual experience in which our sense of self nevertheless stays intact, and ultimately, in the completed (fulfilled) empathic act, that sense of the 'higher we' – of community. However, there is no suggestion here either of the *Mitgefühl* (the fellow-feeling she holds as sympathy), nor of the emotional wave sweeping through the group and infecting its members like a contagious illness. Rather, Stein's assigning of significance to shared feeling in community invokes a further category of feeling *alongside* those arising from interpersonal empathising. This is taken up by Angelika Krebs in her investigation of Max Scheler's conception of *Miteinanderfühlen* – that is, 'joint, shared and common feeling or emotional sharing' (Krebs, 2011, p. 6) which Scheler positioned as *distinct from* 'empathy, compassion, emotional contagion and identification' (ibid). Krebs explicitly calls upon Stein in this discussion, suggesting that 'with Edith Stein building on Max Scheler's foundations we finally have a convincing account of shared feeling' (Krebs, 2011, pp. 6–7). Krebs concludes that:

> shared feeling is a feeling, in which the participants intend their feelings
> as a contribution to a shared feeling and understand the feelings of others
> in the same way. A shared feeling is a **unity of sense** of different feeling
> contributions.
>
> (Krebs, 2011, p. 16)

It is not to be understood as any kind of 'summative' phenomenon, but is 'an irreducible category of feeling' (ibid.).

Contagion

Stein argues that emotional contagion has nothing to do with comprehension of another's feelings, but concerns direct *expression* of feeling, transmitted *non*-cognitively. The experience of the other is not 'announced' and grasped as in empathic comprehension, and contagion differs *quintessentially* not only from empathy, but also from the feeling of oneness and from sympathy, in that these all involve a transfer of *self* into the foreign experience, and not merely of *feeling* from one psyche to another. She goes further:

> It is certain that as we are saturated by such 'transferred' feelings, we live in
> them and thus in ourselves. This prevents our turning toward or submerging ourselves in the foreign experience, which is the attitude characteristic of empathy.
>
> (Stein, 1917/1989, p. 23)[32]

in other words, suggesting that our attention is no longer on the other's 'foreign' experience at all, but entirely self-directed.[33]

Perspective-taking

Stein does not deny the possibility of seeing another's viewpoint, but regards this act separate from empathy (a 'surrogate'):

> if ... we put ourselves in the place of the foreign 'I' and suppress it while we surround ourselves with its situation, we have one of these situations of 'appropriate' experience. If we then again concede to the foreign 'I' its place and ascribe this experience to him, we gain a knowledge of his experience ... Should empathy fail, this procedure can make up the deficiency, but is not itself an experience. We could call this surrogate for empathy an 'assumption' but not empathy itself.
>
> (Stein, 1917/1989, p. 14)

At this point, we can see that the two main tenets informing our current take on empathy – perspective-taking and 'feeling the other's feeling' – are in fact, and remarkably perhaps, both sidelined by Stein, as is also contagion.[34]

Similarity

Stein's concluding topic, the fundamental significance of perceived similarity between empathiser and empathised-with other, recalls Hume's contingent 'vivacity' with which the other person's emotion is 'enlivened' in the observer according to the degree of resemblance (see above). Hume observes also that:

> We sympathize more with persons contiguous to us, than with persons remote from us: With our acquaintance, than with strangers: With our countrymen, than with foreigners.
>
> (Hume, 1739–40/ 2009, p. 763)

This idea recurs constantly in ensuing discussions of empathy, discipline-wide, including, for example, the respective approaches of Davis and Hoffman (see above). Davis places similarity in the 'antecedent' category of his model of the empathic 'episode' (Davis, 1994); Hoffman locates it as a core construct in his theory of empathy-based morality (Hoffman, 2000). Similarity has been found to be a point of consonance across theories (Katz, 1963), with subsequent empirical research consistently and numerously producing clear correlations between empathic responses and behaviour (whatever strand of empathy is being examined), and perceptions by the empathiser of the other's similarity.

Stein takes her notion of 'fulfilment', mentioned above, which can, as we have seen, be impeded by the traits of the would-be empathiser, and to these now adds the degree of perceived similarity, arguing that while it *is* possible empathically to understand a very different other, this is only to an *unfulfilled* extent – via an imagining of another's experience rather than through the fulfilled empathic process, which fulfilment depends upon sufficient extant shared experience and view of the world:

> … I cannot fulfill what conflicts with my own experiential structure.
> (Stein, 1917/1989, p. 115)

In other words, empathiser and 'empathised-with' need, in the empathiser's perception, to be like *enough* for empathising to be possible.

If we can really only empathise the experience of the alike-enough other, and there is, as we have seen, plenty of evidence that this is so, then we have a dilemma. I conclude this light portrayal of Stein's thesis with an earlier (minutely amended) musing on this paradox to which her own investigation brought her, and us:

> For where empathy strengthens *intra-group* connection there is the spectre not only of a concomitant lessening in empathy with those *outside* the group, but of the increasingly active construction of the latter's foreignness. The more we discover our intra-group commonality, the less like us those outside our group may seem. The irony of this extrapolation is cruelly sharp in view of her own ultimate fate; gassed in Auschwitz as an *Untermensch* – less than fully human, unempathisable and ultimately disposable.
> (Laurence, 2008, p. 21)

Empathy and music: reflections

In this brief sampling of thoughts and analyses from the beginnings of empathy's passage into our own conceptual world, and thereafter into the various disciplines in which it now resides, if restlessly, I hope to have highlighted number of cross-currents and reverberations. Stein's narrowing down of empathy and her positioning of what we now generally see as its main components to one side or other of what she is conjecturing as its real nature and purpose is intriguing; in her delineation of perspective-taking we may, for example, see some kind of pre-echo of Goldie's fine distinction between 'in-his-shoes' and 'empathetic' perspective-shifting. Likewise, her positioning of a cognitive act before the affective response may be called to mind by subsequent explications of what it is to empathise.[35] Holding up the concept this way and that to its various scrutinisers (of whom of course there is room here for only a few) can bring shifts in insight and point us to areas of caution.

There are a myriad questions of sharp salience facing us as we look at empathy and musical experience. In this newly burgeoning field, two main strands appear – as indeed vividly exemplified in the chapters that follow: one strand concerned with a specific notion of 'musical empathy', and the other explicitly seeking music's affordance of general empathic response. However, in the former category there is also a tendency to extrapolate, even if only in mild con-jecture, to the latter – that is, to try to connect empathising *within* the musical experience to empathising *beyond* it, even when that is not our primary focus. In moving from nuanced accounts of intersubjective experience in musical in-teraction to assumptions of its effect upon a rather more amorphous 'general' or 'social' empathy, we may risk losing the ground just gained. We can mitigate this kind of 'slippage', and the current diffuseness of the concept, by articulating precisely the specific facet with which we are dealing at any given moment, and its non-synonymity with other facets.[36] We might also consider in cases where we have direct utterances from musicians the ways in which these may afford specificity.

'Musical empathy' might eventually be described as a separate concept with its own phenomenological structure; its relationship with 'general' empathy may be found to be contingent upon exactly which account of empathy is being invoked. But inasmuch as we do seem to yearn so for more empathy, here we must return to our earlier question: is empathy always in fact a 'good thing' to promote? This doubt has gradually presented itself in my own forays into these matters, which are located first in the classroom, often in contexts where there are issues of emotional neediness, or intercultural dissonance (for example, where there have been fairly sudden increases in populations of refugee children), and second in the wider area of the arts in conflict resolution (Cross, Laurence, & Rabinowitch, 2012; Laurence, 2008, 2010, 2011a; 2011b).[37] In both spheres exists a buoyant rhetoric (if sparsely grounded) of music's 'power' to overcome interhuman bar-riers including the geopolitical barricades that proliferate as I write, and I have been exploring the role of empathy in this discourse (my research thus located in the second 'strand' of the music–empathy field) – and finding reason to be pretty cautious the more I probe.

In a long classroom-based study using ethnographic methodology and draw-ing specifically upon Christopher Small's finely wrought concept of 'musicking' (Small, 1998) and a 'working definition' of what it is to empathise, I sought to tease out conceptual resonances between musicking and empathising.[38] I found not only *intentionality* to be pivotal in increasing empathic response and process, that is, the children's *wanting* to find ways of becoming more empathic with each other in the first place, but also *consensus* among them that it *was* indeed a 'good thing', and furthermore, that the children's sense of *agency* was crucial in their taking an empathic stance. These aspects were at least as germane to empathis-ing as the musical experiences (of singing and composing songs together) around which our empathic project centred, and although there occurred instances of emotional contagion in response to certain events in the musicking, there was no automaticity in the relation between musicking and empathising.

The school in which I carried out my research undoubtedly developed an al-most palpable 'empathic climate', the concept explicit in the children's vocabu-lary and a reference point over time for their ways of conducting relationships with each other. But there were many vulnerable children among the group and the question gradually emerged of whether they were being 'seduced' by the musicking, the sense of oneness this increasingly provided, and the general blossoming of thought and agency, to reveal more of their own inner states than was 'right' – or 'appropriate'. And that very agency the children acquired in 'tuning in' to empathic patterns of response also eventually resulted in their becoming demanding of a democratic 'say' in the running of school, 'troubling' the head's role to an extent (notwithstanding her participation in the underpinning consensus and commitment to inter-child empathic concern). The question of 'appropriate' empathy arose too at a deeper level; was this engagement with empathy in fact 'unfitting' the children for the world awaiting them beyond primary school?

In more recent work, now situated in the mire of the Middle Eastern arena, I have been investigating what might be 'going on' in a series of musical encounters between some Israeli and (West Bank-located) Palestinian children. Here, there has arisen a perhaps unique kind of 'connecting', in which a *musical* empathising might well be argued, but I have concluded that the only *general* empathic aspect that could legitimately be construed was the *pre-existing* concern (the Steinian 'what is already in me') of the former for the latter. This seemed to arise from an extant fellow-feeling and moral stance rather than from any initial empathic 'grasping', and motivated these (politically almost impossible) meetings in the first place. The Israeli children were cautious about empathy, and made no suggestion that the *musicking* affected what they had already brought to the encounter. In these glimpses of their subsequent responses, 'Noa' seems to be echoing Goldie, while 'Jonathan' – a little miraculously – catches the 'entering into' of Stein's *Einfühlung*.

> We have this *idea*, this theory, to see it how they see it. Not in very clear way, just in theory, and not really – we never, we *will never* can see how they see it.
>
> ('Noa')

> I think there is a way. And it's usually with solidarity. Then we can *enter to*, when you're, when you, when there are things, specific things that you can empathise with. But we're not there yet. Maybe we will be, maybe...
>
> ('Jonathan')

'Hamed' from the Palestinian group considers their stance, and seems to stand in their shoes for a moment:

> There is a conflict between the two nations. Some people choose to be part of the conflict, and some people don't. 'They' chose *not* to be a part of the conflict. That's why 'they' are here! I saw them, and said they are friends, not enemies.
>
> ('Hamed')

But in any case, empathising between the children, whether in a Steinian sense, or taking my own more general view (see endnote 37), could have provoked a charge of 'normalisation' from fellow citizens of the Palestinian children (the perceived effect of such cross-occupation fraternising as in fact consolidating the occupation). Again, in hot conflicts like the one these children are caught up in, seeking intracultural empathy – through music or any other means – may take us along that doomed road paved with good intentions.

Our novel music–empathy field is strewn with notions, as with empathy itself, that need constant turning on their heads: the very nature of music – how we construe its meaning, expressivity, role – within and indeed beyond the Western classical canon or jazz practice to which much of the inquiry in this volume is addressed; what constitutes human musicality; the ever-lurking assumption (and often explicit argument) of music's inherent virtue – which holds (the right kind of) music as an instrument of civility – a notion that can swiftly be 'made strange' as we contemplate the manifold instances of beautiful music serving terrible purposes.

In what follows arises also the core question of commonality of response to music, invoked every time we speak of 'pleasant' music, or assume shared feelings about music's meaning. I leave the reader at this point with some astute observations from Thomas Wright in 1604 about the diverse responses to the same music that different persons may have according to their disposition, situation, or personality, foreseeing perhaps the thoughts about the sovereignty of individual feeling surveyed in this Prologue. It seems that we cannot rely upon music's 'power' always to move us in the same way, to bring about empathic, or indeed sympathetic resonance between us.

> Let a good and a Godly man heare musicke, and hee will lift up his heart to heaven: let a bad man heare the same, and hee will convert it to lust; Let a souldiour heare a trumpet or a drum, and his bloud will boile and bend to battell; let a clowne heare the same, and he will fall a dauncing; if the common people heare the like, and they will fall a gazing, or laughing, and many never regard them. ... True it is, that one kind of musicke may be more apt to one passion than another [but] I cannot imagine, that if a man never had heard a trumpet or a drum in his like, that he would be at the first hearing be moved to warres.
>
> (Wright, 1601–04/1986, p. 208)

Notes

1 *The Age of Empathy: Nature's Lessons for a Kinder Society* by Frans de Waal and *The Empathic Civilization* (Rifkin, 2009), the latter a particularly solid tome, both appeared in the same year, seeming to catch, and seeking to substantiate, the hopeful and clearly persistent empathic Zeitgeist already flourishing at that time. (Note; references to de Waal's volume within this prologue are taken from the *Souvenir Press* 2010 edition).

2 A more comprehensive discussion of mirror neurons is undertaken in Chapter 3 (Molnar-Szakacs, this volume). See also Dan Zahavi's examination (2011) of mirror neurons in relation to earlier theories of empathy (for example, the 'inner imitation' explanation as given in Theodor Lipps' exposition). Zahavi's main foci are Husserl's phenomenological account of empathy (intersubjectivity), and the arguments of

Gallese, one of the original discoverers of mirror neurons, who claims a continuity with the earlier phenomenological accounts of empathy. While agreeing in the end that there are some strong resonances, Zahavi pinpoints serious problems in drawing a straight line from mirror neurons to any kind of nuanced concept of empathy, and indeed alludes to Gallese's own acknowledgement of the limits of 'what the mirror neuron model can explain' (Zahavi, 2011, p. 248).

3 For example, Will Hutton's assumption of empathy's apparently instantaneous effect in addressing the profound predicaments of our lopsided society – here equating empathy with perspective-taking, but also attributing to it an inherent ethic of caring – in his discussion of empathy's role in Rawls's 'just society': '[Rawls] wants us to make a thought-leap about what it might be like to be in someone else's skin … The instant empathy enters the equation … hatred and the justification for palpable inequity become impossible' (Hutton, 2002).

4 Goldie ups the ante with the upper case in implicitly tackling this mantra: 'surely empathy is so obviously a Good Thing that if someone is against it, either there must be something wrong with him, or he must be confused as to what it is' (Goldie, 2011, p. 302).

5 Hoffman, while arguing the necessity of strengthening empathy in general, does argue that 'promiscuous' or 'diffuse' empathy may cause societal breakdown if everyone, empathically but impossibly, tried to help everyone else all the time (Hoffman, 2000). I am to an extent hijacking the term to try to catch the sense of empathy's current apparent ability to mean anything we want it to mean.

6 Three accounts which collectively offer a diverse and rich overview are Eisenberg and Strayer's seminal volume *Empathy and its Development* (1987) which situates the concept in a (then) recent historical context; Coplan and Goldie's much more recent collection *Empathy: Philosophical and Psychological Perspectives* (2011) of wonderfully picky delvings into intricacies of meaning; and Hollan and Throop's special journal issue *Whatever Happened to Empathy* (2008) which brings into the picture new and sharp anthropological perspectives. The burgeoning neuroscientific research further glosses this overview; for an excellent, detailed look at 'where we are' with this aspect (at the time of writing) see Lamm and Majdandžić's review 'The role of shared neural activations, mirror neurons, and morality in empathy – A critical comment' (2015).

7 Frans de Waal (though hardly alone in doing so) appears to interchange the terms 'sympathy' and 'empathy' (for example, de Waal, 2010, p. 91) – in this instance having just explained that they are different ('sympathy is a separate process under quite different controls', ibid., p. 90). He also more or less conflates compassion and empathy in one or two sentences (ibid, pp. 224–225).

8 See Baron-Cohen, for example his *Zero Degrees of Empathy* (2011) and his contention of empathy's absence in a person – not 'having' it – as equating with moral deficit.

9 For example, de Waal's (2010) immediate harnessing of 'empathy' and kindness in the subtitle of *The Age of Empathy* – 'Nature's Lessons for a Kinder Society' – although he appears to review this implication himself in various ways throughout the book.

10 Writing at a time when in his view the field had been 'balkanised' Davis suggests that theorists had in fact been studying its discrete facets, investigating one while simultaneously peripheralising and even denying the validity of others; the resulting ways of researching empathy, and attempts to measure it, developed along accordingly different paths, each deriving from and appropriate to whichever definition is being invoked.

11 See Chapter 5 (Wöllner, this volume).

12 In any case, where self-report stands at the centre of experimental work, then that in turn stands or falls upon the quality and veracity of any questionnaires used, as well as and whatever the underpinning concepts of empathy, and also ways in which people respond to questions.

13 For a number of theorists of empathy, prominent among these, W. Ickes, empathic accuracy is a central concern. See, for example, Eisenberg, Murphy and Shephard (1997) in *Empathic Accuracy* edited by Ickes.

14 Goldie mentions also a third kind of 'imagining', to be understood as essentially *other* than 'perspective-shifting'. This is what he describes as *'imagining-how-it-is'* (Goldie, 2011, pp. 305–306) which doesn't require any imagining *'from the inside'*: he gives the example of imagining how it is for his wife in a meeting with a tricky person, and her feelings and actions and so on. But 'imagining how it is for her' is conceptually different from 'imagining *from the inside* what it is like for her' (ibid., p. 306); perspective-shifting, while possible, is not required here. Goldie points to confusion arising from conflation of 'imagining-how-it-is' and perspective-shifting, in areas such as literary interpretation and also social psychology (ibid., p. 306).

15 However, this is exactly what Amy Coplan (Coplan, 2011, pp. 9–10) gives as her own understanding of empathy, and moreover, she suggests that what Goldie's construes as 'in-his-shoes' perspective-taking be *excluded* (my italics) from the concept of empathy if it does not also include his 'empathetic perspective-shifting' – what Coplan terms 'other-oriented perspective-taking' (ibid., p. 10). Intensely elaborate webs of meaning apart, these profoundly different positions among prominent theorists of empathy highlight the immense complexity of the task undertaken as we bring 'empathy' into the field of musical experience.

16 Here, Goldie footnotes Stueber's (2006) discussion of the 'limits' of empathy, where Stueber refers to 'what Gadamer called "the prejudicial structure of understanding"'. Goldie's citation of Stueber bears repeating here.

> understanding another persons' reasons for his actions or grasping his thoughts cannot merely be understood as re-enactment or as a form of inner imitation because the manner in which we "think" that thought is always already – to use one of the signature phrases of hermeneutic thinkers – colored by our system of beliefs and values, which can differ considerably from that of the interpretee.
>
> (Stueber, 2006, p. 205)

17 See also Wispé's chapter in Eisenberg and Strayer's *Empathy and its Development* (1987) and her detailed examination of sympathy *The Psychology of Sympathy* (1991). Rae Greiner notes that empathy and sympathy were 'overlapping terms' even while conceptual distinction was being sought for empathy. For a succinct but insightful view of the sympathy versus empathy question, see Greiner's sketching out of some of the initial and persisting snags in the intersection of the two concepts, in which she suggests that the early understandings of empathy 'represent[s] a continuation of, rather than a radical break from, [a] sympathy ...', concluding that 'Empathy does not supplant a naïve, outmoded sympathy but seeks to answer different questions or to answer old ones in new ways' (Greiner, 2012).

18 As with Hoffman's seminal theory, based around a core concept of 'empathic distress'. Hoffman's empathy is 'the spark of human concern for others, the glue that makes social life possible' (Hoffman, 2000, p. 3).

19 See Geoffrey Sayre-McCord's (2015) lucid discussion of these differences in his chapter *Hume and Smith on Sympathy* in the volume *Sympathy* (Schliesser, 2015).

20 See Debes's (2015) excellent discussion 'From *Einfühlung* to Empathy' in *Sympathy* (Schleisser, 2015).

21 See above and in subsequent chapters for accounts of Vischer's introduction of the concept of *Einfühlung*. Debes notes that Vischer also carefully distinguished various other 'feeling' concepts including *Anfühlung* (attentive feeling), *Nachfühlung* (responsive feeling) and *Zufühlung* (immediate feeling) – 'all in explicit addition to *Mitfühlung* or "sympathy"' (Debes, 2015, p. 296).

22 In an informal personal exchange some years ago, Trevarthen lambasted Titchener's translation as deeply flawed and calling upon the Greek term with no real justification, Trevarthen robustly deriding the very idea of 'empathy' as a concept. Trevarthen notes the derivation of 'sympathy' from the Greek *sympatheia* that connotes 'moving and feeling with'.

23 As Debes tartly puts it: 'Titchener's blasé tone foreshadows his eventual obscurity on the subject' (Debes, 2015, p. 291).

24 See Chapter 5 (Wöllner, this volume).

25 McDaniel notes Husserl's seemingly half-hearted recommendation for Stein, when she applied for a university position at Göttingen, and his refusal to support her habilitation (McDaniel, 2016).

26 See Chapter 7 (Rahaim, this volume).

27 I have previously suggested (Laurence, 2008) that it was a 'hot' concept in the early twentieth century (oddly enough given the political horrors getting going at that point), but then again, it's much hotter now.

28 Hollan and Throop speak of the 'flip side of empathy' (2008, p. 391) in their discussion of the cruciality of the feelings, intentions and stance of the person who is being empathised; empathising becomes thus dependent upon 'what others are willing or able to let us understand about them' (ibid., p. 392) and therefore concerns itself too with the experience of being understood – thus a *dialogical* process, and different from projection.

29 Zahavi translates this as 'originary'.

30 Zahavi notes that Lipp's account was one 'from which all the phenomenologists to varying degrees distanced themselves' (Zahavi, 2011, p. 222).

31 It is interesting, when we consider the posited prosocial outcomes of empathy, to consider the educational philosopher Nel Noddings's echo of Stein in her declaration that in caring 'I do not relinquish myself' (Noddings, cited in Verducci, 2000, p. 89).

32 This echoes Katz's caution about *sympathy*, that in sympathising we are more concerned with our *own* feelings and needs (than, as in empathising, with the other's), and with our presumption of the other person's reflection of our own experience and reality. He goes as far as suggesting that sympathy in fact 'blunts' our perception of the other's self and situation (Katz, 1963).

33 I have suggested elsewhere (Laurence, 2008) that contagion in musical experience may in some circumstances indeed be antithetical to empathic understanding of others – as for example when an 'emotional bath' engulfs a crowd who, now losing that vital sense of their own 'self' and its boundaries with the next 'self', might then be driven by the musical forces of synchrony towards a feeling or action determined by those using the music precisely to accomplish this work.

34 As noted above, Davis posits both 'cognitive role taking' and 'affective reactivity to others' (Davis, 1994, p. 9) as facets of his composite model of empathy; the distinct notions of 'cognitive' and 'affective' empathy have characterised investigation into the topic and continue to do so, as evident from the following chapters, with 'perspective-taking' generally held as in some way correlating or being equivalent to the former, and 'feeling the other's feeling' likewise related to the latter. As we have seen, Stein's conception of the nature of empathising positions cognitive processes and affective responses differently, rejecting any direct synonymity or even relation between the former and perspective-taking, or the latter and 'feeling the other's feeling' – itself relegated in her view to the realm of the emotional contagion she roundly dismisses as any part of the phenomenon of empathy.

35 See, for example, Waddington's allusion to Baron-Cohen's definition of empathy in Chapter 10 (Waddington, this volume).

36 'Contending with [its] multiple meanings and plurality of frames' as Sharma suggested some time ago (Sharma, 1993, p. 7), a thought mirrored more recently by

Coplan (Coplan, 2011) as noted in Chapter 10 (Waddington, this volume); see also Chapter 5 (Wöllner, this volume) and Chapter 4 (Miu & Vuoskoski, this volume).

37 These publications, all chapters in edited collections, cover sections of the exploration described here.

38 My 'working definition' drew principally on Stein and Davis. Here is the first section; in the light of my ensuing work, I would now amend 'virtually the same' to clarify that this does not mean 'the same'.

> In empathizing, we, while retaining fully our sense of our own distinct consciousness, enter actively and imaginatively into others' inner states to understand how they experience their world and how they are feeling, reaching out to what we perceive as similar while accepting difference, and experiencing upon reflection our own resulting feelings, appropriate to our own situation as empathic observer, which may be virtually the same feelings or different but sympathetic to theirs, within a context in which we care to respect and acknowledge their human dignity and our shared humanity.
>
> (Laurence, 2008, p. 24)

References

Baron-Cohen, S. (2011). *Zero degrees of empathy.* London: Penguin.

Blake, W. ([1789–1794]/1970). *Songs of innocence and of experience: Shewing the two contrary states of the human soul* (Ed. G. Keynes). London: Oxford University Press.

Coplan, A. (2011). Understanding empathy: Its features and effects. In A. Coplan & P. Goldie (Eds.), *Empathy: Philosophical and psychological perspectives* (pp. 3–18). Oxford: Oxford University Press.

Coplan, A., & Goldie, P. (Eds.) (2011). *Empathy: Philosophical and psychological perspectives.* Oxford: Oxford University Press.

Cross, I., Laurence, F., & Rabinowitch T. (2012). Empathy and creativity in musical group practices: Towards a concept of empathic creativity. In G. MacPherson & G. Welch (Eds.), *Oxford handbook of music education* (pp. 337–533). Oxford: Oxford University Press.

Davis, M. (1994). *Empathy: A social psychological approach.* Madison, WI: Brown and Benchmark.

Davis, M. H. (1983). Measuring individual differences in empathy: Evidence for a multidimensional approach. *Journal of Personality and Social Psychology, 44,* 113–26.

Debes, R. (2015). From *Einfühlung* to empathy: Sympathy in early phenomenology and psychology. In E. Schliesser (Ed.), *Sympathy: A history* (pp. 286–322). New York: Oxford University Press.

de Waal, F. B. (2010). *The age of empathy: Nature's lessons for a kinder society.* London: Souvenir Press.

Eisenberg, N., & Strayer, J. (1987). (Eds.) *Empathy and its development.* Cambridge: Cambridge University Press.

Eisenberg, N., Murphy, B., & Shepard, S. (1997). The development of empathic accuracy. In W. Ickes (Ed.), *Empathic accuracy* (pp. 73–116). New York: Guilford Press.

Goldie, P. (2011). Anti-Empathy. In A. Coplan & P. Goldie (Eds.), *Empathy: Philosophical and psychological perspectives* (pp. 302–17). Oxford: Oxford University Press.

Greiner, R. (2012). 1909: The introduction of the word 'empathy' into English. *BRANCH: Britain, Representation, and Nineteenth-Century History,* online-only journal.

34 *Felicity Laurence*

Herbstrith, W. (1985). *Edith Stein: A biography.* San Francisco, CA: Harper and Row.

Hoffman, M. L. (2000). *Empathy and moral development.* Cambridge: Cambridge University Press.

Hollan, D. (2012). Emerging issues in the cross-cultural study of empathy. *Emotion Review, 4*(1), 70–78.

Hollan, D., & Throop, C.J. (2008). Whatever happened to empathy?: Introduction. *Ethos, Journal of the Society for Psychological Anthropology, 36*(4), 385–401.

Hume, D. (1739–1740/ 2009). *A treatise of human nature.* Auckland: The Floating Press.

Hutton, W. (2002, April 7). Reason with your heart, Mr Sharon. *The Observer,* www.theguardian.com/world/2002/apr/07/guardiancolumnists (accessed 5 January 2016).

Ickes, W. (Ed.) (1997). *Empathic accuracy.* New York: Guilford Press.

Katz, R. L. (1963). *Empathy: Its nature and uses.* New York: Free Press of Glencoe.

Krebs, A. (2011). Phenomenology of shared feeling. *Appraisal, 8*(3) 6–21.

Krebs, A. (2015). *Zwischen Ich und Du. Eine dialogische Philosophie der Liebe.* Berlin: Suhrkamp Verlag.

Lamm, C., & Majdandžić, J. (2015). The role of shared neural activations, mirror neurons, and morality in empathy – A critical comment. *Neuroscience Research, 90,* 15–24.

Laurence, F. (2008). Music and empathy. In O. Urbain (Ed.), *Music and conflict transformation: Harmonies and dissonances in geopolitics* (pp. 13–25). London: I. B. Tauris.

Laurence, F. (2010). Listening to children: Voice, agency and ownership in school musicking. In R. Wright (Ed.), *Sociology and music education* (pp. 243–62). Farnham: Ashgate.

Laurence, F. (2011a). Introduction. In F. Laurence & O. Urbain (Eds.), *Music and solidarity: Questions of universality, consciousness, and connection* (pp. 1–15). New Brunswick: Transaction Publishers, Rutgers University.

Laurence, F. (2011b). Musicking and empathic connections. In F. Laurence & O. Urbain (Eds.), *Music and solidarity: Questions of universality, consciousness, and connection* (pp. 171–83). New Brunswick: Transaction Publishers, Rutgers University.

McDaniel, K. (2016). Edith Stein: On the problem of empathy. In E. Schliesser (Ed.), *Ten Neglected Classics of Philosophy.* Oxford: Oxford University Press.

Penelhum, T. (1992). *David Hume: An introduction to his philosophical system.* West Lafayette, IN: Purdue University Press.

Rifkin, J. (2009). *The empathic civilization.* New York: Tarcher/Penguin.

Sayre-McCord, G. (2015). Hume and Smith on sympathy, approbation, and moral judgment. In E. Schliesser (Ed.), *Sympathy: A history* (pp. 208–46). New York: Oxford University Press.

Schertz, M. V. (2004). *Empathic pedagogy* (Unpublished doctoral dissertation). Montclair State University, USA.

Schliesser, E. (2015). *Sympathy: A history.* Oxford: Oxford University Press.

Sharma, R. M. (1993). *Understanding the concept of empathy and its foundations in psychoanalysis.* Lewiston, NY: E. Mellen Press.

Small, C. (1998). *Musicking: The meanings of performing and listening.* Hanover, NH: Wesleyan University Press.

Smith, A. (1759/1790). *The theory of moral sentiments.* London: A. Millar Library of Economics and Liberty, www.econlib.org/library/Smith/smMSCover.html (accessed 7 January 2016).

Stein, E. (1917/1989). *On the problem of empathy.* Washington, DC: ICS Publications.

Stein, E. (1922/2000). *Philosophy of psychology and the humanities* (Ed. M. Sawicki). Washington, DC: ICS Publications.

Stueber, K. (2006). *Rediscovering empathy: Agency, folk psychology, and the human sciences*. Cambridge, MA: MIT Press.

Trevarthen, C. (2010, 10 November). *Confidence, confiding and acts of meaning: Infant's moral feelings and philosophers in Scotland*. Paper presented at The 2010 Theology & Therapy Day Conference, The Churches, Pastoral Care and Counselling: Recent Traditions and Current Prospects, University of Edinburgh, www.theologyandtherapy. div.ed.ac.uk/Trevarthen.pdf (accessed 5 January 2016).

Verducci, S. L. (2000). A moral method?: Thoughts on cultivating empathy through method acting. *Journal of Moral Education, 29*(1), 87–99.

Wispé, L. (1968). Sympathy and empathy. *International Encyclopedia of the Social Sciences*, www.encyclopedia.com/doc/1G2-3045001233.html (accessed 5 January 2016).

Wispé, L. (1987). History of the concept of empathy. In N. Eisenberg & J. Strayer (Eds.), *Empathy and its development* (pp. 17–37). Cambridge: Cambridge University Press.

Wispé, L. (1991). *The psychology of sympathy*. New York: Plenum Press.

Wright, T. ([1601–1604]/1986). *The passions of the mind in general* (Ed. W. Webster). London: Garland.

Zahavi, D. (2011). Empathy and mirroring: Husserl and Gallese. In R. Breeur & U. Melle (Eds.), *Phaenomenologica 201: Life, subjectivity, & art – essays in honor of Rudolf Bernet* (pp. 217–54). Netherlands: Springer Netherlands.

Part I

Empathy and musical engagement

1 Towards a developmental model of musical empathy using insights from children who are on the autism spectrum or who have learning difficulties

Adam Ockelford

Introduction

This chapter interrogates the notion of 'musical empathy' (Livingstone & Thompson, 2009), and considers whether it is distinct from the widely acknowledged 'emotional' and 'cognitive' forms of empathy that function for most people in everyday life (Davis, 1996): that is, whether it is possible for one person, as a listener or a performer, to discern and appreciate others' musical perspectives, without necessarily being able to identify more generally with their thoughts or feelings. It is suggested that musical empathy may itself be of two types, affective and cognitive, and that these pertain to the 'content' and 'structure' of music that, according to zygonic theory (Ockelford, 2005, 2012), make up the warp and the weft of the musical fabric. A challenge of this line of thinking is being able to identify contexts in which musical empathy may potentially be isolable from 'everyday' empathic thoughts and feelings, and a novel approach is adopted here, which considers case studies of children who are on the autism spectrum or who have learning difficulties (or both). This is because while research shows that children with autism generally find it difficult to grasp how others think and feel, typically lacking 'theory of mind' (Baron-Cohen, 1997), there is evidence to suggest that, in some cases, music may have the capacity to act as a vehicle through which they can relate empathically to other people (Greenberg, Rentfrow, & Baron-Cohen, 2015; Ockelford, 2013).

Previous research – the *Sounds of Intent* project – that sought to map the musical development of children with intellectual disabilities (Cheng, Ockelford, & Welch, 2009; Vogiatzoglou *et al.*, 2011; Welch *et al.*, 2009), suggests that, while these young people tread essentially the same music-developmental path as their 'neurotypical' peers, the stages of musical understanding that they attain take longer to evolve and so are easier to capture, facilitating their identification. The research has had to address certain difficulties, however, including the fact that such children may be non-verbal, or at least have little or no capacity for metacognition. As a consequence, data tend to be in the form of musical rather than verbal products, requiring the specialised music-analytical tools offered by zygonic theory to track musical intentionality and influence (Ockelford, 2012).

The results of such analysis undertaken in this study provide evidence that musical empathy may indeed exist as a discrete phenomenon, with distinct stages of development that run in parallel to the six music-developmental levels identified in *Sounds of Intent*. These entail traversing an ontogenetic path that potentially ranges from a state in which one has no sense of self or of other people (Level 1) to the position of having the (intuitive) notion of a proto-musical self and other (Level 2); thence having the recognition that there are others who are musically 'like me', in the moment, (Level 3); to those who are 'like me, yet different', to whom one can relate beyond the perceived present (Level 4); and so to an awareness that it is possible to share a musical journey with another or others through taking a common structural path (Level 5); and finally to a realisation that two musicians or more can work together to create a blended cognitive–emotional narrative in sound (Level 6). Here, musical empathy can extend beyond an understanding of the thinking and feelings of the individuals concerned to having a sense of the musical psyche of a wider cultural community.

What is empathy?

Through introspection and observation, philosophers and psychologists have identified two types of empathy: the kind through which we directly come to share the emotions of others, through an extension of 'emotional contagion' ('catching' the emotional states of others through being in their presence when they are showing how they feel), and the sort that enables us figuratively to put ourselves in others' shoes, and appreciate their situation on an intellectual level (mental activity that may well also have an affective component) – the capacity for theory of mind (see, for example, Coplan, 2011; de Waal, 2008; Håkansson, 2003). In recent years, this dual classification has received some neuroscientific support (for example, Goldman, 2011; Shamay-Tsoory, Aharon-Peretz, & Perry, 2009).

A good deal of theoretical and empirical attention has also been devoted to the related issue of how empathy arises in human development (McDonald & Messsinger, 2011), in particular exploring Andrew Meltzoff's contention that infant imitation (which starts in neonates) leads to the perception of other people as being 'like me', and that others who act in the way that I do are likely to have internal states that are 'like mine' (Meltzoff, 1990, 1995, 2002, 2007; Meltzoff & Moore, 1983, 1989). Some believe that a system of mirror neurons, which are activated not only when a person undertakes a particular action, but also when the same action is merely observed in another (Cattaneo & Rizzolatti, 2009; di Pellegrino *et al.*, 1992; Gallese *et al.*, 1996; Rizzolatti *et al.*, 1996) may lie at the heart of empathic responses (for example, Carr *et al.*, 2003; Decety, 2004; Gallese, 2003; Iacoboni, 2009; Keysers, 2011; Miall, 2003; Preston & de Waal, 2002). Of particular interest in the current context is the finding that mirror neurons may be triggered by sounds as well as visual images (Kohler, 2002), and that, through this process, auditory input is capable of stimulating empathic reactions too (Gazzola, Aziz-Zadeh, & Keysers, 2006). For further discussion of mirror neurons, see also Molnar-Szakacs (this volume).

It is possible to model a mature empathic response as shown in Figure 1.1, which sets out the potential routes through which one person's feelings or thoughts (or both) may be transferred to another. For example, Person A could convey what she or he thinks or feels (often, though not necessarily, elicited by a given set of external circumstances) through language, observable behaviours or actions. These may be detected by Person B, and the mental imagery so generated evoke similar thoughts and feelings to those of Person A. It is also possible for Person B to observe Person A experiencing a given set of circumstances and for these to elicit thoughts or feelings directly.

This model makes certain assumptions. For the successful transmission of thoughts or feelings to occur and for empathy to be engendered requires that Person B has had a previous experience that has enough in common with that

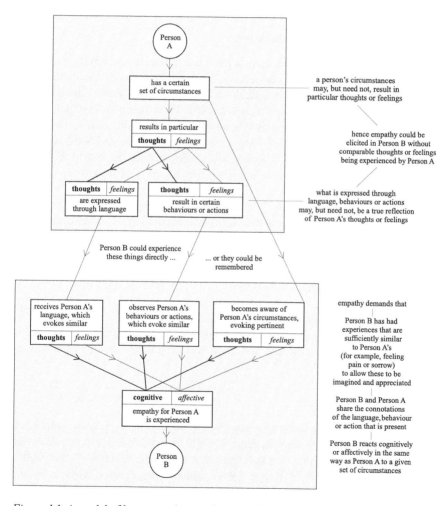

Figure 1.1 A model of how empathy may be engendered in everyday contexts.

encountered by Person A to allow this to be appreciated; that Person B and Person A share the connotations of the language, behaviour or action that are present; that Person B reacts cognitively or affectively in the same way as Person A to a given set of circumstances; and that Person B is aware that his or her thoughts or feelings are elicited by the situation or disposition of Person A.

There are potential complications too. For example, Person B can experience empathy for someone who does not exist (who is purely imagined, or whose persona is conjured up in a novel, play, film or cartoon, for example); Person A may consciously seek to elicit empathic thoughts (where none is actually merited) in Person B through pretence; and Person B may experience empathy for Person A who has no related thoughts or feelings – for example, Person B may be aware that a tragedy is about to befall Person A, who is, however, ignorant of what is shortly going to occur.

Musical empathy: initial questions

Unsurprisingly, perhaps, given music's potential for conveying emotion and creating a sense of interpersonal connection, the notion of empathy has come to the notice of some researchers in the fields of music psychology and education, including, for example, Patrik Juslin (Juslin, 2001, 2009; Juslin & Västfjäll, 2008), who contends that listeners perceive the emotional expression conveyed by musicians in performance then 'mimic' this expression internally, and Seddon (2005) and Cross, Laurence and Rabinowitch (2012), who advance the idea of 'empathic creativity', through which interpersonal attunement may occur in group musical interaction.

But what *is* 'musical empathy'? Is it ultimately the same as everyday empathy, but elicited via a different route (through abstract patterns of sound rather than words or actions, for example)? Or is it a way of sharing thoughts and feelings that is fundamentally different? Or can it be either according to context? Figure 1.2 models these two possibilities: the thicker dotted lines in the lower shaded box indicate the potential route to *musical* empathy; the thinner ones show *everyday* empathy being evoked in response to music. It is suggested that musical empathy may, like everyday empathy, have two strands: cognitive and affective.

To facilitate analysis of this issue, we will consider a group in whom musical empathy and everyday empathy appear to be uncoupled – those on the autism spectrum.

Autism and empathy

Empathy has become a focus of research in the area of autism, since emotional contagion and theory of mind are generally held by psychologists to be two of the principal deficits of those on the spectrum (see, for example, Baron-Cohen, 2005; Boucher, 2008; Frith, 2003; Happé, 1998), though some research (Mazza *et al.*, 2014) has suggested that the deficit in affective empathy is limited to negative emotional valence. The conjecture that a defective mirror neuron system may be

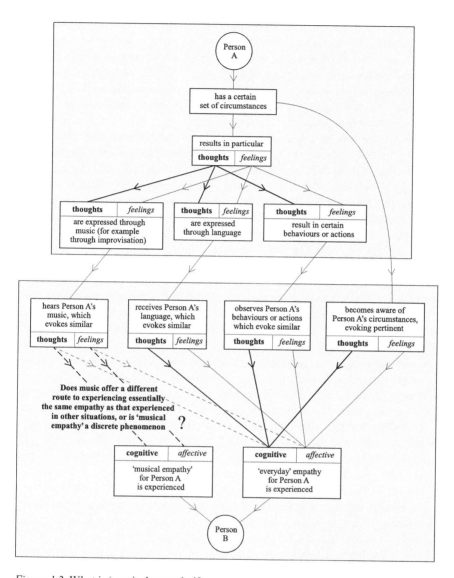

Figure 1.2 What is 'musical empathy'?

a contributory – even primary – factor in this developmental lacuna has found widespread (though not universal) support (see, for instance, Fan *et al.*, 2010; Hadjikhani, 2005; Oberman *et al.*, 2005; Ramachandran & Oberman, 2006; Rizzolatti & Fabbri-Destro, 2010; Williams *et al.*, 2006). At the same time, while there are some accounts of young people on the autism spectrum playing music inexpressively or with scant regard to the aesthetic intent of fellow performers

(Winner, 1996, p. 136), other studies have suggested that autistic children can detect the intended emotional import of music just as well as their neurotypical peers (Heaton, Hermelin, & Pring, 1999), and can perform with great sensitivity, with an awareness of the impact of their playing and singing on others and sensible to the expressive aspirations of other performers in ensembles (Ockelford, 2008, 2013). Indeed, it has been suggested that music-making with others may provide a vehicle for engaging the mirror neuron system in children on the autism spectrum (Wan *et al.*, 2010).

Hence, there may be a mismatch between the degree of empathy exhibited by people with autism in day-to-day life and that which they display (and so presumably experience) during musical engagement with others. Take, for example, Romy (of whom we will hear more later), who, at the time of writing, is 14 years old, severely developmentally delayed, with no formal expressive language, and with many of the characteristics of autism: she appears to be oblivious to the emotional states of those around her (the obverse of her infectious, effervescent egocentricity), and would be wholly unable to appreciate another's point of view on an intellectual level through theory of mind. However, she is a young musician of extraordinary sensitivity, and enjoys playing familiar melodies on the piano with her right hand alone to the author's improvised accompaniments, not only following the tempo, dynamics and articulation that are offered (in accordance with the expressive conventions of Western classical performance), but also *predicting* what her co-performer is likely to do next: delaying the placement of notes at the climaxes of phrases, for example, and even pushing the temporal envelope through *rubato* further than in the model that is provided. Observers comment on how Romy not only appears to have an intuitive understanding of the emotional narrative of the music that is projected from the harmonic framework and rhythm of the accompaniment, but that they find her playing musically persuasive and genuinely moving – a feeling that she seems to share, as she will often vocalise excitedly at the melodic climaxes that she articulates so compellingly and vigorously flaps her left hand (both indicators of a positive affective response), as though intoxicated by the products of a shared musical discourse.

So what is happening here? To reiterate our central question: is the empathy that Romy is able to experience in a musical context different from everyday empathy? Or does music offer a route to empathic engagement with another that she cannot otherwise access? In either case, is this something that is unique to Romy, or to people with autism and learning difficulties more generally, or could it be that many (or all) of us have the potential to experience a distinct, musical form of empathy? And if musical empathy does exist as a mental entity in its own right, does it evolve in line with a child's musical development?

We will address these issues through a series of case studies of children at different stages in the development of their musical abilities. We will structure our discussion in terms of the *Sounds of Intent* framework, which, created through over a decade of research in the field, seeks to map musical development in children and young people with learning difficulties, including those with autism (see, for example, Cheng, Ockelford, & Welch, 2010; Ockelford *et al.*, 2005;

Ockelford *et al.*, 2011; Ockelford & Matawa, 2009; Vogiatzoglou *et al.*, 2011; Welch *et al.*, 2009). Underpinning *Sounds of Intent* is 'zygonic' theory, which sets out to explain how music works as a communicative medium: how it is that abstract patterns of sound are able to convey meaning, and what the nature of that meaning is. And it is to this theory that we now turn our attention.

The zygonic conjecture

In seeking to describe zygonic theory, we will consider first the issue of meaning in language-based art forms, which, as a reflection of an external 'reality' or potential, have a more evident source of meaning construction. According to T. S. Eliot (1933, 1960), literature has three principal sources of meaning (couched in terms of aesthetic response):

- an *objective correlative* – a set of objects, a situation, a chain of events, which shall be the 'formula of a particular emotion';
- the *manner of representation* (including, for example, the use of metaphor);
- the *sound qualities* and *structure* of the language itself.

This thinking may be represented as shown in Figure 1.3. In semiotic terms, the model captures the stages corresponding to the transition from:

- *semantics* (the relationships between signs and the things to which they refer); through
- *syntactics* (the relationships between signs); to
- *pragmatics* (the relationships between the signs and the effects they have on readers or listeners).

However, absolute music (and the abstract component of music with referential meaning) has no objective correlative – no semantic component (see Figure 1.4). In these circumstances, how is meaning constructed and conveyed?

In the absence of semantics, it follows that the meaning of music must derive solely from its syntax – the logical arrangement of its constituent sounds – that has two elements: the qualities of the sounds themselves (in zygonic theory referred to as 'content') and their organisation (termed 'structure').

First, we consider content. Zygonic theory asserts that *all* sounds and the relationships we perceive between them can potentially cause or enable an emotional response (*cf.* Johnson-Laird & Oatley, 1992; Sparshott, 1994, p. 28). There appear to be two main sources of such responses (a) 'expressive non-verbal vocalisations' and (b) 'music-specific' qualities of sound.

'Expressive non-verbal vocalisations' comprise the cues used to express emotions vocally in non-verbal communication and speech (Juslin, Friberg, & Bresin, 2001). They are present cross-culturally (Scherer, Banse, & Wallbott, 2001), suggesting a common phylogenetic derivation from 'non-verbal affect vocalisations' (Scherer, 1991) and apparently embedded ontogenetically in

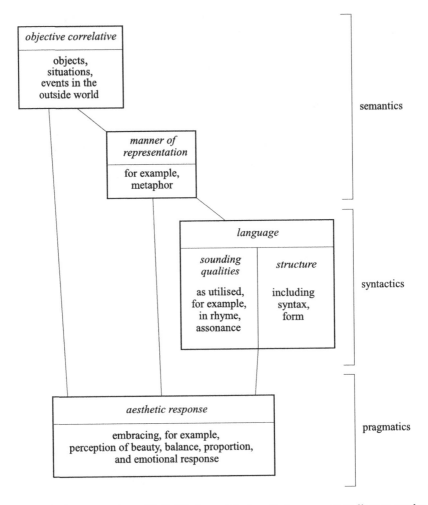

Figure 1.3 Representation of T. S. Eliot's model of aesthetic response to literary works, and its correspondence to semiotic thinking.

early maternal/infant interaction (Malloch, 1999; Trehub & Nakata, 2002). It seems that these cues can be transferred in a general way to music, and music-psychological work from the last 70 years or so has shown that features such as register, tempo and dynamic level do relate with some consistency to particular emotional states (Gabrielsson & Lindström, 2001). For example, passages in a high register can feel exciting (Watson, 1942) or exhibit potency (Scherer & Oshinsky, 1977), whereas series of low notes are more likely to promote solemnity or to be perceived as serious (Watson, 1942). A fast tempo will tend to induce feelings of excitement (Thompson & Robitaille, 1992), in contrast to slow tempi that may connote tranquility (Gundlach, 1935) or even peace (Balkwill &

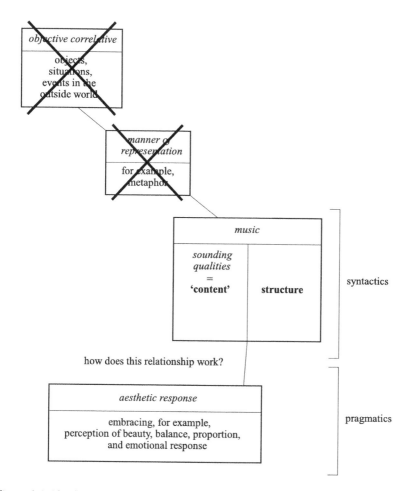

Figure 1.4 Absolute music has no objective correlative – so how is meaning conveyed?

Thompson, 1999). Loud dynamic levels are held to be exciting (Watson, 1942), triumphant (Gundlach, 1935) or to represent gaiety (Nielzén & Cesarec, 1982), while quiet sounds have been found to express fear, tenderness or grief (Juslin, 1997). Conversely, as Leonard Meyer observes (2001, p. 342), 'one cannot imagine sadness being portrayed by a fast forte tune played in a high register, or a playful child being depicted by a solemnity of trombones'.

'Music-specific' qualities of sound, like those identified above in relation to early vocalisation, have the capacity to induce consistent emotional responses, *within* and sometimes *between* cultures. For example, in the West and elsewhere, music typically utilises a framework of relative pitches with close connections to the harmonic series. These are used idiosyncratically, with context-dependent frequency of occurrence and transition patterns, together yielding the sensation of 'tonality' (Krumhansl, 1997; Peretz, 1998). These frameworks of relative pitch can accommodate different 'modalities', each potentially bearing distinct emotional connotations. In Indian music, for example, the concept of the 'raga' is based on the idea that particular patterns of notes are able to evoke heightened states of emotion (Jairazbhoy & Khan, 1971), while in the Western tradition of the last four centuries or so, the 'major mode' is typically associated with happiness and the 'minor mode' with sadness (Crowder, 1985; Hevner, 1936), differences which have been shown to have neurological correlates (Nemoto, Fujimaki, & Wang, 2010; Suzuki *et al.*, 2008).

On their own, however, separate emotional responses to a series of individual sounds or clusters would not add up to a coherent musical message – a unified aesthetic response that evolves over time. So what is it that binds these discrete, abstract experiences together to form a cogent musical narrative? It is my contention that organising force is 'structure', as defined in zygonic theory.

To understand how this works, consider verbal language once more. Eliot's 'objective correlative' is likely to be a series of events, actions, feelings or thoughts that are in some way *logically related*, each contingent on another or others through concepts such as causation. Relationships like these will be conveyed and given additional layers of meaning through language-specific relationships such as metaphor (in the domain of 'manner of representation'), rhyme and meter (in the domain of 'sounding qualities') and syntax (in the domain of 'structure') – see Figure 1.5.

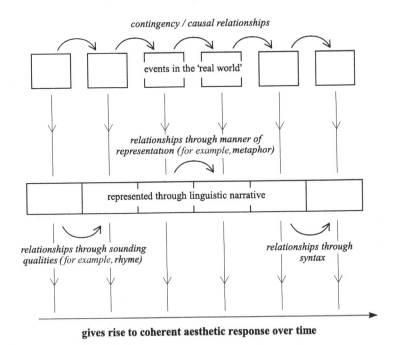

Figure 1.5 The forms of logical relationship underpinning meaning in language.

But how does a comparable sense of coherence and unity – a sense of structure – come about in music, when it cannot borrow a sense of contingency from the external world? In the absence of an objective correlative, musical events can refer only to *themselves* (Selincourt, 1920). Self-evidently, one sound does not *cause* another one to happen (it is performers who do that), but one can *imply* another (Meyer, 1989, p. 84ff) through a sense of derivation. That is, one musical event can be felt to stem from another, and it is my contention that this occurs through imitation: if one fragment or feature of music echoes another, then it owes the nature of its existence to its model. And just as certain perceptual qualities of sound are felt to derive from one another, so too, it is hypothesised, are the emotional responses to each. Hence, over time a metaphorical (musical) narrative, the expression of coherently linked emotional states that exist and can change over time, can be built up through abstract patterns of sound (see Figure 1.6).

The agency through which musical implication occurs is held to be a particular kind of perceived relationship that acknowledges the qualities of separate sounds that are the same or similar. Such relationships – purely mental constructs – are termed 'zygonic', after the Greek 'zygon', meaning a 'yoke' or connection between similar things (Ockelford, 1991). The musical effect of a zygonic relationship is that a second event seems to *derive from* one that precedes, or, conversely, that a given event appears to *generate* one that follows. The underlying imitation can be exact or approximate, and refer to part or the whole of a musical event. Relationships can be of different levels: 'primary', between percepts themselves; 'secondary', between perceptual differences; and 'tertiary', between the relationships between differences (see Figure 1.7).

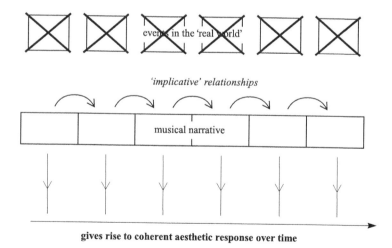

Figure 1.6 Relationships underpinning logic in music.

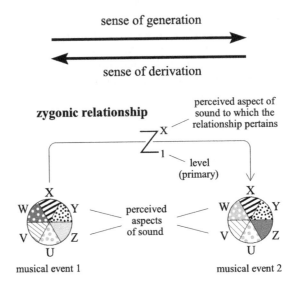

Figure 1.7 Representation of primary zygonic relationship.

The cognition of musical structure

Zygonic theory holds that the cognition of musical structure occurs at three levels in the domains of pitch and perceived time, and that these pertain to 'events', 'groups' and 'frameworks' (Ockelford, 2006, 2011). Essentially the same conjecture pertains to groups and frameworks as to events: that musical structure will be cognised when one musical element or feature is heard as imitating another. Given young children's propensity to copy sounds and to relish being copied, it seems that the neural correlates of zygonic relationships must emerge early in the development of cognition, with the capacity to function both reactively (that is, *recognising* the imitation of one musical event by another) and proactively (*creating* one musical event by copying another). How this ability subsequently evolves to enable young listeners to gauge the similarities between groups of sounds and between the imaginary, probabilistic frameworks of pitch and perceived time within which pieces of music are typically cast, is the subject of other research (Ockelford & Voyajolu, 2016). For example, the way in which zygonic relationships of pitch can function reactively between events, groups and frameworks to create perceived coherence at different structural levels, and the cognitive demands that each is hypothesised to pose on listeners (see Figure 1.8) will be illustrated in relation to the opening bars of Beethoven's 5th Symphony.

Recognising imitation between *events* is postulated to take the least mental processing power, requiring (at least) two items of musical information (which comprise notes in the current example) to be held in working memory and compared. The temporal envelope within which such structures occur and are

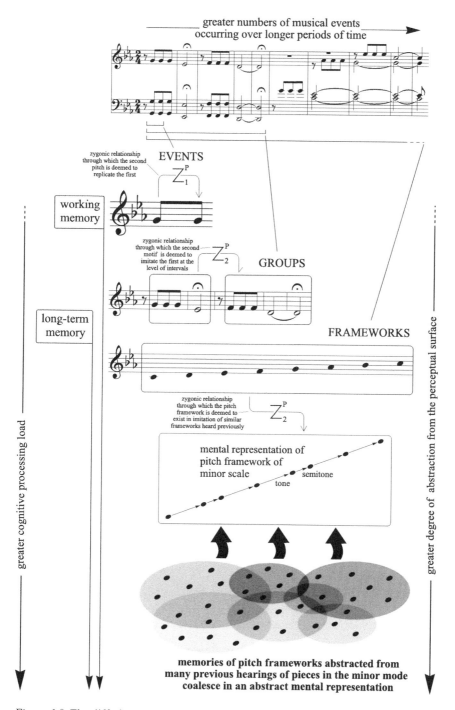

greater numbers of musical events
occurring over longer periods of time

EVENTS

zygonic relationship
through which the second
pitch is deemed to
replicate the first

Z_1^P

working
memory

zygonic relationship
through which the second
motif is deemed to
imitate the first at the
level of intervals

Z_2^P

GROUPS

long-term
memory

FRAMEWORKS

zygonic relationship
through which the pitch
framework is deemed to
exist in imitation of similar
frameworks heard previously

Z_2^P

mental representation of
pitch framework of
minor scale

semitone

tone

greater cognitive processing load

greater degree of abstraction from the perceptual surface

memories of pitch frameworks abstracted from
many previous hearings of pieces in the minor mode
coalesce in an abstract mental representation

Figure 1.8 The differing cognitive demands of processing musical structure at the level
of events, groups and frameworks.

perceived is generally constrained, sometimes extending to little more than the perceived present. Zygonic connections between *groups* necessarily involve four events or more (Ockelford, 2006, p. 109), whose temporal disposition is potentially far more variable, possibly implicating long-term memory. Here, there may also be a greater degree of abstraction from the perceptual 'surface', when it is relationships between the events within each group that are being compared (as in the example shown – see Figure 1.9). Imitative links between *frameworks* appear to be the most cognitively demanding of all. They depend on the existence of long-term 'schematic' memories (Bharucha, 1987) – in the case of a listener stylistically attuned to the Beethoven symphony, for example, built up from substantial exposure to other pieces in the minor mode. Here, it is assumed that the details of the perceptual surface and individual connections perceived between musical events are not encoded in long-term memory discretely or independently, but are combined with many thousands of other similar data to create probabilistic networks of relationships between notional representations of pitch and perceived time. That is, large amounts of perceptual information are merged to enable the requisitely parsimonious deep level of cognitive abstraction to occur.

In summary, then, it is hypothesised that the cognitive correlates of musical structure grow in complexity as one moves from events to groups and frameworks, reflecting an increasing amount of perceptual input, experienced over longer periods of time, and processed and stored using progressively more abstract forms of mental representation. Moreover, the logic of the music-theoretical model suggests that the cognitive operations pertaining to higher levels of structure must build on and incorporate those required to process lower levels, since connections between groups comprise a series of relationships between events (see Figure 1.9), and links between frameworks are established by acknowledging the correspondences that exist between groups.

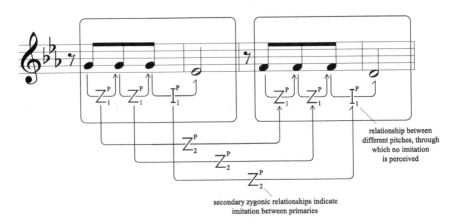

Figure 1.9 Zygonic connections between groups of notes frequently involve the cognition of relationships *between* relationships.

The *Sounds of Intent* project

The existence of the cognitive correlates of musical structure (postulated above from the point of view of an enculturated listener of Western classical music) was first corroborated empirically in the *Sounds of Intent* studies, which were designed to explore the musical development of children with learning difficulties (for example, Cheng, Ockelford, & Welch, 2009; Ockelford *et al.*, 2005; Ockelford *et al.*, 2011; Vogiatzoglou *et al.*, 2011; Welch *et al.*, 2009). Here, the evidence of music-structural processing pertaining to events, groups and frameworks comes from hundreds of observations of young people engaging with music in a range of everyday contexts.

For example, an appreciation of imitation at the level of *events* is implied by Zeeshan's laughing and rocking 'when he hears his teacher imitating Tom's vocal sounds', an understanding that is translated into action by Xavier, who 'distinctly tries to copy high notes and low notes in vocal interaction sessions' (Ockelford, 2012, pp. 130, 133). Lottie seems to be able to recognise *group* structures, since she 'cries whenever she hears the "goodbye" song. It only takes the first two or three notes to be played on the keyboard, and she experiences a strong emotional reaction'. This capacity is realised in sound by Lottie, who 'hums distinct patterns of notes and repeats them. Her favourite sounds rather like a playground chant, and she repeats it from one day to the next' (Ockelford, 2012, pp. 129–130). Quincy, who 'knows that when his music teacher plays the last verse of *Molly Malone* in the minor key it signifies sadness' shows some non-conceptual understanding of how pitch *frameworks* work in the Western musical vernacular, while Janet, with severe learning difficulties, has taken Quincy's intuitive grasp of mode a stage further, having 'developed the confidence to introduce new material on her saxophone in the school's jazz quartet' (Ockelford, 2012, pp. 129–130).

Although much of the data gathered in the course of the *Sounds of Intent* project comprised 'snapshots' of children's musical engagement at a single point in time, rather than offering longitudinal accounts, two developmental features of music-structural cognition did become apparent. First, as one would expect, it appeared that the successively more extensive cognitive abilities required to process musical structure at the level of events, groups and frameworks arise sequentially in development. The evidence for this stemmed from the observation that there were no instances of children showing music-structural engagement at the level of frameworks who were not also able to recognise or create imitative patterns involving groups, nor of children who could process or produce group structures who could not also operate cognitively at the level of events. Second, it became evident that the cognitive capacities pertaining to each structural level do not emerge fully functioning, but themselves evolve incrementally: that is to say, as well as music-structural processing developing *between* levels, there also appeared to be development *within* each of them.

In addition, the *Sounds of Intent* data suggested precursors to the three stages of music-structural cognition whose postulated existence they substantiated. To frame these developmental antecedents theoretically, consider that imitation, which lies at the heart of zygonic theory, can only have significance in the context of potential *variety*. This is because for one sound (or aspect of sound) to be heard as deriving from another – for the concept of agency in repetition to exist – requires a (hypothetical) range of options to be available. That is to say, before children can appreciate or make imitatively generated patterns in sound, they need to be able to process or create a range of sonic alternatives. This in turn implies that they will have had many, diverse listening experiences and sound-making opportunities. Examples of children functioning at this level who were observed in the course of the *Sounds of Intent* project include Rick, whose 'eye movements intensify when he hears the big band play' and Oliver, who 'scratches the tambourine, making a range of sounds … whenever he plays near the rim and the bells jingle, he smiles' (Ockelford *et al.*, 2011, pp. 179–180).

A few of the children who were involved in the *Sounds of Intent* research appeared to be at a stage before this one of developing auditory perception, when the processing of sound had yet to get underway at all. Examples included Anna, who

> sits motionless in her chair. Her teacher approaches and plays a cymbal with a soft beater, gently at first, and then more loudly, in front of her and then near to each ear. She does not appear to react.

and Yerik, who

> usually makes a rasping sound as he breathes. He seems to be unaware of what he is doing, and the rasping persists, irrespective of external stimulation. His class teacher has tried to see whether Yerik can be made aware of his sounds by making them louder (using a microphone, amplifier and speakers), but so far this approach has met with no response.
>
> (Ockelford, 2012, p. 129)

It seemed that nothing could precede this pre-perceptual stage, so it was termed (*Sounds of Intent*) Level 1. The pre-structural stage, referred to above, of which Rick and Oliver provided examples, was called Level 2. The three stages of structural cognition, pertaining to events, groups and frameworks, were designated respectively Levels 3, 4 and 5. These five levels, while covering a vast range of musical development, did not seem to present a complete picture, however, as there were examples of children engaging with music who were more or less consciously manipulating the parameters of sound – pitch, timing, loudness and timbre – to achieve particular expressive ends. For instance, Ciara

> who is a good vocalist despite having severe learning difficulties, is learning how to convey a range of different emotions in her singing through using techniques such as vibrato, rubato, consciously using a wider range of dynamics, and producing darker and lighter sounds.

And Ruth,

> who sings well, and is used to performing in public, although she has severe learning difficulties and autism. She can learn new songs just by listening to

her teacher (who is not a trained singer) run through them, and as she gets to know a piece, she intuitively adds expression as she feels appropriate. … Later, when she listens to other people singing the songs she knows, she clearly prefers some performances to others. Her teacher believes this shows that she has a mature engagement with pieces in mid-to-late twentieth-century popular style.

(Ockelford, 2012, p. 129)

This stage of musical development, in which young people appeared to be aware of the culturally determined rules of expressive performance, was labelled Level 6.

The six *Sounds of Intent* levels, and the core cognitive abilities associated with each, can be summarised as follows (Ockelford, 2012, p. 148). See Table 1.1.

The *Sounds of Intent* research further divided the universe of potential musical engagement into three domains: 'reactive' (R), which entailed listening and responding to sounds; 'proactive' (P), which involved causing, creating or controlling sounds; and 'interactive' (I), which meant participating in sound-making activity in the context of others. Conceptually, the three domains and six levels were orthogonal, implying that they could be represented as a matrix with 18 cells. This was represented visually as a series of concentric circles divided into segments, ranging from the centre (Level 1), with its focus on self, to the outermost ring (Level 6), with its reference to wider communities of others. The convention of denoting each segment by its domain (R, P or I) followed by its level (1, 2, 3, 4, 5 or 6) was used. Hence 'R.1' refers to 'Reactive Level 1', 'P.3' to 'Proactive Level 3', and 'I.6' to 'Interactive Level 6'. Brief descriptors were developed for the segments, which sought to summarise the nature of the musical engagement that each involved – see Figure 1.10.

Table 1.1 The six levels underpinning the *Sounds of Intent* framework (acronym 'CIRCLE').

Level	Description	Acronym	Core cognitive abilities
1	Confusion and Chaos	C	No awareness of sound
2	Awareness and Intentionality	I	An emerging awareness of sound and of the variety that is possible within the domain of sound
3	Relationships, repetition Regularity	R	A growing awareness of the possibility and significance of relationships between sonic *events*
4	Sounds forming Clusters	C	An evolving perception of *groups* of sounds and of the relationships that may exist between them
5	Deeper structural Links	L	A growing recognition of whole pieces, and of the *frameworks* of pitch and perceived time that lie behind them
6	Mature artistic Expression	E	A developing awareness of the culturally determined 'emotional syntax' of performance that articulates the 'narrative metaphor' of pieces

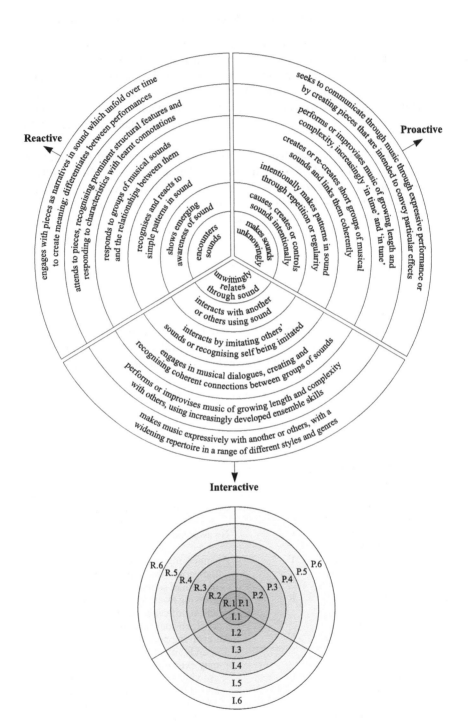

Reactive

engages with pieces as narratives in sound which unfold over time to create meaning; differentiates between performances

attends to pieces, recognising prominent structural features and responding to characteristics with learnt connotations

responds to groups of musical sounds and the relationships between them

recognises and reacts to simple patterns in sound

shows emerging awareness of sound

encounters sounds

Proactive

seeks to communicate through music through expressive performance or by creating pieces that are intended to convey particular effects

performs or improvises music of growing length and complexity, increasingly 'in time' and 'in tune.'

creates or re-creates short groups of musical sounds and links them coherently

intentionally makes patterns in sound through repetition or regularity

causes, creates or controls sounds intentionally

makes sounds unknowingly

unwittingly relates through sound

interacts with another or others using sound

interacts by imitating others' sounds or recognising self being imitated

engages in musical dialogues, creating and recognising coherent connections between groups of sounds

performs or improvises music of growing length and complexity with others, using increasingly developed ensemble skills

makes music expressively with another or others, with a widening repertoire in a range of different styles and genres

Interactive

R.6 R.5 R.4 R.3 R.2 R.1 P.1 P.2 P.3 P.4 P.5 P.6

I.1
I.2
I.3
I.4
I.5
I.6

Figure 1.10 Visual representation of the *Sounds of Intent* framework.

Implications of the *Sounds of Intent* music-developmental model for our understanding of the evolving sense of self in children with learning difficulties

Ockelford and Welch (2012) and Ockelford and Vorhaus (2016) explored the connection between the music-developmental levels identified in the *Sounds of Intent* framework and the evolving sense of self found in children with learning difficulties. To do this, the *Sounds of Intent* levels were matched to an extended version of the model of early expressive communication set out in Ockelford (2002). The result is shown in Table 1.2.

This composite developmental map was aligned with the notion of an evolving self through reference to Shaun Gallagher's distinction between the *minimal* self, considered as a 'consciousness of oneself as an immediate subject of experience, unextended in time', and the *narrative* self, considered as 'self-image that is constituted with a past and a future in the various stories that we and others tell about ourselves' (Gallagher, 2000, p. 15). The outcome is shown in Figure 1.11.

The discussion that follows extends this thinking (which conceives of musical engagement as a proxy indicator of a sense of self): conceptualising musical reactivity, proactivity and interactivity at different development levels as a window onto the evolving empathic mind of children with learning difficulties and autism. To this end, we present six vignettes of musical engagement at each of the six *Sounds of Intent* levels, with reflections on each of these in terms of their implications for the children's awareness of and sensitivity to others' musical thinking and feeling, and for our understanding of musical empathy more generally.

Six vignettes

1. **Amelia** A teaching assistant pushes Amelia in her wheelchair into the music room to join her class for their weekly session with the music therapist. All six children in the group, who are 13 or 14 years of age, have profound and multiple learning difficulties, meaning that they are in the very early stages of cognitive, emotional and social development. In previous sessions, the therapist has been unable to discern any response from Amelia to the wide range of musical sounds – particularly vocal sounds – that have been presented. And today is the same: Amelia reclines motionless in her chair, gaze fixed, apparently not making sense of visual stimuli. She makes no discernible response to any of the sounds that are presented, nor any observable attempt to make sound deliberately with her voice or by moving her fingers against a lightweight wind chime that is placed next to her hand. Although she sometimes wheezes as she exhales, the therapist's efforts to make Amelia aware of this by using a microphone and amplification system do not elicit a response or change in her breathing pattern. Amelia makes no noticeable attempts to interact with her assistant who, as the session progresses, sensitively tries to engage her through touch, sight and sound, emulating and complementing the breathy sounds that Amelia makes.

Table 1.2 The *Sounds of Intent* levels mapped onto the developmental stages of expressive communication.

Phase of expressive communication	Vocal/verbal level of development	Corresponding Sounds of Intent proactive levels	Corresponding Sounds of Intent interactive levels
non-intentional	cries in response to need	P.1 makes sounds unknowingly	I.1 unwittingly relates through sound
intentional	deliberately vocalises to show need	P.2 causes, creates or controls sound intentionally	I.2 interacts with another or others using sound
symbolic	makes personal utterances: for example, says 'mmm', meaning hairdryer	P.3 intentionally makes patterns in sound through repetition or regularity	I.3 interacts by imitating other's sounds or recognising self being imitated
		P.4 creates or re-creates short groups of musical sounds and links them coherently	I.4 engages in musical dialogues, creating and recognising coherent connections between groups of sounds
formal	speaks (using words)	P.5 performs or improvises music of growing length and complexity, increasingly 'in time' and 'in tune'	I.5 performs or improvises music of growing length and complexity with others, using increasingly developed ensemble skills
pragmatic	uses language with appropriate social understanding	P.6 seeks to communicate through music through expressive performance or by creating pieces that are intended to convey particular effects	I.6 makes music expressively with another or others, with a widening repertoire in a range of different styles and genres

Amelia appears to be oblivious to the sounds around her (and of stimuli in other sensory domains), and she seems to be unaware of her capacity to make noises as a product of her own bodily functions such as breathing. Inevitably, then, she is unable to interact knowingly through sound. Hence, we can assume that she is functioning at *Sounds of Intent* Level 1. What does this mean in terms of empathy? As have seen, according to Meltzoff (2007), having a sense of other requires first a sense of self. Yet there are no indications that Amelia

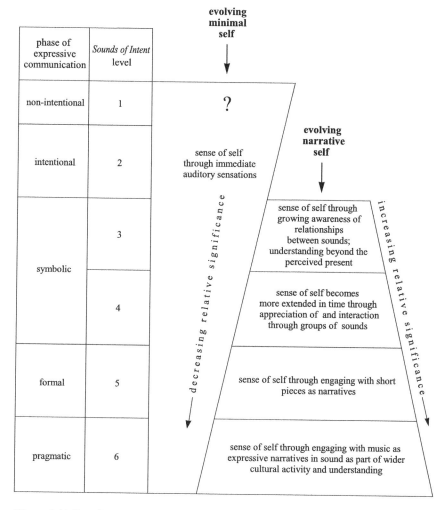

Figure 1.11 Putative parallels between stages of musical development and an evolving sense of self.

has reached this stage of awareness, let alone a notion of self and other. Hence, we must conclude that she is not yet capable of experiencing musical empathy, either affectively or cognitively (see Figures 1.12 and 1.13). The music therapist, however, intuitively interprets Amelia's sounds in the context of communication, and responses are musically empathic. The teaching assistant too, by responding sensitively to Amelia's sounds is exhibiting musical empathy, or, as Cross, Laurence and Rabinowitch (2012) would have it, being 'creatively empathic'.

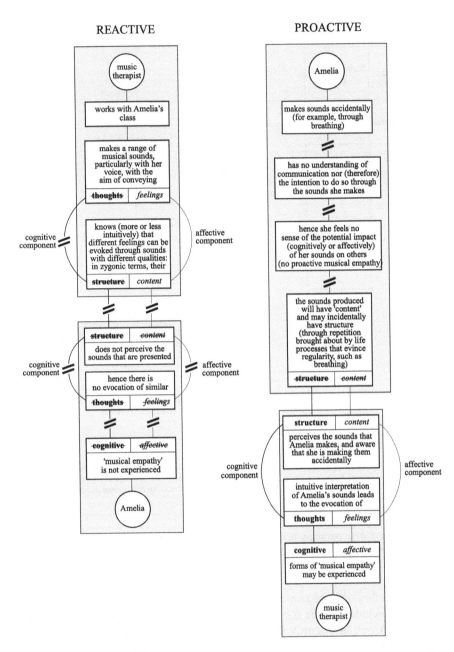

REACTIVE

- music therapist
- works with Amelia's class
- makes a range of musical sounds, particularly with her voice, with the aim of conveying | ~~thoughts~~ | *feelings*
- cognitive component ⪯ knows (more or less intuitively) that different feelings can be evoked through sounds with different qualities: in zygonic terms, their | ~~structure~~ | *content* ⪰ affective component
- ⪯ | ~~structure~~ | ~~content~~ does not perceive the sounds that are presented ⪰
- cognitive component ⪯ hence there is no evocation of similar | ~~thoughts~~ | ~~feelings~~ ⪰ affective component
- ⪯ | ~~cognitive~~ | ~~affective~~ 'musical empathy' is not experienced ⪰
- Amelia

PROACTIVE

- Amelia
- makes sounds accidentally (for example, through breathing)
- has no understanding of communication nor (therefore) the intention to do so through the sounds she makes
- hence she feels no sense of the potential impact (cognitively or affectively) of her sounds on others (no proactive musical empathy)
- the sounds produced will have 'content' and may incidentally have structure (through repetition brought about by life processes that evince regularity, such as breathing) | ~~structure~~ | ~~content~~
- cognitive component ⪯ | structure | *content* perceives the sounds that Amelia makes, and aware that she is making them accidentally ⪰ affective component
- intuitive interpretation of Amelia's sounds leads to the evocation of | **thoughts** | *feelings*
- | **cognitive** | *affective* forms of 'musical empathy' may be experienced
- music therapist

Figure 1.12 Amelia shows no signs of reactive or proactive musical empathy (Level 1).

INTERACTIVE

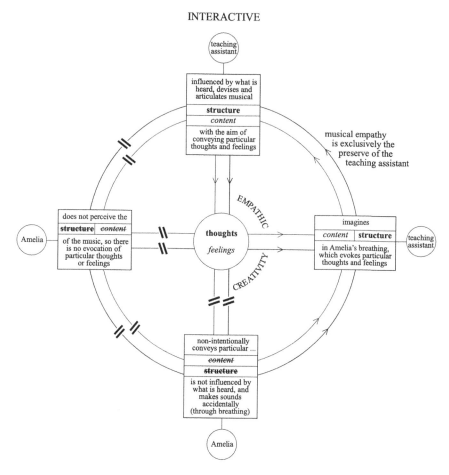

Figure 1.13 Amelia shows no signs of interactive musical empathy (Level 1).

2. **Ethan** Ethan is six. He has profound global developmental delay, functioning physically, cognitively, emotionally and socially as though he were around four or five months old. His mother notices that he is becoming more aware of the sounds around him, and he appears to respond in particular to the female human voice, sometimes picking up on the emotions that are expressed. He tends to find it upsetting when he hears someone cry, for example – particularly other children, such as his baby brother – and will occasionally smile when others laugh. Ethan can himself make a range of vocal sounds, which he uses to express how he is feeling: happy, sad, excited, frustrated, angry or quietly content. He is beginning to

realise that his vocalisations can have an effect on other people, and when he sees someone he knows, he will often try to engage them through making a sound, and waiting for a response. He will also vocalise when people speak or sing to him, though there is no evidence of deliberate imitation on his part.

This account of Ethan suggests that he has an emerging awareness of sound and of the variety that is possible within the auditory domain. He has a sense of his own capacity to make a range of sounds, and interacts through sound with other people. Hence it is reasonable to assert that he is functioning at *Sounds of Intent* Level 2. In terms of the development of musical empathy, we can assume that Ethan's sense of agency, derived from his ability to create sound, and his capacity to externalise his feelings through sound, must contribute to an evolving sense of self – of his own identity in relation to others. This is shown by his realising that he can affect others through his sound-making, and his desire for other people to reciprocate when he vocalises. His sense of other is evident too in the emotional contagion he experiences when those around him cry or laugh. By having the capacity to be stimulated through sounds expressive of emotion to feel what others feel (rather as newborns do – see Martin and Clark (1982), Sagi and Hoffman (1976); Simner (1971)) and despite (presumably) being unable to reflect on this process, it seems reasonable nonetheless to assert that Ethan is capable of experiencing a basic form of affective (though not yet cognitive) empathy in the domain of sound (McDonald & Messinger, 2011; Zahn-Waxler & Radke-Yarrow, 1990). Strictly speaking, this cannot be considered to be 'musical empathy', since, according to zygonic theory, the characteristic that distinguishes music from other forms of sound (such as speech and everyday noise) is the presence of repetition deemed to be brought about through imitation. Hence a more accurate term might be 'proto-musical empathy' – see Figures 1.14 and 1.15.

3. **Chloe** Chloe has severe learning difficulties. She is eight years old. She has a vocabulary of around ten words that she uses to communicate some of her basic needs, and, beyond this, her family and the staff at her school have learnt to interpret a range of idiosyncratic gestures that she makes, such as flapping her hand for 'more'. In day-to-day life, Chloe gives little or no sense of being aware of, or concerned about, other people's circumstances, thoughts or feelings. However, she loves it when people copy the sounds that she produces – when they do it makes her laugh – and she never seems to get bored, flapping her hand enthusiastically. Sometimes she tries to copy other people too, especially the funny sounds that they make with their voices, and she can become excited when she gets it right. Chloe also likes banging things loudly on hard surfaces (such as her kitchen table at home or the wooden floor in her classroom), using anything she has to hand, making regular beats that go on and on, and if her class teacher

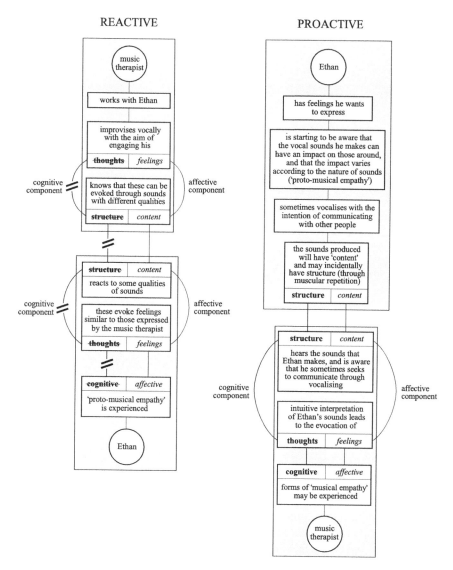

Figure 1.14 Ethan shows signs of reactive and proactive proto-musical empathy (Level 2).

starts clapping or tapping a steady pulse, she can anticipate what comes next and join in. The nature of the sound that is made seems less important to Chloe than the regularity of the beat. She also enjoys listening to any pieces with a strong rhythmic drive – especially the relentless uniformity of dance music.

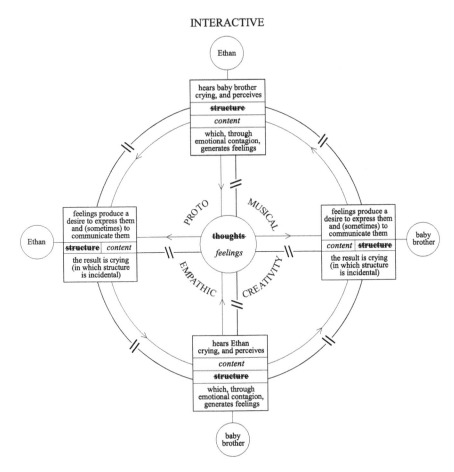

Figure 1.15 Ethan shows signs of interactive proto-musical empathic creativity (Level 2).

It seems that Chloe appreciates simple patterns of repetition and imitation in sound, in relation to listening, to her own production and through interaction with other people. Hence, she appears to be functioning at *Sounds of Intent* Level 3, which has a number of implications for her capacity to think and feel music-empathically. For instance, her ability to copy some of the sounds that other people make (and the pleasure that she takes in doing so) suggests that she has some sense of 'being like them' (Meltzoff, 2007). Moreover, the fact that she is aware of being imitated means that she may have a notion, at some level, of those people 'being like her' (see Figure 1.16). Hence, in Meltzoff's terms, Chloe intuitively knows that there is someone else out there who is 'like her but isn't her' – the first step towards her having a fully-fledged theory of mind. Beyond this, since Chloe can sustain a regular beat, which requires both memory and anticipation, we can surmise that (albeit non-consciously)

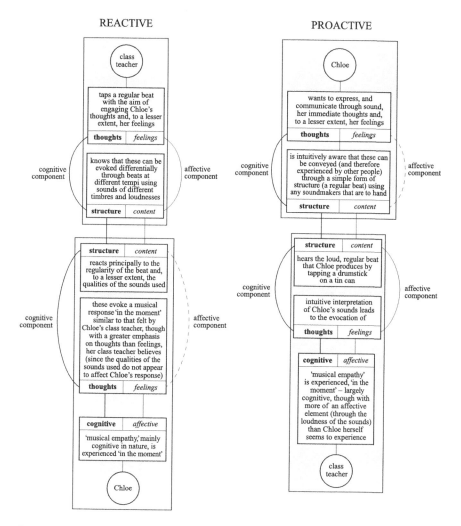

Figure 1.16 Chloe shows reactive and proactive musical empathy in the moment (Level 3).

her sense of self, in the form of her thoughts and feelings expressed in sound, extends from the perceived present into the recent past and the immediate future. Furthermore, her capacity to continue simple patterns started by others shows that she has moved beyond *reacting* to what they think and do to *predicting* their thoughts and actions: a further development in her evolving theory of mind (Figure 1.17). The fact that it is the regularity of the beat that is made (as opposed to the nature of its constituent sounds) suggests that musical structure is more significant to her than content – in empathic terms, that thoughts are more important than feelings, that cognition is of more consequence than affect.

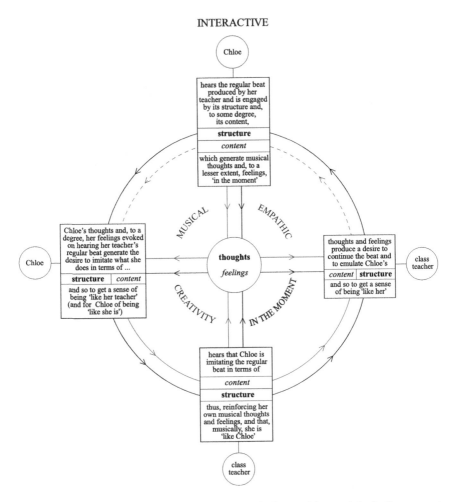

INTERACTIVE

Figure 1.17 Chloe and her class teacher share musical empathic creativity in the moment through playing a common regular beat: 'she is like me' and 'I am like her' (Level 3).

4. **Drew** Drew is 14. He has severe learning difficulties, and functions in many ways at an early years level. He can communicate effectively, if idiosyncratically, using his vocabulary of around 100 words, which he tends to combine in short bursts of meaningful speech when he is motivated to do so. He likes noodling on the keyboard, playing scraps of tunes that he has heard – often the short 'hooks' from pop songs, some of which he appears to like partly through their association with his father, who plays in a band. He will repeat simple jazz riffs too, apparently relishing the fact that he can create an ongoing stream of sound. Although processing and producing verbal language appears to be something of an effort for Drew, he relaxes and evidently enjoys

it when his music teacher sits down with him at the keyboard, and the two of them have extended conversations in sound, using short bursts of melodic material, sometimes copying exactly what the other has just done, and sometimes engaging in 'call and response' patterns, where ideas are changed as they bounce back and forth. During these interactions, Drew makes frequent eye contact with his teacher, and smiles from time to time, seeming to delight in the engagement with another person that music enables him to make.

Drew's preoccupation with 'chunks' of musical material suggests that he is functioning in music-developmental terms at *Sounds of Intent* Level 4. His capacity not only to repeat motifs but to develop them when interacting with his music teacher suggests, in terms of musical empathy, that he has moved beyond Meltzoff's notion of understanding that he is 'like his teacher yet *not* him' (*Sounds of Intent* Level 3) to acknowledging (albeit intuitively) that he is 'like his teacher yet *different* from him' (see Figure 1.18). That is, although Drew's

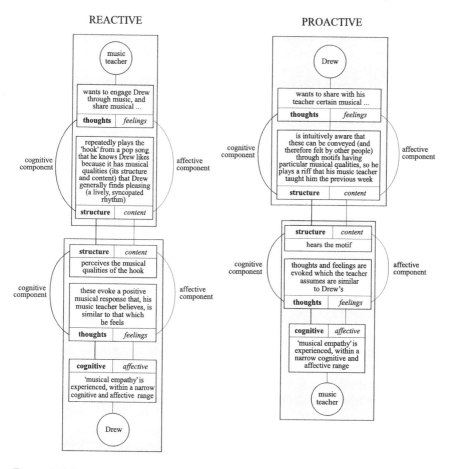

Figure 1.18 Drew shows reactive and proactive musical empathy through sharing a musical motif with his teacher, which has associative memories (Level 4).

empathic capacity lies within a relatively narrow cognitive and affective range, his musical theory of mind appears to have developed to the point where he can grasp that another person's ideas about a fragment of music may be congruent with his own, yet distinct from them. There is a sense too that his appreciation of another's musical perspective extends beyond the immediate present (as experienced by Chloe), and that he recognises that other people's musical thinking may change over time: his music teacher does not always give the same response when Drew plays a particular riff, yet Drew is aware, at some level, that each of his teacher's distinct musical rejoinders arises from the same musical mind. The more extensive temporal envelope of conscious thought that is open to Drew (compared with Chloe) means that longer-term memories can feature in his music-empathic thoughts and feelings too: in particular, he is aware that the thinking and emotion that he associates with particular chunks of music may also be experienced by his music teacher. Yet outside the context of music-making, Drew struggles to get inside other people's heads; his language is too limited for him to convey or understand anything beyond information pertaining to his own immediate circumstances, needs or wants. Paradoxically, it is when he is freed from the constraints and frustrations of trying to use sounds with propositional meaning (words), and interacts instead using sounds with *no* symbolic meaning (notes), that Drew is able to glean insights into other people's minds – thoughts and feelings that the adults around him resort to describing with verbal language (see Figure 1.19).

5.   **Freddie** Freddie, nine years old, is on the autism spectrum and has severe learning difficulties. Although his receptive language enables him to glean, from what he is told, most of what is about to occur in everyday life, he rarely speaks, and when he does it is almost invariably to ask for something that he wants or to check what is going to happen next. Although Freddie is very affectionate and physically demonstrative with his family and the other familiar adults around him, his desire for human contact seems driven more by hedonism than a concern for other's thoughts and feelings. He has a narrow range of interests, including music, in which domain he has exceptional talents (including absolute pitch) and is highly motivated, in a reactive way, spending a good deal of his leisure time listening to a wide range of music on his iPad – often the same piece over and over again. Proactively, however, he is rather more reluctant to engage in music-making, and, despite having been learning the piano for around two years, he still usually displays an initial reluctance to get involved in lessons. Once he is over the participation threshold, though, he will sing and play with enthusiasm, often rocking vigorously to the beat. Freddie loves music that is, in every way, repetitive – the more highly structured the better, it seems – preferably with repeated notes, repeated phrases, and repeated sections, characteristic of such 1970s classics as *Eye Level* (popularly known as the Van der Valk TV theme) and *Rockin' All Over the World* (Status Quo), which he enjoys. He will improvise

INTERACTIVE

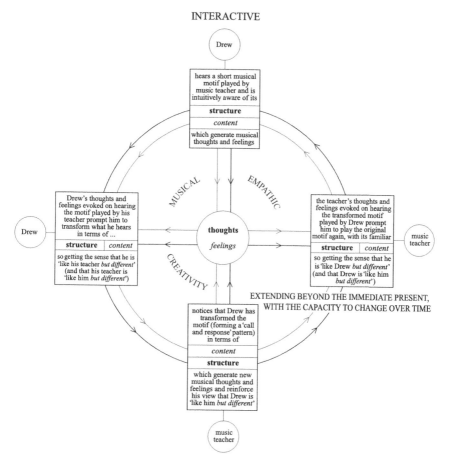

Figure 1.19 Drew and his music teacher share musical empathic creativity beyond the immediate present, that changes over time through a 'call and response' sequence using a short motif (Level 4).

melodies over renditions of pieces that he knows, such as *Twinkle, Twinkle*, singing (wordlessly) or playing the keyboard. However, his productions of musical material, with or without other people, come across as having a 'mechanical' quality, which privileges repetition over change, precision over nuance – in the language of zygonic theory, structure over content.

In music-developmental terms, Freddie's capacity to improvise a tune over a familiar series of harmonies indicates that he has an intuitive grasp of typical Western intervallic and metrical frameworks (an ability that characterises of *Sounds of Intent* Level 5; see Figures 1.20 and 1.21). With regard to musical empathy, Freddie has a somewhat lopsided profile in which the cognitive element is

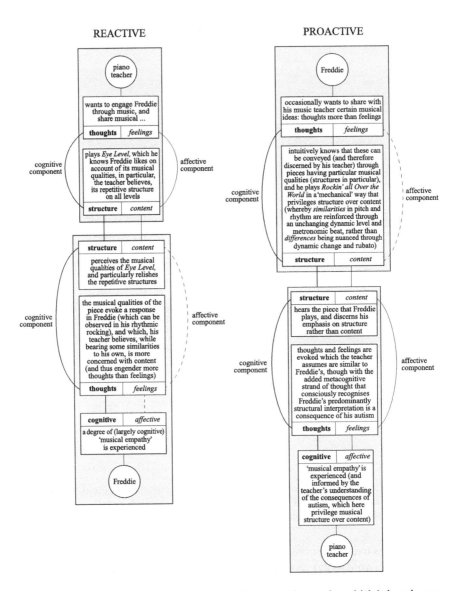

Figure 1.20 Freddie shows reactive and proactive musical empathy, which is largely cognitive in nature (Level 5), and reveals an asymmetrical pattern of empathy with his piano teacher (who appreciates Freddie's playing both cognitively and affectively).

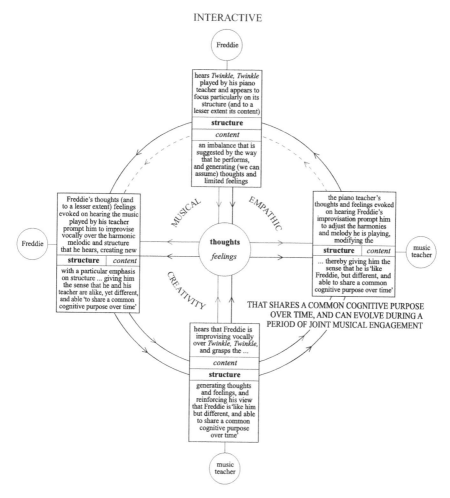

Figure 1.21 Freddie and his piano teacher share an asymmetrical musical empathic creativity through engaging in a common cognitive purpose over time in the domain of music (Level 5).

predominant. However, this is sufficient for him to have a sense of engaging with other people in a common musical purpose over time – sharing a given melodic and harmonic framework and producing either the same or complementary material. Hence we can surmise that Freddie is aware at some level that he and another person can experience periods of shared musical attention in which both parties make distinct contributions to a coherent musical whole; that is, someone else may have thoughts that differ from his yet are nonetheless congruent with them. This level of understanding appears to show that Freddie's capacity for empathy in the domain of music is considerably more advanced than that available to him in everyday life.

6. **Romy** As we noted above, Romy, aged 14, has a severe developmental delay and is unable to speak. She is also left hemiplegic. Romy has a diagnosis of autism, and seems to be largely unaware of (or at least unconcerned by) the thoughts or feelings of other people. Musically, though, she shows great sensitivity, and enjoys playing pieces – including, for example, Stevie Wonder's *I Just Called to Say I Love You* – in the form a melody and a rudimentary bass line (on account of the relative weakness of her left hand), articulating the structure and content using devices such as *rubato* and changes in dynamics, improvising fills, and delighting in the impact that her performance has on listeners in close proximity. Romy likes to be entertained too, and will listen intently to renditions of favourite works, such as Bach's little *Prelude in F*, BWV 928, relishing the climaxes that are marked out with *ritardandi* and *crescendi*, jumping up, flapping her hands and sometimes shrieking with pleasure as a physical embodiment of the strong emotions that she feels. Interactively, in piano duets improvised on pieces such as the *Cavatina* from the film the *Deer Hunter*, Romy, playing the melody, will not only follow the tempo, articulation and dynamic contours that her co-performer offers, but she will also predict, with some accuracy, the expressive devices that her accompanist is likely to use. These include holding back the onsets of notes at the top of phrases, sometimes to an even greater extent than her fellow performer, and exaggerating the dynamics. Romy is increasingly comfortable in interacting with a range of other musicians, and she seems to enjoy testing the limits of their capabilities (by deliberating changing key) and challenging their aesthetic sensibilities (by pushing the expressive envelope even further than usual).

Despite her technical limitations on the piano, Romy's expressive playing and her sophisticated interactions with other musicians suggest that she has a mature understanding of several styles of music within her culture, implying that she is functioning at *Sounds of Intent* Level 6 (see Figures 1.22 and 1.23). Of course, one could contend that Romy has merely learnt to emulate the elements of expressive performance without herself feeling the emotions of which they were originally an expression – an argument that is occasionally levelled at musical savants such as Derek Paravicini (Ockelford, 2008). This line of reasoning can be difficult to counter since neither Romy nor, indeed, Derek are able to reflect verbally on their responses to music. However, the fact that Romy's feelings are embodied in movement and conveyed through screams of delight, and that these correspond to what would generally be acknowledged as emotional peaks in the music, suggest that here is something more than mere imitation of the nuances of another's performance. And Romy's tendency on occasion to push expressivity beyond that of her co-performers also hints at a genuinely advanced level of musicality. In terms of musical empathy, it appears that Romy has the capacity and the desire to share a common musical narrative with another person: as a listener, understanding her

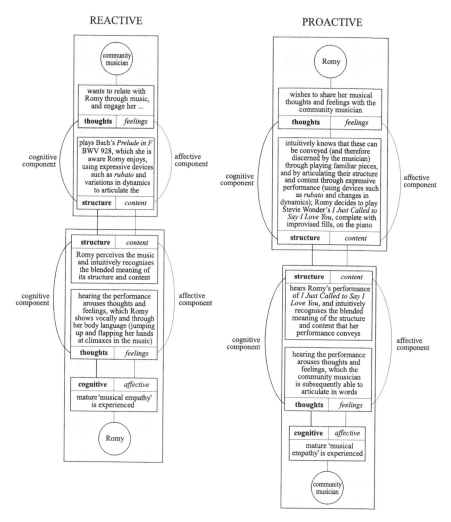

Figure 1.22 Romy shows mature reactive and proactive musical empathy (Level 6).

or his metaphorical emotional–cognitive journey in sound; as a player, knowing how (and wanting) to convey her own interpretations to those around; and as a co-performer, engaging discerningly in empathic creativity. Since Romy is capable of improvising coherently and expressively with musicians with whom she has not worked before, she evidently has musical empathy beyond a few known individuals: she possesses what may be termed 'cultural empathy' in the domain of music (a term coined in the context of multicultural counselling by Ridley and Lingle in 1996).

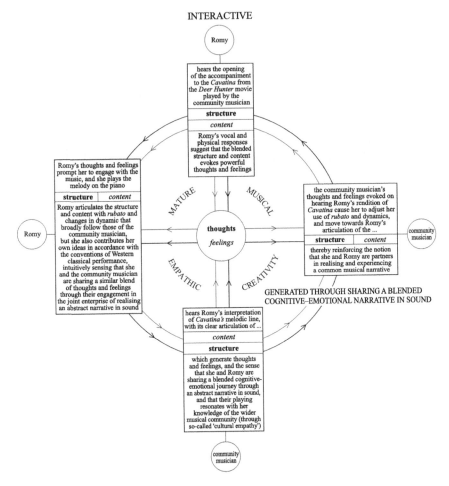

Figure 1.23 Romy and a community musician share a mature empathic creativity (Level 6).

Discussion

What do these six scenarios and the analyses tell us?

1. Musical empathy appears to develop as musicality evolves

The scenarios suggest that there is a correlation between people's developing ability to process, understand and make music and their capacity for behaving empathically in musical terms. Is this a necessary connection, though? The vignettes and corresponding analyses pertain to young people who are consciously *not* neurotypical, since, as we noted above, it is believed that those on the autism spectrum or who have learning difficulties (or both) may, by their very atypicality (including spiky developmental profiles in which the growth of everyday empathy is often inhibited), offer insights that may be obscured in those with a more even spread of intellectual and personality traits. However, the notion of musicality is blind to cerebral 'otherness' (or, indeed, disability): irrespective of individuals' general levels of mental functioning, for them to engage with music is, by definition, for them to engage with the products of other minds. That is to say, one cannot understand music without understanding (albeit intuitively) how other minds work – that is, without musical empathy – whether that manifests itself through joining in with a regular beat (*Sounds of Intent*, Level 3), chanting on the football terraces (Level 4), singing along with a favourite track on the car radio (Level 5), or anticipating (and relishing) the expressive shifts in tempo of a performance of Elgar's cello concerto (Level 6). What the scenarios suggest is that as musical understanding becomes more advanced, so does musical empathy. Moreover, it is worth noting that it is not so much musical *content* that changes between levels but *structure*, which in empathic terms implies that it is not so much *feelings* that are likely to evolve as *thoughts*.

It is of interest to observe that, just as musical engagement moves in broad terms from connection with significant others at Levels 3 and 4, to interaction with increasingly wide groups of peers and fellow music-makers at Levels 4 and 5, and in due course to participation in music-cultural activity at Levels 5 and 6, so musical empathy follows a similar path: from sharing musical thoughts and feelings with other individuals (what may be termed "interpersonal" musical empathy) to more diverse and less familiar sets of people ('group' musical empathy) and eventually to those within wider society, who may even be strangers ('cultural' musical empathy – a feeling for and understanding of the musical heritage and habits of large groups of people with shared values over time). The similarity of this conceptualisation with Bronfenbrenner's ecological systems theory (1979) seems inescapable – see Figure 1.24.

2. *Musical empathy has two strands: 'affective' and 'cognitive'*

It appears that musical empathy, like everyday empathy, has two distinct strands: cognitive and affective, pertaining to thinking and feeling. It is asserted that these in turn relate to the structure and content of music, as defined in zygonic theory. Both are required in order to create a coherent musical message, through which, metaphorically speaking, empathy can flow. Content – the sheer qualities of sounds – can exist without structure, but such irregular features of the auditory landscape do not comprise music, as we saw in the example of Ethan, functioning at Level 2 of the *Sounds of Intent* framework of musical development, and experiencing proto-musical empathy. By the same token, musical structure – the sense of imitation through repetition – requires content in order to be reified. Structure can, however, exist in isolation as an abstract concept (as in the notion of sonata form, for example), and, in terms of styles of listening and performance, as we saw in the case of Freddie (who functions at *Sounds of Intent* Level 5), attention

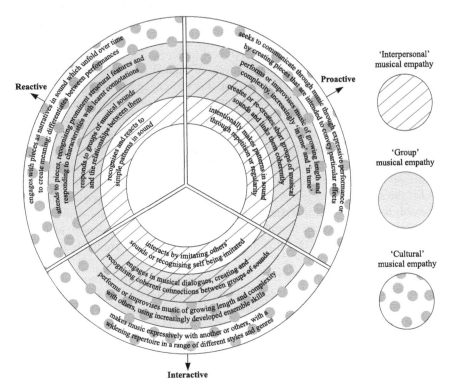

Figure 1.24 Musical empathy extending further into communities of others with maturation.

can largely be devoted to structure at the expense of content: in simple terms, Freddie appears to have a love of repetition for its own sake.

But for most listeners, musical 'thoughts' (as opposed to feelings) apparently exist most if not all of the time beneath the surface of awareness: people can un-thinkingly enjoy the emotional narrative of a piece as it flows by in their stream of consciousness without being sensible of its structure. Hence, a conceptually naïve though perceptually experienced listener of Mozart's *Jupiter* symphony may intuitively delight in the sense of return that the recapitulation brings in the fourth movement, and feel an empathy for the way that, for example, the Chamber Orchestra of Europe under Nikolaus Harnoncourt ushers it in with the subtlest use of *rubato* in the preceding bar, without consciously being aware that this constitutes a restatement of the opening material. In reality, of course, the feeling of 'coming home' after the peregrinations of the development section is due to the *fusion* of structure and content generating a *blend* of thoughts and feelings, and evoking a response that evolves as a *combination* of affect and cognition. It is just that, in the case of the wholly intuitive listener, the former is fore-grounded in consciousness while the latter is less salient. Yet it is safe to assume that Harnoncourt and the musicians of the orchestra, with their advanced musical training, would have recognised the recapitulation on an intellectual level (as well as 'feeling' it). Hence there seems to be an asymmetry in the way that the musicians and many audience members may be perceiving the music. But surely such a mismatch creates difficulties for the notion of musical empathy as defined here? This is the issue to which we next turn our attention.

3. Since those engaging in a common musical activity may do so in different ways and at different levels, so the nature of the musical empathy they experience may differ too

In the scenarios presented above, those engaging with the children tended to use materials that were intended to match their levels of musical development. For example, Chloe's class teacher tapped a regular beat for her to hear and imitate; Drew's music teacher enticed him to participate in musical activity with hooks from his favourite pop songs; and Freddie's piano teacher played him pieces, such as *Eye Level*, that were saturated with repetition. However, there were also occasions when the adults concerned sensed that their own perception of the music may have differed from that of the children's: Freddie's teacher suspected that he himself paid more attention to the content of the music than did his pupil, for example (for whom, as we have seen, structure appeared to be all important). In fact, it seems almost certain that most of the many thousands of hours of music that the children described in the scenarios are likely to have encountered incidentally in everyday life comprised pieces that were not designed with their music-developmental levels in mind, since they are likely largely to have been created and performed by professional musicians functioning at *Sounds of Intent* Level 6. And of the six children mentioned, only Romy has the capacity to appreciate fully the musical messages that are being conveyed and to experience a mature empathic response. But what of Amelia, Ethan, Chloe, Drew and Freddie? What reasonable assumptions can we make about their understanding of and reactions to the music they hear, and what musical empathy are they likely to feel?

As we saw in relation to the zygonic analysis of the first movement of Beethoven's 5th Symphony shown in Figure 1.8, an important feature of the way music works is that structure typically functions on several different levels at once. For instance, we observed that a prerequisite of the cognition of groups of notes (Level 4) is to hear patterning at Level 3 (imitative relationships between individual events), and an awareness of organisation at Level 5 (frameworks) is predicated on the experience of previously having processed the interconnections in the domains of pitch and perceived time between numerous groups (Level 4). Investigation of the ways in which young children engage with music (Ockelford & Voyajolu, n.d.; Voyajolu & Ockelford, 2016) suggests that the developing brain is capable of extracting simpler musical information from the more complex. For example, a two-and-a-half-year-old may dance in time to the beat of a song without grasping its overall structure, while a three-year-old may sing along with a repeated motif without being able to reproduce the whole melody of which it forms a part. It seems that, in developmental terms, the brain first searches for simple patterns of repetition and regularity that may exist on a moment-to-moment basis in the music, before seeking out groups, which require a process of education somewhat removed from the perceptual surface, and make greater demands on attention and memory. Frameworks require the most mental activity of all, with the abstraction of wholly abstract, probabilistic patterns of intervals that we can assume reside deep in long-term memory. Hence, it seems reasonable to assume that, reactively, in relation to a given performance of a particular piece, children will feel musical empathy in a form that accords with their capacity to process the music, rather than necessarily being at the level of those who composed and performed it. And similarly, as youngsters proactively produce music themselves, or interactively make a contribution to a joint musical enterprise, any empathy they experience will be limited by their music-developmental level rather than by what the musical materials potentially have to offer.

For example, let us imagine that Amelia, Ethan, Chloe, Drew, Freddie and Romy are all played a recording of 'When I am laid in earth' from Purcell's *Dido and Aeneas*, sung by Emma Kirkby. What musical empathy is each of them likely to feel? *Given that none of them has fully functioning expressive language, the strongest source of evidence is likely to be found in the musical responses that they may make.* In Amelia's case, her lack of any reaction to the lament (as to all other sound and music) suggests that she derives nothing from the musical exposure nor, therefore, experiences any empathy. Through emotional contagion, Ethan may feel sadness at points in the melody such as those at which Dido sings 'ah!' in a kind of musical wail and respond with his own cries (see Figure 1.25). Chloe may show her empathy for Kirkby's performance (at the level of 'here is someone like me') through short busts of entrained moving or tapping to the underlying pulse, particularly when the beat is set out clearly in the vocal line (as in the opening two bars, for example). Drew may pick up on the repeated iambic pairs of descending semitones in the bass and subsequently use these as a resource for improvising, implying a realisation, at some level, that 'here is someone like me who is nonetheless distinct'. Freddie may well recognise the minor mode, though he is not likely to engage with it on an emotional level. However, he may observe that the bass line is repeated throughout, and later enjoy playing this over and over again while he listens to the recording. Freddie's contribution is likely to be loud and boisterous, apparently trying to push the tempo forward in an effort to get to the next iteration as soon as possible! In empathic terms, we can assume that he has an intuitive sense that Kirkby and her fellow performers are 'like him but different' and able to share a common musical purpose over time. Similarly, after several hearings of the recording, Romy may wish to perform the melody herself on the piano. She is likely to have developed an implicit understanding of the metaphorical narrative of the piece, leading her, like Kirkby, to linger on the climactic top G for expressive effect, as well as emphasising it through a louder dynamic, and reducing the tempo at the end of the (originally instrumental) coda. Hence she will empathise with the performance in a musically mature way.

Musical empathy

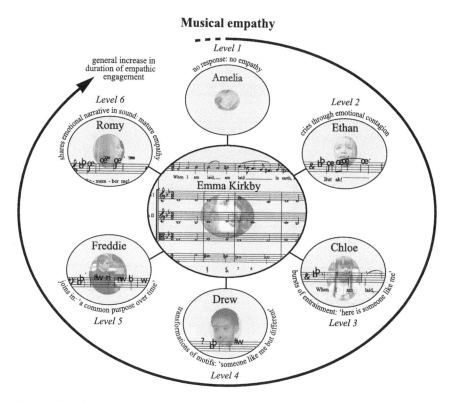

Figure 1.25 Six levels of musical empathy.

In summary, then, it appears that there are six distinguishable stages of musical empathy, which are inherent in developing musicality, and that the *Sounds of Intent* levels can potentially function as proxy music-empathic measures – offering a 'music-empathic quotient' along the lines of the so-called 'Empathy Quotient' (EQ) developed by Baron-Cohen and Wheelwright (2004) and Wakabayashi *et al.* (2006). It is also worth noting that, generally speaking, there is an increase in the duration of empathic engagement as musicality matures.

4. Musical empathy is distinct from and can exist in isolation from everyday empathy

The examples of children and young people on the autism spectrum and with learning difficulties indicate that empathy that arises from music's structure and content (through '*intra*-musical' factors) is distinct from everyday empathy, and can exist in isolation from it (see Figure 1.26). That is not to say, of course, that such a disconnect is the norm: experience suggests that most people, insofar

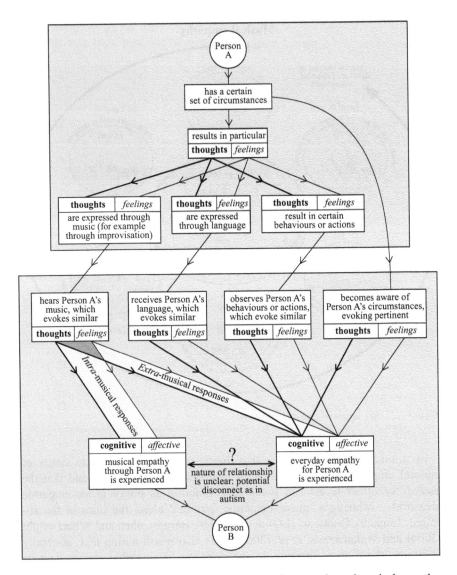

Figure 1.26 Modelling the relationship between everyday empathy and musical empathy.

as they can appreciate music, have musical empathy *in addition* to the general kind. Whether, and if so how, these two mental phenomena interact should be the subject of future research, which could be of particular value for those working with children on the autism spectrum, since it may facilitate the development of pedagogical strategies through which musical empathy could be used to promote empathy in other-than-musical contexts. Conversely, it may also be the case, to the extent that there are some people who do not appear to like music or wish to engage with it at all, for musical empathy to be limited or even absent. Again, this is an area requiring further research.

Finally, to the extent that musical meaning can be generated through the association of particular pieces or excerpts with events, places or people ('*extra-musical*' factors), it is possible for everyday empathy to be elicited through music on account of an extra-musical symbolic connection (rather in the way that verbal narratives can evoke empathy through the *meaning* of the words rather than their *sounds*, although onomatopoeia may play a subsidiary role). This was the case with Drew's music teacher (see Figure 1.18) who played him the hook of a pop song since he was aware that this had pleasant associations for Drew on account of his father's band playing it. One could imagine other cases in which one was cognisant of people's likely reactions to pieces that had been played at a happy occasion (their wedding, for example), or a sad one, such as a close friend's funeral.

Conclusion

The foregoing case studies and discussion enable us to construct a general model of musical empathy, by detailing the nature of the relationship between composer and performer (or improviser) and listener. This is shown in Figure 1.27, where the following sequence of events is illustrated. First, a composer creates music, by producing particular structure and content in the domain of sound, which he or she will be aware can convey certain thoughts and feelings. Sometimes, the desire to express (and communicate) particular musical thoughts and feelings may dictate the choice of structure and content (in the case of composers of film music, for example). Performers take the information about the new music provided by the composer (either indirectly through notation or directly through hearing it played or sung) and add their own layer of interpretation through expressive devices such as *rubato*, *vibrato* and variations in timbre and dynamics. The result is a fusion of structure and content, which elicits a blend of thoughts and feelings that makes up an 'aesthetic response'. In the case of improvisation, this synthesis (and the creation of an aesthetic response) occurs in the moment.

Listeners perceive the integrated flow of musical structure and content over time, which in turn evokes a combination of thoughts and feelings that constitutes their own aesthetic response. To the extent that this is similar to that which the composer and performer (or improviser) intended to be conveyed, so the listener can be said to have musical empathy with the creator and re-creator of the music.

In the case of two people (or more) improvising together, the model may be modified as shown in Figure 1.28. As we noted above, the result is empathic creativity (Cross, Laurence, & Rabinowitch, 2012).

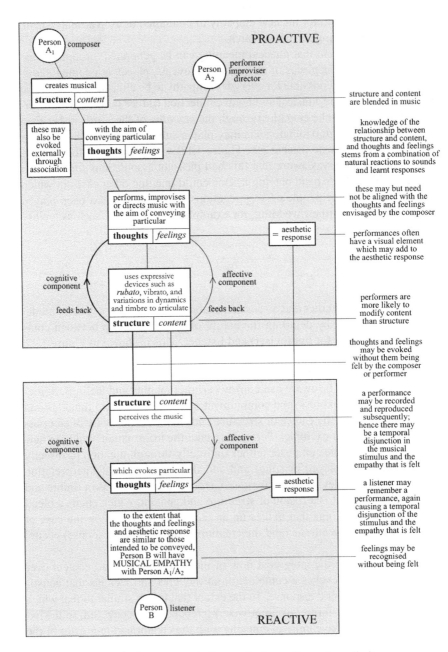

Figure 1.27 A model of mature musical empathy (proactive and reactive).

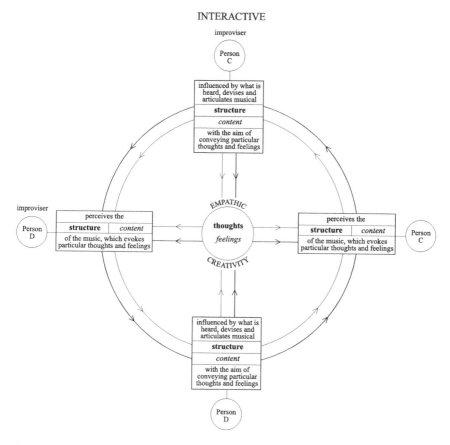

Figure 1.28 A model of mature musical empathy (interactive).

References

Balkwill, L., & Thompson, W. (1999). A cross-cultural investigation of the perception of emotion in music: Psychophysical and cultural cues. *Music Perception: An Interdisciplinary Journal*, *17*(1), 43–64.

Baron-Cohen, S. (1997). *Mindblindness*. Cambridge, MA: MIT Press.

Baron-Cohen, S., Knickmeyer, R. C., & Belmonte, M. K. (2005). Sex differences in the brain: Implications for explaining autism. *Science 310*, 819–823.

Baron-Cohen, S., & Wheelwright, S. (2004). The Empathy Quotient: An investigation of adults with Asperger Syndrome or high functioning autism, and normal sex differences. *Journal of Autism and Developmental Disorders*, *34*(2), 163–175.

Bharucha, J. (1987). Music cognition and perceptual facilitation: A connectionist framework. *Music Perception: An Interdisciplinary Journal*, *5*(1), 1–30.

Boucher, J. (2008). *Characteristics, causes and practical issues*. London: Sage Publications Ltd.

Bronfenbrenner, U. (1979). *The ecology of human development.* Cambridge, MA: Harvard University Press.

Carr, L., Iacoboni, M., Dubeau, M., Mazziotta, J., & Lenzi, G. (2003). Neural mechanisms of empathy in humans: A relay from neural systems for imitation to limbic areas. *Proceedings of the National Academy of Sciences, 100*(9), 5497–5502.

Cattaneo, L., & Rizzolatti, G. (2010). The mirror neuron system. *Archives of Neurology, 66*(5), 557–560.

Cheng, E., Ockelford, A., & Welch, G. (2009). Researching and developing music provision in special schools in England for children and young people with complex needs. *Australian Journal of Music Education, 2,* 27–48.

Coplan, A. (2011). Understanding empathy: Its features and effects. In A. Coplan & P. Goldie (Eds.), *Empathy: Philosophical and psychological perspectives* (pp. 3–18). Oxford: Oxford University Press.

Cross, I., Laurence, F., & Rabinowitch, T. (2012). Empathic creativity in musical group practices. In G. McPherson & G. Welch (Eds.), *The Oxford handbook of music education* (pp. 337–353). New York: Oxford University Press.

Crowder, R. (1985). Perception of the major/minor distinction: III. Hedonic, musical, and affective discriminations. *Bulletin of the Psychonomic Society, 23*(4), 314–316.

Davis, M. (1996). *Empathy.* Boulder, CO: Westview Press.

de Selincourt, B. (1920). Music and duration. *Music and Letters, 1*(4), 286–293.

de Waal, F. (2008). Putting the altruism back into altruism: The evolution of empathy. *Annual Review of Psychology, 59*(1), 279–300.

Decety, J. (2004). The functional architecture of human empathy. *Behavioral and Cognitive Neuroscience Reviews, 3*(2), 71–100.

di Pellegrino, G., Fadiga, L., Fogassi, L., Gallese, V., & Rizzolatti, G. (1992). Understanding motor events: A neurophysiological study. *Experimental Brain Research, 91*(1), 176–180.

Eliot, T. (1933). *The use of poetry and the use of criticism.* Cambridge, MA: Harvard University Press.

Eliot, T. (1960). *The sacred wood.* London: Methuen.

Fan, Y., Decety, J., Yang, C., Liu, J., & Cheng, Y. (2010). Unbroken mirror neurons in autism spectrum disorders. *Journal of Child Psychology and Psychiatry, 51*(9), 981–988.

Frith, U. (2003). *Explaining the enigma.* Oxford: Blackwell.

Gabrielsson, A., & Lindström, S. (2000). The influence of musical structure on emotional expression. In P. Juslin & J. Sloboda, (Eds.), *Music and emotion: Theory and research* (pp. 223–248). New York: Oxford University Press.

Gallagher, S. (2000). Philosophical conceptions of the self: Implications for cognitive science. *Trends in Cognitive Sciences, 4*(1), 14–21.

Gallese, V. (2003). The roots of empathy: The shared manifold hypothesis and the neural basis of intersubjectivity. *Psychopathology, 36*(4), 171–180.

Gallese, V., Fadiga, L., Fogassi, L., & Rizzolatti, G. (1996). Action recognition in the premotor cortex. *Brain, 119*(2), 593–609.

Gazzola, V., Aziz-Zadeh, L., & Keysers, C. (2006). Empathy and the somatotopic auditory mirror system in humans. *Current Biology, 16*(18), 1824–1829.

Goldman, A. (2011). Two routes to empathy: Insights from cognitive neuroscience. In A. Coplan & P. Goldie (Eds.), *Empathy: Philosophical and psychological perspectives* (pp. 31–44). Oxford: Oxford University Press.

Greenberg, D. M., Renfrew, P. J., & Baron-Cohen, S. (2015). Can music increase empathy? Interpreting musical experience through the empathizing-systematizing (E-S) theory. *Empirical Musicology Review, 10*(1), 79–94.

Gundlach, R. (1935). Factors determining the characterization of musical phrases. *The American Journal of Psychology, 47*(4), 624.

Hadjikhani, N. (2005). Anatomical differences in the mirror neuron system and social cognition network in autism. *Cerebral Cortex, 16*(9), 1276–1282.

Håkansson, J. (2003). *Exploring the phenomenon of empathy* (Unpublished doctoral dissertation). Department of Psychology, Stockholm University, Sweden.

Happé, F. (1998). *Autism: An introduction to psychological theory.* Cambridge, MA: Harvard University Press.

Heaton, P., Hermelin, B., & Pring, L. (1999). Can children with autistic spectrum disorders perceive affect in music? An experimental investigation. *Psychological Medicine, 29*(6), 1405–1410.

Hevner, K. (1936). Experimental studies of the elements of expression in music. *The American Journal of Psychology, 48*(2), 246.

Iacoboni, M. (2009). Imitation, empathy, and mirror neurons. *Annual Review of Psychology, 60*(1), 653–670.

Jairazbhoy, N., & Khan, V. (1971). *The rāgs of North Indian music.* Middletown, CT: Wesleyan University Press.

Johnson-Laird, P., & Oatley, K. (1992). Basic emotions, rationality, and folk theory. *Cognition & Emotion, 6*(3), 201–223.

Juslin, P. (1997). Perceived emotional expression in synthesized performances of a short melody: capturing the listener's judgement policy. *Musicae Scientiae, 1*(1), 225–256.

Juslin, P. (2001). Communicating emotion in music performance: A review and a theoretical framework. In P. Juslin & J. Sloboda (Eds.), *Music and emotion: Theory and research* (pp. 309–337). New York: Oxford University Press.

Juslin, P. N. (2009). Emotion in music performance. In S. Hallam, I. Cross, & M. Thaut (Eds.), *Oxford handbook of music psychology* (pp. 377–389). New York: Oxford University Press.

Juslin, P., Friberg, A., & Bresin, R. (2001). Toward a computational model of expression in music performance: The GERM model. *Musicae Scientiae, 5*(1 suppl), 63–122.

Juslin, P., & Västfjäll, D. (2008). Emotional responses to music: The need to consider underlying mechanisms. *Behavioral and Brain Sciences, 31*(6), 751.

Keysers, C. (2011). *The empathic brain.* Lexington, KY: Social Brain Press.

Kohler, E. (2002). Hearing sounds, understanding actions: Action representation in mirror neurons. *Science, 297*(5582), 846–848.

Krumhansl, C. (1997). An exploratory study of musical emotions and psychophysiology. *Canadian Journal of Experimental Psychology/Revue Canadienne de Psychologie Expérimentale, 51*(4), 336–353.

Livingstone, R. S., & Thompson, W. F. (2009). The emergence of music from the theory of mind. *Musicae Scientiae, 13*(2 Suppl), 83–115.

Malloch, S. (1999). Mothers and infants and communicative musicality. *Musicae Scientiae, 3*(1 suppl), 29–57.

Martin, G., & Clark, R. (1982). Distress crying in neonates: Species and peer specificity. *Developmental Psychology, 18*(1), 3–9.

Mazza, M., Pino, M., Mariano, M., Tempesta, D., Ferrara, M., De Berardis, D., Masedu, F., & Valenti, M. (2014). Affective and cognitive empathy in adolescents with autism spectrum disorder. *Frontiers in Human Neuroscience, 8*(791).

McDonald, N., & Messinger, D. (2011). The development of empathy: How, when, and why. In J. Lombo, A. Acerbi, & J. Sanguineti (Eds.), *Free will, emotions and moral actions: Philosophy and neuroscience in dialogue* (pp. 333–361) Rome: IF Press.

Meltzoff, A. (1990). Foundations for developing a concept of self: The role of imitation in relating self to other and the value of social mirroring, social modeling, and self practice in infancy. In D. Cicchetti & M. Beeghly (Eds.), *The self in transition: Infancy to childhood* (pp. 139–164). Chicago, IL: University of Chicago Press.

Meltzoff, A. (1995). Understanding the intentions of others: Re-enactment of intended acts by 18-month-old children. *Developmental Psychology, 31*(5), 838–850.

Meltzoff, A. (2002). Elements of a developmental theory of imitation. In A. Meltzoff & W. Prinz (Eds.), *The imitative mind: Development, evolution, and brain bases* (pp. 19–41). Cambridge: Cambridge University Press.

Meltzoff, A. (2007). The 'like me' framework for recognizing and becoming an intentional agent. *Acta Psychologica, 124*(1), 26–43.

Meltzoff, A., & Moore, M. (1983). Newborn infants imitate adult facial gestures. *Child Development, 54*(3), 702–709.

Meltzoff, A., & Moore, M. (1989). Imitation in newborn infants: Exploring the range of gestures imitated and the underlying mechanisms. *Developmental Psychology, 25*(6), 954–962.

Meyer, L. (1989). *Style and music.* Philadelphia, PA: University of Pennsylvania Press.

Meyer, L. (2001). Music and emotion: Distinctions and uncertainties. In P. Juslin & J. Sloboda (Eds.), *Music and emotion: Theory and research* (pp. 341–360). New York: Oxford University Press.

Miall, R. (2003). Connecting mirror neurons and forward models. *NeuroReport, 14*(17), 2135–2137.

Nemoto, I., Fujimaki, T., & Wang, L. (2010). fMRI measurement of brain activities to major and minor chords and cadence sequences. *2010 Annual International Conference of the IEEE Engineering in Medicine and Biology,* 5640–5643.

Nielzén, S., & Cesarec, Z. (1982). Emotional experience of music as a function of musical structure. *Psychology of Music, 10*(2), 7–17.

Oberman, L., Hubbard, E., McCleery, J., Altschuler, E., Ramachandran, V., & Pineda, J. (2005). EEG evidence for mirror neuron dysfunction in autism spectrum disorders. *Cognitive Brain Research, 24*(2), 190–198.

Ockelford, A. (1991). The role of repetition in perceived musical structures. In P. Howell, R. West, & I. Cross (Eds.), *Representing musical structure,* 1st ed. (pp. 129–160). London: Academic Press.

Ockelford, A. (2002). *Objects of reference.* 3rd ed. London: Royal National Institute for the Blind.

Ockelford, A. (2005). Relating musical structure and content to aesthetic response: A model and analysis of Beethoven's Piano Sonata Op. 110. *Journal of the Royal Musical Association, 130*(1), 74–118.

Ockelford, A. (2006). Implication and expectation in music: A zygonic model. *Psychology of Music, 34*(1), 81–142.

Ockelford, A. (2008). *Music for children and young people with complex needs.* Oxford: Oxford University Press.

Ockelford, A. (2011). Another exceptional musical memory: Evidence from a savant of how atonal music is processed in cognition. In I. Deliège (Ed.), *Music and the mind: A book to honour the achievements of John Sloboda* (pp. 237–288). Oxford: Oxford University Press.

Ockelford, A. (2012). *Applied musicology.* Oxford: Oxford University Press.

Ockelford, A. (2013). *Music, language and autism.* London: Jessica Kingsley Publishers.

Ockelford, A., & Matawa, C. (2009). *Focus on music 2*. London: Institute of Education, University of London.

Ockelford, A., & Vorhaus, J. (2016). Identity and musical development in people with severe or profound and multiple learning difficulties. In R. MacDonald, D. Hargreaves, & D. Miell (Eds.), *The Oxford handbook of musical identities*. New York: Oxford University Press.

Ockelford, A. and Voyajolu, A. (n.d.). The emergence of musical abilities in the early years: A perspective using the Sounds of Intent model. In A. Ockelford & G. Welch (Eds.), *New approaches to analysis in music psychology and education research using zygonic theory*. Farnham: Ashgate.

Ockelford, A., & Welch, G. (2012). What can musical engagement in children with cognitive impairment tell us about their sense of self? In S. O'Neill (Ed.), *Personhood and music learning: Connecting perspectives and narratives* (pp. 216–237). Waterloo, Ontario: Canadian Music Educators' Association.

Ockelford, A., Welch, G., Jewell-Gore, L., Cheng, E., Vogiatzoglou, A., & Himonides, E. (2011). Sounds of Intent, phase 2: Gauging the music development of children with complex needs. *European Journal of Special Needs Education, 26*(2), 177–199.

Ockelford, A., Welch, G., Zimmermann, S., & Himonides, E. (2005). 'Sounds of Intent': Mapping, assessing and promoting the musical development of children with profound and multiple learning difficulties. *International Congress Series, 1282*, 898–902.

Peretz, I. (1998). Music and emotion: Perceptual determinants, immediacy, and isolation after brain damage. *Cognition, 68*(2), 111–141.

Preston, S., & de Waal, F. (2002). Empathy: Its ultimate and proximate bases. *Behavioral and Brain Sciences, 25*(1), 1–20.

Ramachandran, V., & Oberman, L. (2006). Broken mirrors: A theory of autism. *Scientific American, 295*(5), 62–69.

Ridley, C., & Lingle, D. (1996). Counseling across cultures. In P. Pedersen, J. Draguns, W. Lonner, & J. Trimble (Eds.), *Cultural empathy in multicultural counseling: A multidimensional process model*, 4th ed. (pp. 21–46). Thousand Oaks, CA: Sage.

Rizzolatti, G., & Fabbri-Destro, M. (2009). Mirror neurons: From discovery to autism. *Experimental Brain Research, 200*(3–4), 223–237.

Rizzolatti, G., Fadiga, L., Gallese, V., & Fogassi, L. (1996). Premotor cortex and the recognition of motor actions. *Cognitive Brain Research, 3*(2), 131–141.

Sagi, A., & Hoffman, M. (1976). Empathic distress in the newborn. *Developmental Psychology, 12*(2), 175–176.

Scherer, K. (1991). Emotion expression in speech and music. In J. Sundberg, L. Nord, & R. Carlson (Eds.), *Music, language, speech and brain*, 1st ed. (pp. 146–156). London: MacMillan.

Scherer, K., Banse, R., & Wallbott, H. (2001). Emotion inferences from vocal expression correlate across languages and cultures. *Journal of Cross-Cultural Psychology, 32*(1), 76–92.

Scherer, K., & Oshinsky, J. (1977). Cue utilization in emotion attribution from auditory stimuli. *Motivation and Emotion, 1*(4), 331–346.

Seddon, F. (2005). Modes of communication during jazz improvisation. *British Journal of Music Education, 22*(1), 47–61.

Shamay-Tsoory, S., Aharon-Peretz, J., & Perry, D. (2009). Two systems for empathy: A double dissociation between emotional and cognitive empathy in inferior frontal gyrus versus ventromedial prefrontal lesions. *Brain, 132*(3), 617–627.

Simner, M. (1971). Newborn's response to the cry of another infant. *Developmental Psychology, 5*(1), 136–150.

Sparshott, F. (1994). Music and feeling. *Journal of Aesthetics and Art Criticism, 52*(1), 23–35.

Suzuki, M., Okamura, N., Kawachi, Y., Tashiro, M., Arao, H., Hoshishiba, T., Gyoba, J., & Yanai, K. (2008). Discrete cortical regions associated with the musical beauty of major and minor chords. *Cognitive, Affective, & Behavioral Neuroscience, 8*(2), 126–131.

Thompson, W. F., & Robitaille, B. (1992). Can composers express emotions through music? *Empirical Studies of the Arts, 10*(1), 79–89.

Trehub, S., & Nakata, T. (2002). Emotion and music in infancy. *Musicae Scientiae, 5*(1 suppl), 37–61.

Vogiatzoglou, A., Ockelford, A., Welch, G., & Himonides, E. (2011). Sounds of Intent: Interactive software to assess the musical development of children and young people with complex needs. *Music and Medicine, 3*(3), 189–195.

Voyajolu, A., & Ockelford, A. (2016). Sounds of Intent in the early years: A proposed framework of young children's musical development. *Research Studies in Music Education, 38*(1), 93–113.

Wakabayashi, A., Baron-Cohen, S., Wheelwright, S., Goldenfeld, N., Delaney, J., Fine, D., Smith, R., & Weil, L. (2006). Development of short forms of the Empathy Quotient (EQ-Short) and the Systemizing Quotient (SQ-Short). *Personality and Individual Differences, 41*(5), 929–940.

Wan, C., Demaine, K., Zipse, L., Norton, A., & Schlaug, G. (2010). From music making to speaking: Engaging the mirror neuron system in autism. *Brain Research Bulletin, 82*(3–4), 161–168.

Watson, K. (1942). The nature and measurement of musical meanings. *Psychological Monographs, 54*(2), i–43.

Welch, G., Ockelford, A., Carter, F., Zimmermann, S., & Himonides, E. (2009). 'Sounds of Intent': mapping musical behaviour and development in children and young people with complex needs. *Psychology of Music, 37*(3), 348–370.

Williams, J., Waiter, G., Gilchrist, A., Perrett, D., Murray, A., & Whiten, A. (2006). Neural mechanisms of imitation and 'mirror neuron' functioning in autistic spectrum disorder. *Neuropsychologia, 44*(4), 610–621.

Winner, E. (1996). *Gifted children*. New York: Basic Books.

Zahn-Waxler, C., & Radke-Yarrow, M. (1990). The origins of empathic concern. *Motivation and Emotion, 14*(2), 107–130.

2 Synchronisation – a musical substrate for positive social interaction and empathy

Tal-Chen Rabinowitch

Empathy

At its full breadth a capacity for empathy is a capacity to notice, to understand, to internalise, to experience and to adequately respond to another's feelings. Whether empathy is unique to humans is not clear (for example, Bartal, Decety, & Mason, 2011; Langford *et al.*, 2006), but it is definitely a prominent human proficiency. Empathy plays an important part in human life from infancy. For example, in its most essential form empathy constitutes an integral part of parent–infant relations (Elicker, Englund, & Sroufe, 1992; Winnicott, 1960). Parents are constantly striving to unravel their child's needs, wishes and moods and to provide support and consolation as well as direction. At the same time, infants are highly aware of their parents' state of mind and feelings and continuously attempt to adjust to them. As the child develops and grows, he or she exhibits a progressively comprehensive capacity for empathy towards other children and adults (Borke, 1971; Knafo *et al.*, 2008; Rieffe, Ketelaar, & Wiefferink, 2010). Ultimately, full-blown human communities and societies rely on empathy to bring people together, to instill a sense of mutual support among individuals, to enable cooperation and collaboration, and to promote overall social progress.

Empathy is thus an innate human capacity, important for proper social interaction, and may have been essential also for establishing the earliest of human societies. Interestingly, the term empathy was coined only in the beginning of the twentieth century, after the German *Einfühlung*, literally 'feeling into' (Wispé, 1986), originally denoting not interpersonal empathy but rather aesthetic empathy (for a more comprehensive discussion of empathy, see Laurence, this volume). The notion of aesthetic empathy was developed to describe the cognitive and emotional processes characterising aesthetic experience, which consists of a person's projection into nature or a work of art and their perception of the emotions embedded in them. Although interpersonal and aesthetic empathy seem to be distinct, historically they were almost interchangeable. Feeling into another person was likened, if not equated, to an aesthetic experience (Greiner, 2012). But even from a contemporary perspective, it is easy to find similarities between empathy towards another person and empathy or emotional perception of a work of art. A particularly good example for unravelling these links is music, one of the most interactive and emotionally abounding forms of art.

Music and empathy

Music is a rather general term that can mean several different things. Here, music is considered as a form of interaction. Even just listening to music (intently) is an active engagement. The listener experiences the music in his or her own personal way attributing to it meaning, communicating with it, and even guiding it. In fact, it is quite difficult to listen to appealing music without moving, joining in, or occasionally becoming a pretend conductor (Repp, 2002). Listening to music together with other people may further enhance the interaction. It establishes an additional subtle connection among listeners based on the shared experience that they undergo together and on the agreement in taste and enjoyment that they discover. This is even more pronounced in live music performances, in which audience and performers interact and augment each other's experience. Ultimately, playing music together is a full-scale, rich and dynamic interaction whereby participants become highly tuned to one another in an all-immersing experience.

I have previously described in detail how several of the motor, cognitive and emotional processes that take place during musical interaction and determine the quality and character of the interaction may also underlie the capacity to empathise with another person (Cross, Laurence, & Rabinowitch, 2012; Rabinowitch, Cross, & Burnard, 2013). In the current chapter I focus on one of these: synchronisation. First, I will describe synchrony as a general phenomenon of the human experience, then I will consider how in the long-term synchrony might contribute to the acquisition of specific skills that promote empathy, and how in the short-term synchronous interaction might modulate empathic behaviour. Finally, I will outline a rather speculative hypothesis linking synchrony and interpersonal empathy through an aestheticist perspective.

Rhythm and synchrony

The structure and composition of music is highly complex. It comprises a manifold of interleaved sounds and beats, harmony and melody. The backbone of all this is rhythm, the temporal arrangement of beats, which determines the direction, the speed and the temperament of the unfolding music. Consequently, a key component of musical interaction is synchronisation, the temporal aligning of action between two or more interacting individuals. In a broader sense, rhythm and synchrony are not unique to music. In fact, they seem to be fundamental features of our entire world. From the recurring seasons of the year, the repeated succession of lunar phases, the cycle of day and night, to the waves of sound, of heat and light, we are surrounded by rhythm. To these rhythms the human body is tightly tuned, sensing them, responding to them, and producing also rhythms of its own, the rhythms of walking, talking, chewing and breathing. In a sense, music reflects this central role of rhythm in our existence, and synchronised musical interaction is rooted in our deep predisposition to respond to rhythm, to align to it and to create new rhythms of our own.

Synchrony and acquired empathy

Long-term habitual participation in musical interaction is expected, like any practice, to improve the quality of the musical interaction itself. If musical interaction and interpersonal empathy are indeed related, then training in musical interaction might also enhance the capacity for interpersonal empathy (Clarke, DeNora, & Vuoskoski, 2015; Cross, Laurence, & Rabinowitch, 2012; Rabinowitch, Cross, & Burnard, 2013). But could one's capacity for empathy be at all modified? On the face of it, since the capacity for empathy depends on individual personality traits (Dymond, 1950; Knafo *et al.*, 2008), which are largely constant, one might expect the capacity for empathy to be fixed (for example, Meltzoff & Moore, 1997). However, empathy depends also on certain acquired skill sets, abilities and attitudes (Alligood, 1992), rendering the capacity for empathy amenable to change (for example, Heyes, 2011). I term such long-term learned changes in empathy, 'acquired empathy' (see also Ockelford, this volume, for a consideration of the acquisition of musical skills and musical empathy).

I have previously tested experimentally whether long-term musical interaction might contribute to acquired empathy (Rabinowitch, Cross, & Burnard, 2013). To this end, I conducted a one-year study consisting of weekly sessions of a specially tailored musical group interaction programme for elementary school children. The children's scores on several tasks designed to measure their capacity for empathy showed a clear and significant increase in the music group's capacity for empathy compared to the control groups who participated in a parallel story-telling programme or no programme at all (Rabinowitch, Cross, & Burnard, 2013). These results provide evidence for the overall positive long-term effects of musical group interaction on empathy, presumably attained through skill transfer.

Evidence determining whether specifically training in synchronisation can generalise to acquired empathy is still lacking. However, synchronisation was also one of the key ingredients of the musical group interaction programme (Rabinowitch, Cross, & Burnard, 2013). Some of the tasks presented to the children in the study intended to emphasise synchronisation within the musical interaction. One task, for example, consisted of children taking turns in imitating or matching each other's rhythms when tapping on drums. Another example was a game, in which the group composed a certain rhythmic theme, which everybody played together on different instruments. It is hard to tell what the differential contribution of the synchronisation tasks was towards enhancing participants' capacity for empathy, since the programme also included other components of musical interaction in addition to synchronisation. Thus, the degree to which synchronisation played a prominent role in enhancing participants' capacity for empathy and whether their capacity for synchronisation was enhanced as well will have to be examined more closely in the future. Nevertheless, it is worth noting the striking similarities between interpersonal empathy and synchronisation. Empathy and synchronisation rely on the ability to notice, to understand, to internalise, to experience, to connect with and to adequately respond to another's feelings or another's rhythm, respectively. These parallels suggest that synchronisation and empathy might involve similar cognitive processes, and are therefore potentially amenable to skill transfer.

Synchronisation and empathy modulation

In addition to lifelong innate empathy and to long-term acquired empathy, certain real-time factors such as context, mood and various physiological variables may transiently alter the extent and quality of one's capacity for empathy (for example, Bal & Veltkamp, 2013). I refer to such short-term effects as 'empathy modulation'. Does synchronisation lead to empathy modulation? A rapidly growing body of studies indicate that even brief sessions of interpersonal synchronisation are sufficient to modulate a host of prosocial-related behaviours and attitudes such as affiliation, collaboration and willingness to help (for a recent comprehensive survey of this literature refer to Clarke, DeNora, & Vuoskoski, 2015).

Although none of these studies tested directly whether synchronisation might lead to a short-term modulation of participants' capacity for empathy, the expansive effects of synchronisation on multiple aspects of social and emotional interaction that are closely related to empathy, such as a sense of similarity, closeness and affiliation, and the propensity to collaborate, suggest that empathy itself might also be modulated by synchronisation. A few studies have tried to address this issue somewhat more directly. Piercarlo Valdesolo and David DeSteno (2011) showed that synchronous others elicit more compassion and altruistic behaviour than asynchronous others. In addition, it has been shown that in some cases, synchrony may elevate one's inclination to offer help to an interacting partner (Kokal et al., 2011) and that infants as young as 14 months display more helpful behaviours towards an adult who moves in synchrony with them when compared to an adult who moved asynchronously with them (Cirelli, Einarson, & Trainor, 2014). Other studies have demonstrated the relative contribution of synchrony in creating greater affiliation (Hove & Risen, 2009), greater similarity and closeness (Rabinowitch & Knafo-Noam, 2015) as well as enhanced person perception (Macrae et al., 2008) and cooperation (Valdesolo, Ouyang, & DeSteno, 2010; Wiltermuth & Heath, 2009). It will be important to further test the modulatory capacity of synchronisation on empathy.

It is also worth considering potential mechanisms that might underlie empathy modulation by synchronisation. First, when two or more individuals synchronise with each other, their movements become physically aligned. Therefore, if they are to stop actively synchronising, but try and continue the interaction, for example, by executing a joint task together, they will be able to better coordinate their actions in space, but most importantly, they will probably be able to form better eye contact and physical rapport with each other following synchrony, which may in turn lead to enhanced positive social interaction and possibly empathy. Second, Emma Cohen et al. (2010) showed that there is possibly higher secretion of endorphins following extensive synchronised activity (such as rowing), which may be related to social bonding (for example, Dunbar, 2010). Third, the coupling between one's own actions and the perception of another performing a similar action has been suggested to underlie theory of mind and empathy in general (reviewed in Clarke, DeNora, & Vuoskoski, 2015). Synchronisation readily affords such coupling, causing us to embody and internalise a person that is synchronised with us, and regard that person as if from a first-person perspective, facilitating empathy towards that person (see, for example, Decety & Jackson, 2006; Jackson, Meltzoff, & Decety, 2005).

Synchronised intensive interactions such as musical interaction might even go beyond empathy. Although empathy consists of stepping into another's shoes, the interpersonal boundary is never broken. In contrast, 'merged subjectivity' (for a detailed account see Rabinowitch, Cross, & Burnard, 2012) comprises a hypothetical condition whereby individuals playing music together might at some point lose track of who is playing what, as their individual subjectivities merge into one (for a detailed account see Rabinowitch, Cross, & Burnard, 2012, as well as Clarke, DeNora, & Vuoskoski, 2015).

Interpersonal synchronisation as a form of aesthetic empathy

To conclude, I wish to entertain an alternative and speculative idea about synchronisation and interpersonal empathy. This entails some reconsideration of the obsolete concept of *Einfühlung* and the resemblance between interpersonal and aesthetic empathy. A key question that the notion of aesthetic empathy raises is, 'why would anyone imbue a lifeless object, such as music, with emotions?' We can clearly distinguish between live emotional human beings and other entities in the world, including other animals, plants, natural objects, artefacts and works of art. A strong basis for this distinction is provided by theory of mind, the realisation that another person has a mental life comprising intentions, desires, knowledge and emotions (Baron-Cohen, Leslie, & Frith, 1985). Despite this ability, we readily anthropomorphise non-human animals and objects. We ascribe them with human-like characteristics, including emotions, thoughts and intentions. For certain animals, this might be adequate, but less so for physical objects such as cars, clouds or paintings. The term anthropomorphisation itself assumes implicitly that attributing human qualities, such as emotionality to objects is an expansion of theory of mind. First we learn that other people have emotions, and then we imagine that other objects are like other people and therefore may also have emotions.

From this perspective stems a natural inclination to view aesthetic empathy as perhaps an extension of a more fundamental interpersonal empathy. According to this account, humans have a capacity to empathise with other humans, and they use this capacity also when engaging with a work of art. In this sense, they regard the art as if it were another person. Thus, when engaging in music, for example, we notice, understand, internalise and respond to the richness of emotions that we find embedded in the music, in a similar manner to when we empathise with another human. We anthropomorphise music in order to aesthetically empathise with it (Kivy, 1980).

There is no reason, however, to rule out the alternative converse outlook suggested by *Einfühlung*, whereby interpersonal empathy is actually an instance of aesthetic empathy, or that at least the two are closely related (Greiner, 2012). What if generally ascribing emotions to objects outside ourselves, be they other people, or not, precedes theory of mind rather than expands it? It is a valid possibility that before learning to attribute intentions, emotions, and so on to other humans, we initially learn to attribute them to objects in our surroundings. This includes people, but also animals, trees, toys and works of art. Only later do we learn to refine the scope of other-mindedness to humans, singling them out as the true bearers of emotion. According to this account, interpersonal empathy might indeed stem from a more basic aesthetic empathy and not the other way around, or they might be the same altogether. Our capacity to understand, internalise and respond to the emotions of another person may be essentially part of a more fundamental capacity to sense and attribute emotions to objects in general, and in particular to aesthetic objects, such as works of art, which are especially prone to evoke in us emotions.

'The world is a work of art' wrote Nietzsche, expressing an aestheticist ontology (Megill, 1987; Nehamas, 1985) that invites us to view everything in the world and every event that takes place as part of an intricate and vibrant enormous work of art. From this perspective, when interacting with another person, one may regard that other person to some extent as an aesthetic object, and perceive emotions in that other person in a similar manner to perceiving emotions in a piece of music, exhibiting an aesthetic empathy towards that person.

Considering that rhythmic synchronisation is a fundamental element of music, then the experience of acting in synchrony with another person may be equivalent to the experience of engaging in music. Furthermore, from an aestheticist perspective, the aesthetic experience of rhythmically synchronising with another person may actually evoke the sensation that that other person is music. This is because, as mentioned above, playing music with another person and playing music alone are similar forms of interaction, both of which are capable of eliciting aesthetic empathy.

Whether or not the world is a work of art is mostly a question of taste and conviction. Whether or not we regard other humans not just functionally but also from an aesthetic perspective, similar to our perception of landscapes and works of art, is an open empirical question deserving attention and consideration. If it is true, then a new and aesthetic link can be drawn between interpersonal synchronisation and empathy.

Conclusions

The concepts of interpersonal and aesthetic empathy share a long and intertwined history. Current work focuses mainly on the interpersonal aspects of empathy. Of particular interest is how interpersonal empathy may be boosted. Synchronisation, a fundamental component of musical interaction, is emerging as a powerful enhancer of prosocial attitudes and behaviour. Very scant and indirect evidence suggests that synchronisation might also have a positive impact on interpersonal empathy through long-term skill transfer and real-time modulation. New experimental data will be necessary to establish this.

References

Alligood, M. R. (1992). Empathy: The importance of recognizing two types. *Journal of Psychosocial Nursing and Mental Health Services, 30*(3), 14–17.

Bal, P. M., & Veltkamp, M. (2013). How does fiction reading influence empathy? An experimental investigation on the role of emotional transportation. *PloS One, 8*(1), e55341.

Baron-Cohen, S., Leslie, A. M., & Frith, U. (1985). Does the autistic child have a 'theory of mind'?. *Cognition, 21*(1), 37–46.

Bartal, I. B. A., Decety, J., & Mason, P. (2011). Empathy and pro-social behavior in rats. *Science, 334*(6061), 1427–1430.

Borke, H. (1971). Interpersonal perception of young children: Egocentrism or empathy?. *Developmental Psychology, 5*(2), 263–269.

Cirelli, L. K., Einarson, K. M., & Trainor, L. J. (2014). Interpersonal synchrony increases prosocial behavior in infants. *Developmental Science, 17*(6), 1003–1011.

Clarke, E., DeNora, T., & Vuoskoski, J. (2015). Music, empathy and cultural understanding. *Physics of Life Reviews, 15*, 61–68.

Cohen, E., Ejsmond-Frey, R., Knight, N., & Dunbar, R. (2010). Rowers' high: Elevated endorphin release under conditions of active behavioural synchrony. *Biology Letters, 6*(1), 106–108.

Cross, I., Laurence, F., & Rabinowitch, T. C. (2012). Empathy and creativity in group musical practices: Towards a concept of empathic creativity. In G. McPherson & G. Welch (Eds.), *The Oxford handbook of music education* (pp. 337–353). Oxford: Oxford University Press.

Decety, J., & Jackson, P. L. (2006). A social-neuroscience perspective on empathy. *Current Directions in Psychological Science, 15*(2), 54–58.

Dunbar, R. I. (2010). The social role of touch in humans and primates: Behavioural function and neurobiological mechanisms. *Neuroscience & Biobehavioral Reviews, 34*(2), 260–268.

Dymond, R. F. (1950). Personality and empathy. *Journal of Consulting Psychology, 14*(5), 343–350.

Elicker, J., Englund, M., & Sroufe, L. A. (1992). Predicting peer competence and peer relationships in childhood from early parent-child relationships. In M. England & L. A. Sroufe (Eds.), *Family-peer relationships: Modes of linkage* (pp. 77–107). Hillsdale, NJ: Erlbaum.

Greiner, R. (2012). 1909: The introduction of the word 'empathy' into English. *BRANCH: Britain, Representation, and Nineteenth-Century History*, online-only journal.

Heyes, C. (2011). Automatic imitation. *Psychological bulletin, 137*(3), 463–483.

Hove, M. J., & Risen, J. L. (2009). It's all in the timing: Interpersonal synchrony increases affiliation. *Social Cognition, 27*(6), 949–960.

Jackson, P. L., Meltzoff, A. N., & Decety, J. (2005). How do we perceive the pain of others? A window into the neural processes involved in empathy. *NeuroImage, 24*(3), 771–779.

Kivy, P. (1980) *The corded shell: Reflections on musical expression*. Princeton, NJ: Princeton University Press.

Knafo, A., Zahn-Waxler, C., Van Hulle, C., Robinson, J. L., & Rhee, S. H. (2008). The developmental origins of a disposition toward empathy: Genetic and environmental contributions. *Emotion, 8*(6), 737–752.

Kokal, I., Engel, A., Kirschner, S., & Keysers, C. (2011). Synchronized drumming enhances activity in the caudate and facilitates prosocial commitment – if the rhythm comes easily. *PloS One, 6*(11), e27272.

Langford, D. J., Crager, S. E., Shehzad, Z., Smith, S. B., Sotocinal, S. G., Levenstadt, J. S., Chanda, M. L., Levitin, D. J., & Mogil, J. S. (2006). Social modulation of pain as evidence for empathy in mice. *Science, 312*(5782), 1967–1970.

Macrae, C. N., Duffy, O. K., Miles, L. K., & Lawrence, J. (2008). A case of hand waving: Action synchrony and person perception. *Cognition, 109*(1), 152–156.

Megill, A. (1987). *Prophets of extremity: Nietzsche, Heidegger, Foucault, Derrida.* Berkeley, CA: University of California Press.

Meltzoff, A. N., & Moore, M. K. (1997). Explaining facial imitation: A theoretical model. *Early Development and Parenting, 6*, 179–192.

Nehamas, A. (1985). *Nietzsche: Life as literature.* Boston, MA: Harvard University Press.

Rabinowitch, T. C., Cross, I., & Burnard, P. (2012). Musical group interaction, intersubjectivity and merged subjectivity. In D. Reynolds & M. Reason (Eds.), *Kinesthetic empathy in creative and cultural practices* (pp. 109–120). Bristol: Intellect.

Rabinowitch, T. C., Cross, I., & Burnard, P. (2013). Long-term musical group interaction has a positive influence on empathy in children. *Psychology of Music, 41*(4), 484–498.

Rabinowitch, T. C., & Knafo-Noam, A. (2015). Synchronous rhythmic interaction enhances children's perceived similarity and closeness towards each other. *PloS One, 10*(4).

Repp, B. H. (2002). The embodiment of musical structure: Effects of musical context on sensorimotor synchronization with complex timing patterns. In W. Prinz & B. Hommel (Eds.), *Common mechanisms in perception and action: Attention and performance XIX* (pp. 245–265). Oxford: Oxford University Press.

Rieffe, C., Ketelaar, L., & Wiefferink, C. H. (2010). Assessing empathy in young children: Construction and validation of an Empathy Questionnaire (EmQue). *Personality and Individual Differences, 49*(5), 362–367.

Valdesolo, P., & DeSteno, D. (2011). Synchrony and the social tuning of compassion. *Emotion, 11*(2), 262–266.

Valdesolo, P., Ouyang, J., & DeSteno, D. (2010). The rhythm of joint action: Synchrony promotes cooperative ability. *Journal of Experimental Social Psychology, 46*(4), 693–695.

Wiltermuth, S. S., & Heath, C. (2009). Synchrony and cooperation. *Psychological Science, 20*(1), 1–5.

Winnicott, D. W. (1960). The theory of the parent-infant relationship. *International Journal of Psychoanalysis, 41*(6), 585–595.

Wispé, L. (1986) The distinction between sympathy and empathy: To call forth a concept, a word is needed. *Journal of Personality and Social Psychology, 50*(2), 314–321.

3 Music

The language of empathy

Istvan Molnar-Szakacs

Introduction

> if I had to live my life again, I would have made a rule to read some poetry
> and listen to some music at least once every week; for perhaps the parts of
> my brain now atrophied would thus have been kept active through use. The
> loss of these tastes is a loss of happiness, and may possibly be injurious to
> the intellect, and more probably to the moral character, by enfeebling the
> emotional part of our nature.

> (Darwin, 1887, p. 139)

Music listening is an unparalleled experience – it allows our imagination to
travel, to feel, regulate and express emotion, to experience a feeling of belonging
and identification. Music is the most abstract of arts, and yet music is a ubiquitous element in all human cultures, a pervasive part of social life – present
in weddings, funerals and many other 'rite-of-passage' ceremonies (Wallin,
Merker, & Brown, 2000). Empirical research has shown that both children and
adults can readily identify four basic emotions – joy, fear, sadness and anger – as
conveyed by music (Dolgin & Adelson, 1990; Terwogt & Van Grinsven, 1988).
Furthermore, it has also been found, through self-report measures, that music
can elicit emotion in listeners (Garrido & Schubert, 2011). In addition to eliciting
and intensifying emotions (Vuoskoski & Eerola, 2012), music can also act as
a powerful cue to recall emotional memories back into awareness (Sloboda &
Juslin, 2001; Zentner, Grandjean, & Scherer, 2008). It is the ability of music to
convey, elicit and recall emotion that makes it such a powerful stimulus. Through
these emotions, music has the potential to create empathic connections among
humans across cultures, places and time.

A variety of reasons for the existence and evolution of music have been proposed, including that it evolved as part of our hominid mating strategy (Darwin,
1871), from animal territorial signals (Hagen & Hammerstein, 2009), or simply
because of the pleasure it produced (Wallin, Merker, & Brown, 2000). Music
production involving the use of the human body (singing, drumming, stomp-
ing and so on) has been a part of human history and evolution for millennia
in ritual dances, hunting songs, religious hymns, nursery rhymes and concerts.

In fact, recent findings show that the earliest bone flutes date to approximately 40,000 years ago (Conard, Malina, & Munzel, 2009), meaning that forms of music-making possibly existed even before this period.

Music is often thought of as a social activity, reported to unite us, to promote self-awareness and self-esteem, mutual tolerance, sense of spirituality, intercultural understanding, the ability to cooperate and healing (Clarke, DeNora, & Vuoskoski, 2015; Cross & Morley, 2008; Laurence, 2008). However, music today is often experienced as an asocial phenomenon as we put on our headphones to go jogging or turn up the car stereo while driving home from work. In this chapter, I will suggest that our brain has a built-in neural network, anchored by the human mirror neuron system (MNS), that allows abstract musical signals to be attributed with agency, thus turning an asocial experience into a social one (Launay, 2015; Molnar-Szakacs, 2015). I will also discuss how music's inextricable relationship with action allows music to create intense and powerful communicative links among us at the individual or group level.

Music's ability to create strong, emotionally charged experiences within and among us, is based in interacting neural systems for embodiment and emotion. Abstract musical sounds are able to simultaneously activate these neural systems, giving music a privileged path to empathy. Several theories of music-induced emotions suggest that empathy may be involved in the emotional responses induced by music (Juslin, 2013; Juslin & Västfjäll, 2008; Livingstone & Thompson, 2009; Scherer & Zentner, 2001). The human capacity for embodied representation allows an individual to relate to music on an intimate level, and empathy allows music's powerful effects on emotion to become shared and magnified to the group level. Thus, music may act as a universal language of empathy, whereby a series of abstract sounds can communicate emotion among individuals who do not speak the same language or share the same culture (for a recent perspective, see Clarke, DeNora & Vuoskoski, 2015).

I will begin this chapter by discussing evidence for the existence of a human MNS, a proposed neural architecture for embodiment and empathy (Gallese, 2001, 2003b; Rizzolatti & Craighero, 2004). Using the framework of the Shared Affective Motion Experience (SAME) model of music perception (Molnar-Szakacs, Green Assuied, & Overy, 2012; Molnar-Szakacs & Overy, 2006; Overy & Molnar-Szakacs, 2009), I describe how the human MNS may support a mechanism by which listeners can experience music through a pre-reflective, automatic resonance mechanism, rather than through an effortful, top-down cognitive process. I summarise support for the hypothesis that the perception of action and language share neural resources with music perception (Koelsch et al., 2013; Molnar-Szakacs & Overy, 2006), providing support for the role of music as 'the language of empathy'. I then discuss persuasive new neuroimaging evidence that has revealed the involvement of brain regions associated with emotion and reward processing in emotional responses to music, particularly, the mesolimbic dopaminergic system (Salimpoor et al., 2011, 2013). I conclude by briefly discussing how different neural networks may interact to provide our fullest experience of music, its power to connect individuals and even heal, using as an example musical therapy settings (Molnar-Szakacs, Green Assuied & Overy, 2012).

The neural bases of embodiment

The 'shared manifold hypothesis' proposes that interpersonal relations fundamentally depend upon a 'shared space' – a pre-reflective understanding that others are 'like us' (Gallese, 2001, 2003b). This shared space is functionally characterised by automatic, unconscious, embodied simulation routines. Simulation has been defined as the 'attempt to replicate, mimic or impersonate the mental life of the target' (Gallese & Goldman, 1998, p. 497), and may include representing the basic motor behaviours of others, but also the more complex emotional states of others, to understand and predict their behaviour (Adolphs, 2009). Indeed, many neuroscientific studies show that the same neural mechanisms involved in processing one's own actions, sensations and emotions are also involved in perceiving and understanding the actions, sensations and emotions of others (Gallese & Goldman, 1998; Gallese, Keysers, & Rizzolatti, 2004; Keysers & Gazzola, 2009; Keysers, Kaas, & Gazzola, 2010). For example, observing someone make an action (for example, hammer a nail) has been shown to activate brain regions such as the pre-motor cortex and the posterior parietal cortex (PPC) that are also related to generating actions (Gallese, Keysers, & Rizzolatti, 2004; Rizzolatti & Craighero, 2004). Similarly, watching a spider crawl on James Bond's chest in a movie, may activate somatosensory cortices (SII) for processing tactile sensations in our own brain (Keysers et al., 2004). Furthermore, experiencing disgust and observing someone else experience disgust can activate common areas involved in visceromotor processing in the anterior insula (Jabbi, Bastiaansen, & Keysers, 2008; Wicker et al., 2003). These 'shared circuits' consist of neural circuits active both for processing our own actions, perceptions and feelings and when we see, hear or feel similar things being done by someone else. This 'mirroring' mechanism is believed to allow for pre-reflective, automatic, bottom-up processes in social cognition that do not necessarily require reflective, top-down meta-cognition (Gamez-Djokic, Molnar-Szakacs, & Aziz-Zadeh, 2015).

A commonly proposed neural substrate for this mirroring mechanism are mirror neurons, a class of neurons with the special characteristic that they fire both when an agent performs a particular action such as grasping, and when it observes another agent performing a similar action (Ferrari, Bonini, & Fogassi, 2009; Ferrari et al., 2003; Ferrari, Rozzi, & Fogassi, 2005; Gallese et al., 1996; Rizzolatti et al., 1996). Mirror neurons were first discovered and described in the ventral pre-motor area F5 of the macaque monkey brain (Gallese et al., 1996). Important for our discussion of music, subsets of these pre-motor mirror neurons have also been shown to have audiovisual properties (Keysers et al., 2003; Kohler et al., 2002). Evelyne Kohler and colleagues (2002) found neurons in the monkey pre-motor cortex that discharged when the monkey performed a specific action, when it heard the related sound, and when the monkey observed the same action.

These audiovisual mirror neurons code actions independently of whether the actions are performed, seen or heard.

In the macaque, two major areas containing mirror neurons have been identified: area F5 in the inferior frontal cortex, and area PF/PFG in the inferior parietal cortex (Rizzolatti & Craighero, 2004). It has been suggested that parietal mirror neurons have the special property of coding motor acts as belonging to an action sequence and, thus, are capable of predicting the intended end goal of a complex action (Fogassi et al., 2005; Fogassi & Luppino, 2005). In light of this, it has been proposed that reciprocal connections between area F5 in the pre-motor cortex and parietal area PF (Luppino et al., 1999) form what is called the mirror neuron system (MNS). Research suggests that the MNS may provide the fundamental neural mechanism for action understanding and intention attribution in the macaque brain (Fogassi et al., 2005; Rizzolatti & Craighero, 2004; Rizzolatti, Fogassi, & Gallese, 2001).

Early action observation studies using both transcranial magnetic stimulation (TMS) (Fadiga et al., 1995) and positron emission tomography (PET) (Rizzolatti et al., 1996), provided some evidence for the existence of a human MNS. A few years later, Marco Iacoboni and colleagues (1999) used functional Magnetic Resonance Imaging (fMRI) to show that regions exhibiting mirroring responses – active during both execution of an action and during observation of the same action – were localised to the inferior frontal gyrus (IFG) of the ventral pre-motor cortex (vPMC) and the PPC in the human brain (Iacoboni et al., 1999). Both phylogenetic and cytoarchitectonic evidence suggest a homology of these regions with those found to contain mirror neurons in the macaque brain (Preuss, 1995; Rizzolatti & Arbib, 1998). Furthermore, the investigators found that these regions showed higher activity during execution compared with observation of action, and highest activity during imitation – a process that includes both an observation and an execution component. In addition to these early neuroimaging experiments, a wealth of additional studies have shown that simulation mechanisms are involved in action perception and performance, meaning that overlapping neural systems are recruited during the observation and execution of actions (Aziz-Zadeh et al., 2006; Buccino et al., 2004; Grezes et al., 2003; Johnson-Frey et al., 2003; Koski et al., 2002; Molnar-Szakacs et al., 2005; Nishitani & Hari, 2000).

Important to our discussion of music perception is the finding that a variety of commonly recognised hand action sounds show motor resonant effects, such as fingers typing on a typewriter, hands clapping and paper being ripped (Aziz-Zadeh et al., 2004; Engel et al., 2009; Lewis et al., 2005; Pizzamiglio et al., 2005). Furthermore, studies with dancers and musicians have revealed that the activity of the MNS is modulated by experience (Bangert et al., 2006; Cross, Hamilton, & Grafton, 2006; D'Ausilio et al., 2006; Margulis et al., 2009). For example, there is more mirror activation in pianists than in non-pianists during observation of piano-playing finger movements (Haslinger et al., 2005), as well as during listening to short piano melodies or pressing keyboard keys (Bangert et al., 2006), and more mirror activation in classical ballet dancers than in capoeira dancers during observation of ballet movements (Calvo-Merino et al., 2005).

Based on these findings, it has been proposed that in addition to action under-standing, neural circuits in motor regions may provide a basic mechanism for understanding the intentions behind actions as well. Iacoboni and colleagues (2005) found that observation of hand actions embedded within a context (i.e. with information about both the action and intention) led to more activity in the MNS than hand actions without a context (i.e. information about the action alone). Most importantly, different contexts, implying different intentions, led to differential levels of activation of the MNS. These results showed that the human MNS is sensitive to the context within which actions are embedded, and codes actions that imply different intentions differently. Thus, human mirror areas may play a role in the understanding of the intentions behind others' actions. In an important experimental manipulation, instructions to simply watch the videos versus instructions to infer intention yielded no differences in activity within the MNS, lending support to the theory that the representation of intentions and actions at the level of the MNS may be automatic and pre-reflective (Iacoboni et al., 2005).

Although mirroring was originally thought to be specifically associated with mirror neurons, the phenomenon of shared circuits in the brain constitutes a more general mechanism for mapping our own representations of actions, perceptions and feelings to our observations or auditory perceptions of others' actions, perceptions and feelings (Gallese & Sinigaglia, 2011; Keysers & Gazzola, 2009; Keysers & Perrett, 2004). For instance, a social mirroring mechanism is thought to exist for pain processing, whereby we process and empathise with other people's pain by activating the neural systems that process pain in our own bodies. This 'pain matrix' includes the insula, the anterior and middle cingulate gyrus, and the somatosensory cortices (SI and SII) (Bufalari et al., 2007; Jackson, Rainville, & Decety, 2006; Singer et al., 2004; Singer et al., 2006; Valeriani et al., 2008). In fact, it is thought that empathy for pain is supported by two distinct cerebral processes, enabling us to empathise with others through internal psychological aspects involving the cingulate cortex and insula; and external physical features involving the somatosensory cortices (Avenanti et al., 2007; Valeriani et al., 2008). This latter type of empathic process would be automatic, appear earlier ontogenetically and phylogenetically, and involve shared circuits that would map sensory–motor characteristics in our own body (Avenanti et al., 2007; Preston & de Waal, 2002). Thus, our ability to '*re*-present' through simulation of the pain, the emotions and motor behaviour of others within parts of our brain that are responsible for representing our own pain, emotions and actions, may serve as the foundation for our ability to learn and know about other minds and understand that others are 'like me' (Gallese, 2007).

Embodied empathy

The concept of empathy – the capacity to share others' feelings and emotions – was introduced in aesthetics to indicate the attitude of an observer toward an artist's work. In 1903, Theodor Lipps used the term *Einfühlung* – an understanding, or sensitivity so intimate, that feelings of one person are readily understood by another – to describe the concept of empathy (Lipps, 1903). However, in this original definition the observer was described as having an aesthetic experience, rather than an interpersonal one (for a more comprehensive discussion of empathy, see Laurence, this volume). Music is of course also an aesthetic experience, and indeed has long been considered in such terms by philosophers and musicologists (for example, Langer, 1954; Meyer, 1967). Music has the additional quality though, of requiring human performance for its realisation, involving perfectly executed action in real-time. This multidimensional (temporal, physical, aesthetic) quality of musical experience brings additional layers to our empathic and emotional responses.

The shared manifold hypothesis (Gallese, 2001, 2003b) – or the notion that we possess a kind of immediate understanding of what others are doing or feeling is also rooted in philosophy. Adam Smith, in 1759, proposed the concept of sympathy, defining it as 'fellow-feeling with any passion whatever' (p. 5) – the ability to feel something similar to what others feel, by simply observing others' behaviour (Smith, 1759/1976). Smith argued that people feel pleasure from the presence of others with the *same* emotion as oneself, proposing that such mutual sympathy heightens the original emotion and can 'disburden' the person of sorrow, 'because the sweetness of his sympathy more than compensates the bitterness of that sorrow' (Smith, 1759/1976, p. 14). It is perhaps within this shared space of experience that music has qualities suited for enhancing the feeling of communal experience, providing a non-verbal pathway for empathic communication. In fact, David Freedberg and Vittorio Gallese have proposed that 'a crucial element of aesthetic response consists of the activation of embodied mechanisms encompassing the simulation of actions, emotions and corporeal sensation, and that these mechanisms are universal' (Freedberg & Gallese, 2007).

Humans have a highly developed capacity to deduce, on the basis of observed behaviour, the intentions and emotions of others (Tomasello et al., 2005). This information allows us to survive, learn and thrive in a complex social world by guiding our own intentions, actions and feelings towards others and our environment. For instance, humans have a propensity to automatically and unconsciously align their behaviour to cues in their environment or to individuals around them – a type of behavioural 'mirroring'. In a clever experimental demonstration of this propensity, a group of participants were exposed to words typically associated with the elderly, such as 'Florida', 'bingo', 'grey', and an experimenter timed their walk as they left the lab. These primed participants walked significantly slower, unconsciously imitating the slower speed of the elderly, compared to participants who were not exposed to elderly stereotype words (Bargh, Chen, & Burrows, 1996). Several other studies (Dijksterhuis, 2005; Dijksterhuis, Bargh, & Miedema, 2000; Dijksterhuis & van Knippenberg, 1998) have since demonstrated a similar tendency for people to naturally align their behaviour with others or environmental cues. In other words, humans are able to embody the knowledge that other individuals have intentions that are manifest through bodies that think, feel and move in similar ways to their own.

As I have discussed, observing another person's emotional state activates parts of the neuronal network involved in processing that same state in oneself, whether it is disgust (Wicker et al., 2003), touch (Keysers et al., 2004) or pain (Singer et al., 2004). While this is likely not the only way social cognition occurs, the results from a variety of studies indicate that shared circuits exist in multiple parts of the human brain and constitute one prominent way that we understand the actions of other people and share their sensory and emotional experience (Keysers & Gazzola, 2009). In the musical domain, studies have shown that more empathic listeners seem to experience more intense emotions, especially in response to sad and tender music (Vuoskoski & Eerola, 2011; Vuoskoski et al., 2012). In a recent study by Andrei Miu and Felicia Balteş (2012), asking participants to adopt either an empathic or an objective perspective while listening to opera performances led to differing physiological responses (for example, skin conductance and heart rate) and differing ratings of experienced emotion, with the emotional responses in the high empathy condition being more congruent with the emotions expressed in the opera performances. Furthermore, Tal-Chen Rabinowitch and colleagues (2013) have shown that children involved in rhythmically synchronised music activities subsequently behaved more cooperatively and empathically than did children who were involved in an equivalent but not synchronised activity.

The Shared Affective Motion Experience (SAME) model

In a theory bringing together music and empathy, Istvan Molnar-Szakacs and Katie Overy (2006) hypothesised that the human MNS provides a mechanism by which listeners may experience music through a pre-reflective, automatic resonance mechanism, rather than through an effortful, top-down cognitive process. The authors suggest that music is likely to be interpreted in terms of the action and the potential agent that is implied by the sound rather than as disembodied abstract sounds. That is, music can be interpreted fundamentally as physical gestures emanating from another person – a person with intentions and emotions – resulting in a shared affective motion experience (SAME) (Molnar-Szakacs, Green Assuied, & Overy, 2012; Molnar-Szakacs & Overy, 2006; Overy & Molnar-Szakacs, 2009). The SAME model proposes that a limbic–insular–MNS network is centrally involved in musical experience. According to SAME, an emotional response at the simulation level will include a sense of the motor gestures behind the signal, in relation to personal knowledge or experience of such gestures (Molnar-Szakacs & Overy, 2006; Overy & Molnar-Szakacs, 2009). For musicians, this feeling will be quite specific, for example a pianist is likely to hear a familiar piece of music in terms of the precise motor movements required. For non-musicians the feeling is likely to be more generalised, such as in terms of the vocal requirements of the melodic line, or an impression of the speed and intensity of movements (for example, low-pitched, slow, quiet music can convey low energy states such as calmness or sadness, while high-pitched, fast, loud music can convey high energy states such as joy or anger) (Molnar-Szakacs, Green Assuied, & Overy, 2012).

An fMRI study explored the emotional responses to music in individuals with and without musical experience (Chapin et al., 2010). The authors hypothesised that MNS activity would influence emotional responses in listeners with explicit experience performing music. The neural responses to an expressive performance of a Chopin Etude (Opus 10, no.3) were correlated with emotional valence ratings for the music and compared to those of a mechanical performance of the same piece of music, as a control condition. Results showed that several brain regions including those consistent with the MNS and the limbic system were activated most significantly during moments of strongest emotional valence, which were also the most expressive, temporally dynamic sections of the musical pieces. This result was particularly strong for the participants with musical experience, providing support for the SAME model. Thus, network interactions between the MNS, insula and limbic system may be more readily engaged in those with musical experience. Such individuals have the experience of conveying emotion through music performance and may have a more developed mapping between musical structure, motor experience and emotion.

An unexpected finding of this study was that, for all participants, the tempo fluctuations of the expressive performance correlated with dynamic activation changes in brain regions that are consistent with the human MNS, including bilateral BA 44/45, superior temporal sulcus, ventral PMC and inferior parietal cortex, along with other motor-related areas and with insula (Chapin et al., 2010). Tempo and sound intensity, parameters that are manipulated through emotionally charged movement, are two properties of music that may convey emotion from performer to listener through a process of motor resonance. As the SAME model proposes, the MNS provides a neural mechanism for the communication of emotion during music listening by which emotions in music are perceived by listeners through a pre-reflective resonance process (Molnar-Szakacs & Overy, 2006; Overy & Molnar-Szakacs, 2009). The result of Heather Chapin and colleagues (2010) suggests the possibility that listeners perceive motion in the dynamic fluctuations of music performance, and this results in a form of empathic motor resonance by which listeners are able to feel the emotion communicated by the performer, leading to emotional responses within them.

Further evidence in support of the SAME model can be found in a number of studies of auditory–motor interactions and emotional responses to music. For example, an fMRI study by Stefan Koelsch and colleagues compared non-musicians while listening to 'pleasant' and 'unpleasant' (distorted) music, and found that pre-motor regions in the vocal area were significantly more active during the pleasant music, suggesting some kind of sub-vocal engagement with the melodic line (Koelsch et al., 2006). Others have found that trained pianists show significantly more pre-motor activation than non-musicians while listening to piano music, indicating a well-developed motor representation of the musical sound (Bangert et al., 2006; Haslinger et al., 2005; Haueisen & Knosche, 2001). The specificity of this motor understanding has been shown in a study by Lahav and colleagues, which involved training novices to play short melodies on the piano keyboard. Using fMRI, the researchers found that, after just five daily lessons on a collection of melodies, participants showed significantly stronger pre-motor activation while listening to the practised melodies, compared to unfamiliar melodies involving the same notes (Lahav, Saltzman, & Schlaug, 2007). These results provide evidence of the incredible plasticity of the human MNS, and confirm the inextricable relationship between music and motor function.

Music and motor function

The connection between music and motor function is evident in all aspects of musical activity – we dance to music, we move our bodies to play musical instruments, we move our mouths and larynx to sing. From dancing to singing to the playing of an instrument, the production of music involves well-coordinated motor actions that produce the physical vibrations of sound. The experience of music involves the perception of purposeful, intentional and organised sequences of motor acts as the cause of temporally synchronous auditory information. As Friedrich Nietzsche puts it, 'we listen to music with our muscles' (quoted in Sacks, 2007, p. xi). Thus, according to the theory of embodied simulation, the equivalent motor network is engaged, by those listening to singing and drumming, as by those singing and drumming. This allows for co-representation of the musical experience, emerging out of the shared and temporally synchronous recruitment of parallel neural networks in the sender and the perceiver of the musical message (Molnar-Szakacs & Overy, 2006). This shared musical representation has a similar potential for communication as shared language or action. Numerous studies have relied on this coupling of perception and action in musical experience to investigate the neural organisation of such complex behaviours as sequence learning and temporal production (Janata & Grafton, 2003), and others have shown that specific musical experience or expertise (Bangert et al., 2006; Haslinger et al., 2005), dancing experience (Cross, Hamilton, & Grafton, 2006) and music-related motor learning (Calvo-Merino et al., 2004) can all modulate activity within the human MNS.

Long before the discovery of neural mechanisms of embodiment and mirroring, developmental investigations, psycholinguistic research, cross-species comparison and neuroscientific studies had shown behavioural and neural links between the emergence of hierarchical processing in action and aspects of language, such as hierarchy in linguistic grammar (Greenfield, 1978; Greenfield & Dent, 1982). M. Grossman (1980) used evidence from aphasic patients to suggest that Broca's area is the common neural substrate for processing hierarchy in both language and action (Grossman, 1980). He found that Broca's aphasics who lack hierarchical organisation in their syntactic production were also impaired in recreating hierarchically organised tree structures. In contrast, fluent aphasics, who have hierarchically organised (but semantically empty) speech, were able to reproduce the hierarchical structure of the models (Grossman, 1980). Kimura and colleagues further proposed that sequential operations involved in both language and action might explain the co-occurrence of motor and speech deficits in apraxia (Kimura & Archibald, 1974; Lomas & Kimura, 1976). In summary, hierarchically organised sequential operations are fundamental to both language and action. Thus, language and motor abilities may share cognitive resources and a homologous neural substrate. In fact, recent theoretical developments on the evolution of language propose that language may have evolved from the motor system and the two cognitive functions may still be governed by the same fundamental rules (Arbib, 2005; Greenfield, 1991; Rizzolatti & Arbib, 1998).

Neuroimaging studies of language function and studies of sensory–motor integration have also pointed to links between the MNS and the brain regions involved in linguistic processing (Arbib, 2005; Rizzolatti & Arbib, 1998). For instance, it has been shown that a fronto-parietal network was engaged during comprehension of hierarchically organised language (Bornkessel et al., 2005). Molnar-Szakacs and colleagues further showed this to be the case for hierarchical actions by showing that the sequential manipulation of objects also recruits the fronto-parietal mirror neuron network for action representation (Molnar-Szakacs et al., 2006). Given these findings, Molnar-Szakacs and colleagues have proposed that parallel functional segregation within Broca's area during language and motor tasks may reflect similar computations used in both language and motor control (Molnar-Szakacs et al., 2005). Furthermore, neuroimaging studies show that regions of the action recognition network are also important for a variety of language functions (Fadiga, Craighero, & Olivier, 2005). An overlap of activations was found in these regions for action recognition and language production (Hamzei et al., 2003).

Human language is a communicative signal with a hierarchical structure, in which phonemes are combined to form words, phrases and sentences up to the discourse level of speech structure (Hockett, 1960). Such principles of hierarchical organisation have also been shown to underlie other complex abilities such as problem-solving (Newell & Simon, 1972) and tool-use (Greenfield, 1991; Greenfield et al., 2000). Important parallels exist between music and language. Both are governed by theories of temporal coherence – the sensory input evolves over time in a coherent structure (Lerdahl & Jackendoff, 1983); and both exhibit specific and relatively fixed developmental time courses (Trehub, 2001). Furthermore, as previously discussed (Overy & Molnar-Szakacs 2006), music, like language, is a communicative signal comprised of patterns whose performance and perception are governed by combinatorial rules, or a sort of musical grammar (Sloboda, 1985). As in language, the musical signal is not simply organised in consecutive sequential elements, but involves hierarchical relationships. Hierarchical organisation is the process of integrating lower-level units to form more complex higher-level units and in the case of music this involves combinations of both sequential and simultaneous elements such as notes, rhythms, phrases, chords, chord progressions and keys to form an overall musical structure (Lerdahl & Jackendoff, 1983).

Koelsch and colleagues (2013) recently used neuroimaging to investigate hierarchical processing in music. Their results revealed that a brain mechanism fundamental for syntactic processing is engaged during the perception of music, indicating that processing of hierarchical structure with nested non-local dependencies is not just a key component of human language, but a multi-domain capacity of human cognition (Koelsch et al., 2013). More precisely, their findings indicate that, when listening to music, humans apply cognitive processes that are capable of dealing with long-distance dependencies resulting from hierarchically organised syntactic structures. In the case of music for example, perception of a melody does not proceed in a simple sequential manner, it involves active prediction, such that expectancies are generated based upon a listener's implicit knowledge about musical rules that have been acquired by previous exposure to music of their culture. Thus, hearing a particular set of tones leads one to expect certain specific continuations with greater probability than others (Huron, 2006). There is good evidence that the relevant sequential contingencies are encoded based on a process of statistical learning (Schon & Francois, 2011), which emerges early in life for both speech and music (Saffran, 2003) and continues into adulthood (Loui et al., 2009). The neural substrates associated with musical expectancies and their violation have been measured using electrophysiological markers. These studies show that there is sensitivity to predictions based on a variety of features including contour (Tervaniemi et al., 2001) and interval size (Trainor, McDonald, & Alain, 2002), as well as harmonies (Leino et al., 2007). The localisation of these processes is complex and not fully deciphered, but most likely involves interactions between belt/parabelt auditory cortices and inferior frontal cortices (Opitz et al., 2002; Schonwiesner et al., 2007).

Initial evidence for a shared role for the inferior frontal cortex in linguistic and musical processing, came from event-related potential (ERP) and magnetoencephalography (MEG) studies (Koelsch, Maess, & Friederici, 2000; Maess et al., 2001). Neuroimaging studies on musical syntax (as probed with sequential harmonic or melodic structures) also consistently revealed activation in BA 44/45, typically in both the right and left hemispheres, but sometimes biased to the right side (Brown, Martinez, & Parsons, 2006; Fadiga, Craighero, & D'Ausilio, 2009; Koelsch, Maess, & Friederici, 2000; Maess et al., 2001). Using fMRI to investigate the neural correlates of musical structure, Levitin and Menon (2003) randomised musical excerpts within a piece of music in order to disrupt musical structure. Comparing music to its scrambled counterpart, they found focal activation in the pars orbitalis region (Brodmann Area 47) of the left IFG, a region that has been previously closely associated with the processing of linguistic structure in spoken and signed language (Levitin & Menon, 2003). Thus, finding support for the theory that processing of musical and linguistic syntax share common neural substrates. Furthermore, damage to this area of the posterior inferior frontal gyrus can lead to the conjoint impairments of aphasia and amusia, a selective problem with perceiving and interpreting music (Alajouanine, 1948). Evidence has also shown that aphasic patients with syntactic comprehension difficulties in language exhibit similar syntactic difficulties in the domain of musical harmony (Patel, 2005). In fact, Tecumseh Fitch and Maurício Martins (2014, p. 91) recently concluded that 'The best characterized, and to us most convincing, nonlinguistic function of the IFG is in music processing and memory.'

The range of research findings discussed so far lends support to the hypothesis that the perception of action, language and music recruit shared neural resources. In parallel with the developmental literature on action and language, infants also seem to show implicit knowledge of principles of hierarchical organisation for music. For example, they are able to distinguish different scales and show preferences for consonant over dissonant tonal combinations (Trehub, 2003). It has been shown that children with dyslexia exhibit specific timing difficulties in the domain of music (Overy et al., 2003), motor control (Fawcett & Nicolson, 1995; Wolff, 2002) and language (Goswami et al., 2002; Tallal, Miller, & Fitch, 1993) and that music lessons with dyslexic children can lead to improvements in language skills (Overy, 2003). Taken together, these results support the notion that action, language and music are ontogenetically and phylogenetically linked and share neural resources.

But, as Oliver Sacks put it, 'music itself [that] has something very peculiar about it – its beat, its melodic contours, so different from those of speech, and its peculiarly direct connection to the emotions' (Sacks, 2007, p. 40).

Musical emotion and reward

> The inexpressible depth of music, so easy to understand and yet so inexplicable, is due to the fact that it reproduces all the emotions of our innermost being, but entirely without reality and remote from its pain... Music expresses only the quintessence of life and of its events, never these themselves.
>
>   (Arthur Schopenhauer, quoted in Sacks, 2007, p. xi)

As previously discussed (Molnar-Szakacs & Overy, 2006), one of the defining features of music is its ability to induce an emotional response in listeners (Gabrielsson, 2001). Emotional responses to music are present in early life and across cultures (Balkwill & Thompson, 1999), indicating that the ability to perceive emotions in music may be innate (Trevarthen, 1999; Zentner & Kagan, 1996). Numerous measures of arousal have been used to investigate the emotion-inducing effects of music. Skin conductance responses appear to be useful indicators of musically induced emotional arousal (VanderArk & Ely, 1992, 1993), and 'chills' (goosebumps) can be elicited when participants are allowed to select music they find arousing (Gabrielsson, 2001; Panksepp, 1995).

More recently, a multitude of neuroimaging studies have shown that brain areas associated with emotion and reward processing are also involved in emotional responses to music. Listening to pleasant, relative to unpleasant, music was associated with activation of insula, IFG and the ventral striatum, a key structure in reward and addiction circuits (Berridge & Robinson, 2003; Koelsch et al., 2006). The opposite act of listening to unpleasant compared to pleasant musical excerpts activated parahippocampal gyrus as well as amygdala, and the temporal poles – regions also belonging to limbic and paralimbic circuitry (Koelsch et al., 2006). Similarly, increasing dissonance of short chord sequences led to increased activity in parahippocampus and precuneus, whereas increasing consonance was associated with activation of orbitofrontal and frontopolar cortices and subcal-losal cingulate, regions implicated in emotion processing (Blood et al., 1999; Royet et al., 2000). Activation of emotion- and reward-related networks was found to be associated with increasing pleasurable chill ratings in response to listening to self-selected musical excerpts (Blood & Zatorre, 2001) and while listening to music rated as happy versus sad (Mitterschiffthaler et al., 2007).

Taken together, neuroimaging studies of affective responses to music have revealed activations across a network of brain regions, including frontal pole, orbitofrontal cortex, parahippocampal gyrus, superior temporal gyrus/sulcus, cingulate and the precuneus (Blood & Zatorre, 2001; Blood et al., 1999; Koelsch et al., 2006; Koelsch & Siebel, 2005; Menon & Levitin, 2005). These regions be-long to a network that has traditionally been referred to as the limbic system. The limbic system influences the activity of other brain regions through dopaminer-gic (DA) projections, playing an essential role in motivation, memory formation, processing emotional states and evaluating reward (Adolphs, 1999, 2001, 2003; Adolphs et al., 2000).

Although many different types of rewards exist, among the most fundamental are those relating to food and sex (Cannon & Bseikri, 2004). This is perhaps not a coincidence, as both are biologically necessary for survival and reproduction. It has been widely demonstrated that DA neurons mediate the reinforcing quality of these stimuli (Cannon & Bseikri, 2004; Egerton et al., 2009; Wise, 2002). Many highly addictive drugs of abuse, including cocaine and amphetamines also spe-cifically target this system, increasing DA to create feelings of intense euphoria. Valorie Salimpoor and colleagues (2011) investigated the possibility that music may also be targeting the mesolimbic DA system in a similar way to food and sex. However, music as a stimulus is different from food and sex, because it is not essential to survival, it is abstract, and without meaning. In this study, participants were asked to choose music that they found intensely emotional, and led them to experience chills. They used PET to determine whether DA is released during pleasurable responses to music, as well as the links between peak emotional mo-ments and pleasure. The 'chills response' was used as an objective indicator of peak emotional responses and emotional arousal was further assessed through psychophysiological measurements (heart rate, respiration, temperature). Find-ings revealed that DA release in the nucleus accumbens (NAcc) was positively correlated with emotional arousal (i.e. intensity of the chills response), and DA release in the caudate was positively correlated with the number of chills expe-rienced. Furthermore, the anticipation of chills led to DA release in the dorsal striatum, whereas the chills response itself led to DA release in the ventral stri-atum (Salimpoor et al., 2011). This finding parallels results observed in research on drugs of abuse, where anticipation of a reward is associated with dorsal striatal DA release and reward itself with ventral release (Leyton et al., 2002; Small et al., 2003). Interestingly, 'anticipatory' and 'release' phases in music are often used by composers to manipulate emotional arousal through violation of expectancies or delayed resolution. These results also provided the first direct evidence that listening to highly emotional music can lead to DA release in the limbic system.

This is a significant finding, as it suggests that music, an abstract aesthetic stimulus, can naturally target the DA systems of the brain (Salimpoor et al., 2013). As these neural systems are typically involved in highly reinforcing and addictive behaviours, the fact that they are targeted by music may help explain how music exerts such powerful emotional effects. Thus, in addition to the recruitment of neural networks of embodiment discussed earlier, music listening activates an extensive network of brain regions – the limbic system – important for processing emotion, reward, motivation and memory formation (Morgane et al., 2005). These findings indicate that listening to music we like may be experienced as emotional and rewarding. In fact, one of the main reasons people give for listening to music is to experience or modulate their emotional state (Sloboda & O'Neill, 2001).

An interesting quality of music is its personal nature – whether it is perceived to be rewarding is listener-specific. I might love a song so much that I have it on repeat on my iPod, but you may not like it at all. So what happens in the brain when we hear a song we like, versus one we don't really care for? A recent study investigated this question, by giving individuals a chance to purchase each piece of music they wanted to listen to in an auction paradigm. This meant that the research team could assess the 'reward value' of music – they assumed that the more an individual spent to hear a piece of music, the more they liked it (Salimpoor et al., 2013). Results revealed that activity in the mesolimbic striatal areas, the NAcc in particular, was most associated with reward value of musical stimuli, as measured by the amount participants bid for a piece of music. As you might recall, DA release in the NAcc was associated with the intensity of the chills response, and it has also been implicated in anticipation and reward prediction errors – that is, detecting the difference between what was expected and the actual outcome (O'Doherty, 2004; Schott et al., 2008).

A second and perhaps more important finding was that for the more rewarding pieces of music, the auditory cortices in the superior temporal gyrus (STG), which were equally active during processing of all musical stimuli, showed significantly stronger functional interactions with the NAcc (Salimpoor et al., 2013). The authors propose that the STG may be a 'repository' of an individual's prior experiences with musical sounds, and expectations were compared to information stored in the STG, giving rise to the increased functional connectivity between the subcortical NAcc and cortical STG with more rewarding pieces of music. This functional interaction between subcortical reward circuits and 'person-specific' cortical regions might explain why different people like different music, and how this may be a function of an individual's previous experiences with musical sounds. Thus, the reward value for music is coded by activity levels in the NAcc, whose functional connectivity with auditory and frontal areas increases as a function of increasing musical reward (Zatorre & Salimpoor, 2013). Activation of these brain systems in response to a stimulus as abstract as music may represent a relatively newer property of human cognition. Perhaps, over evolutionary time, music co-opted neural systems of emotion processing, making musical experiences rewarding, and as connections between phylogenetically older, survival-related brain systems and newer, more cognitive systems increased, and our general capacity to assign meaning to abstract stimuli developed, our capacity to derive pleasure from abstract stimuli like music also increased (Blood & Zatorre, 2001).

Implications for music therapy

The effective and efficient expression of emotion is essential to the survival of our species. It has been shown that basic emotions (such as anger, fear, joy and surprise) are expressed in similar ways cross-culturally, and are universally recognised (Biehl et al., 1997). Vocal expressions of basic emotions (for example, sighs, screams, gasps, laughs) show similarly universal recognition across cultures (Scherer & Zenter, 2001). As previously discussed by Molnar-Szakacs, Green Assuied and Overy (2012), the universality of such forms of emotional expression highlights the fact that their production is rooted in human motor behaviour and thus human physio-logy: the possibilities and limitations of human facial muscles and vocal apparatus. Our felt emotions can only be expressed within the means and limitations of our motor system. Manfred Clynes has hypothesised that the human system for express-ing emotion must be based on biologically fixed, universal, primary dynamic forms, and has shown that emotions conveyed by dynamic gestures of touch can be trans-lated into sound and interpreted cross-culturally (Clynes, 1973). Emotional expres-sion is also affected by physiological arousal, for example a heightened emotional state (increased heart rate, increased breathing rate and tense vocal chords) can have an impact on the quality of vocal expressions during that state (high-pitched, fast vocalisations). Since the acoustic parameters of vocal expression are identical to those of music – pitch, timbre, intensity and duration – musical expression can thus approximate, imitate and extend the natural qualities of emotional vocalisations to heightened pitch, dynamic, timbral and temporal ranges (Molnar-Szakacs, Green Assuied, & Overy, 2012). What singing can achieve naturally, musical instruments can expand even further, abstracted in terms of fixed timbres, pitches and scales. For example, an early study by Klaus Scherer and James Oshinsky showed that a variety of specific emotional states can be conveyed by certain characteristics of musical pitch sequences, for example sadness is conveyed most saliently by a slow tempo and low pitch level, while anger is conveyed most saliently by rising pitch sequences, and small pitch variation (Scherer & Oshinsky, 1977).

Of course, there are also cultural differences in emotional signals across vocal, musical and physical gestures. Molnar-Szakacs and colleagues (2007) used TMS to explore neural representations of culturally specific manual gesture vocabular-ies, and found that neural activity was modulated by whether or not the actor and perceiver were from the same cultural group. In addition, it was found that, even when perceiving unfamiliar gestures from an unfamiliar cultural group, there was a stronger neural 'simulation' when the gestures had genuine meaning – that is, when the gesture itself was made in an intentional way (Molnar-Szakacs et al., 2007). Thus suggesting, that it is the intentionality and universality of musical expression that gives it exceptional power and utility in a non-verbal, therapeutic context. An individual can express emotions through music that can be interpreted by others based on their own emotional and musical experiences, without reliance on linguistic expression. The musical exchange among these individuals may become an empathic experience if there is a feeling of shared affect, and this in turn may give rise to feelings of 'togetherness'.

This is the key of musical communication – it relies on sounds and actions rather than words – and in clinical therapeutic settings allows the therapist to establish a connection with a client that is embodied rather than cognitive. Unlike language, in which words refer symbolically to a certain emotion, music can be used to express the feeling of an emotion itself (Ansdell, 1995). 'We communicate with words to convey our meaning, whereas we improvise music to *find* something meaningful between us' (Ansdell, 1995, p. 26). As described in Molnar-Szakacs, Green Assuied and Overy (2012), a therapist and client build a relationship together through spontaneous and purposeful expression (Aldridge, 2005), listening, and reflection: by responding to each other's emotional presence. 'Mirroring' a client's behaviour is considered to be critical in creating an empathic relationship in interactive music therapy.

Interestingly, evidence from music therapy literature indicates that linking a musical sound specifically to the agent or source of the sound can facilitate increased awareness of other individuals and external surroundings. Children on the autistic spectrum, for example, have been found to attend more to music when they are able to observe a musical partner playing an instrument, and to have improved motor skills when imitating and making music themselves (Alvin & Warwick, 1991). While working with children on the autistic spectrum, a therapist may employ a variety of musical interventions to engage them in developing a greater awareness – initially of themselves, then of the person with whom they are creating music, and then by extension, their external surroundings and other people (Molnar-Szakacs & Heaton, 2012). An important aspect of such musical development and interaction is physical coordination in time, involving a developing awareness of the temporal linking of sounds with movements, as well as the potential for temporal synchronisation between client and therapist. Music therapy, although context-dependent and constantly changing, is at its core a powerful empathic and social experience – and neuroscience is beginning to discover the neural scaffolding that supports these behaviours. It is through a fundamental understanding of the biological bases of these behaviours that we can further develop these techniques and develop evidence-based models of their effectiveness.

Conclusion

Music is a unique 'language' without words, an abstract stimulus with complex hierarchical structure present in cultures across the globe, and through time. Music is capable of conveying as well as inducing a wide range of emotions in listeners, and studies of music perception have shown that music can evoke strong emotional responses such as chills and an increased heart rate. Neuroimaging has revealed that music activates more of the brain than any other stimulus – from cortical regions to subcortical limbic structures and from frontal regions to the temporal lobe. The increasing use of music as a research tool has allowed the study of relationships among these regions, the pathways connecting them, and the dynamics of communication within and among networks formed by these brain regions. Studies using musical stimuli have provided us with insights about motor learning, auditory processing, emotion perception, language processing, memory, and so much more (for example, Baird & Samson, 2009; Janata & Grafton, 2003; Koelsch, 2010; Patel, 2003).

Music has such powerful ability to evoke emotions in individuals, that even solo listening to recorded music has been described as a social experience (Launay, 2015; Molnar-Szakacs, 2015) – music imbued with its own form of 'agency'. Building on what is known about language and action representation, it has been proposed that music may also be similarly embodied within fronto-parietal structures of the human MNS (Molnar-Szakacs, Green Assuied, & Overy, 2012; Molnar-Szakacs & Overy, 2006; Overy & Molnar-Szakacs, 2009). Subcortical mesolimbic pathways and limbic structures provide emotional colour to musical experiences (Salimpoor et al., 2011). Music may in fact have co-opted these evolutionarily ancient neural systems through evolutionary time. Culturally acquired experiences and learned preferences represented in temporal cortex can interact with this system to guide an individual's personal responses to a particular piece of music (Blood & Zatorre, 2001).

Music has a universal appeal that is often attributed to its ability to make us feel a certain way or change how we are currently feeling – moving us to tears of joy or sorrow. Music is an integral part of most important of life's events, including graduations, weddings and funerals. Music is also widely used as a therapeutic tool to improve physical and mental health and promote prosocial behaviour. For example, collaborative music-making involving shared affective motion experiences including collaboration, mirroring and imitation can build empathy. There is growing evidence, both behavioural and neural, showing that music can enable us to 'get inside each other's minds', and recognise each other's shared humanity. The abstract sounds of musical signals can communicate universal emotions, creating an empathic connection among individuals. It may be said that music is indeed the language of empathy.

Acknowledgements

I would like to thank Katie Overy, Caroline Waddington and an anonymous reviewer for comments on previous versions of this chapter. Any errors or omissions are my own.

References

Adolphs, R. (1999). Social cognition and the human brain. *Trends in Cognitive Sciences*, *3*(12), 469–479.

Adolphs, R. (2001). The neurobiology of social cognition. *Current Opinion in Neurobiology*, *11*(2), 231–239.

Adolphs, R. (2003). Cognitive neuroscience of human social behaviour. *Nature Reviews Neuroscience, 4*(3), 165–178.

Adolphs, R. (2009). The social brain: Neural basis of social knowledge. *Annual Review of Psychology, 60*(7), 693–716.

Adolphs, R., Damasio, H., Tranel, D., Cooper, G., & Damasio, A. R. (2000). A role for somatosensory cortices in the visual recognition of emotion as revealed by three-dimensional lesion mapping. *The Journal of Neuroscience, 20,* 2683–2690.

Alajouanine, T. (1948). Aphasia and artistic realization. *Brain, 71,* 229–241.

Aldridge, D. (Ed.) (2005). *Music therapy and neurological rehabilitation: Performing health.* London: Jessica Kingsley Publishers.

Alvin, J., & Warwick, A. (1991). *Music therapy for the autistic child.* Oxford: Oxfor University Press.

Ansdell, G. (1995). *Music for life: Aspects of creative music therapy with adult clients.* London: Jessica Kingsley Publishers.

Arbib, M. A. (2005). From monkey-like action recognition to human language: An evolutionary framework for neurolinguistics. *Behavioral and Brain Sciences, 28*(2), 105–124; discussion 125–167.

Avenanti, A., Bolognini, N., Maravita, A., & Aglioti, S. M. (2007). Somatic and motor components of action simulation. *Current Biology, 17*(24), 2129–2135.

Aziz-Zadeh, L., Iacoboni, M., Zaidel, E., Wilson, S., & Mazziotta, J. (2004). Left hemisphere motor facilitation in response to manual action sounds. *European Journal of Neuroscience, 19*(9), 2609–2612.

Aziz-Zadeh, L., Koski, L., Zaidel, E., Mazziotta, J., & Iacoboni, M. (2006). Lateralization of the human mirror neuron system. *The Journal of Neuroscience, 26*(11), 2964–2970.

Baird, A., & Samson, S. (2009). Memory for music in Alzheimer's disease: Unforgettable?. *Neuropsychology Review, 19*(1), 85–101.

Balkwill, L.-L., & Thompson, W. F. (1999). A cross-cultural investigation of the perception of emotion in music: psychophysical and cultural cues. *Music Perception, 17*(1), 43–64.

Bangert, M., Peschel, T., Schlaug, G., Rotte, M., Drescher, D., Hinrichs, H., Heinze, H. J., & Altenmuller, E. (2006). Shared networks for auditory and motor processing in professional pianists: evidence from fMRI conjunction. *Neuroimage, 30*(3), 917–926.

Bargh, J. A., Chen, M., & Burrows, L. (1996). Automaticity of social behavior: direct effects of trait construct and stereotype-activation on action. *Journal of Personality and Social Psychology, 71*(2), 230–244.

Berridge, K. C., & Robinson, T. E. (2003). Parsing reward. *Trends in Neurosciences, 26*(9), 507–513.

Biehl, M., Matsumoto, D., Ekman, P., Hearn, V., Heider, K., Kudoh, T., & Ton, V. (1997). Matsumoto and Ekman's Japanese and Caucasian facial expressions of emotion (JACFEE): Reliability data and cross-national differences. *Journal of Nonverbal Behavior, 21,* 3–21.

Blood, A. J., & Zatorre, R. J. (2001). Intensely pleasurable responses to music correlate with activity in brain regions implicated in reward and emotion. *Proceedings of the National Academy of Sciences of the United States of America, 98*(20), 11818–11823.

Blood, A. J., Zatorre, R. J., Bermudez, P., & Evans, A. C. (1999). Emotional responses to pleasant and unpleasant music correlate with activity in paralimbic brain regions. *Nature Neuroscience, 2*(4), 382–387.

Bornkessel, I., Zysset, S., Friederici, A. D., von Cramon, D. Y., & Schlesewsky, M. (2005). Who did what to whom? The neural basis of argument hierarchies during language comprehension. *Neuroimage, 26*(1), 221–233.

Brown, S., Martinez, M. J., & Parsons, L. M. (2006). Music and language side by side in the brain: A PET study of the generation of melodies and sentences. *European Journal of Neuroscience, 23*(10), 2791–2803.

Buccino, G., Vogt, S., Ritzl, A., Fink, G. R., Zilles, K., Freund, H. J., & Rizzolatti, G. (2004). Neural circuits underlying imitation learning of hand actions: an event-related fMRI study. *Neuron, 42*(2), 323–334.

Bufalari, I., Aprile, T., Avenanti, A., Di Russo, F., & Aglioti, S. M. (2007). Empathy for pain and touch in the human somatosensory cortex. *Cerebral Cortex, 17*(11), 2553–2561.

Calvo-Merino, B., Glaser, D. E., Grezes, J., Passingham, R. E., & Haggard, P. (2005). Action observation and acquired motor skills: An fMRI study with expert dancers. *Cerebral Cortex, 15*(8), 1243–1249.

Cannon, C. M., & Bseikri, M. R. (2004). Is dopamine required for natural reward? *Physiology and Behavior, 81*(5), 741–748.

Chapin, H., Jantzen, K., Kelso, J. A., Steinberg, F., & Large, E. (2010). Dynamic emotional and neural responses to music depend on performance expression and listener experience. *PLoS ONE, 5*(12), e13812.

Clarke, E., DeNora, T., & Vuoskoski, J. (2015). Music, empathy and cultural understanding. *Physics of Life Reviews. 15*, 61–68.

Clynes, M. (1973). Sentics: Biocybernetics of emotion communication. *Annals of the New York Academy of Science, 220*(3), 55–131.

Conard, N. J., Malina, M., & Munzel, S. C. (2009). New flutes document the earliest musical tradition in southwestern Germany. *Nature, 460*(7256), 737–740.

Cross, E. S., Hamilton, A. F. d. C., & Grafton, S. T. (2006). Building a motor simulation de novo: observation of dance by dancers. *NeuroImage, 31*(3), 1257–1267.

Cross, I., & Morley, I. (2008). The evolution of music: Theories, definitions and the nature of the evidence. In S. Malloch & C. Trevarthen (Eds.), *Communicative musicality* (pp. 61–82). Oxford: Oxford University Press.

D'Ausilio, A., Altenmuller, E., Olivetti, B.M., & Lotze, M. (2006). Cross-modal plasticity of the motor cortex while listening to a rehearsed musical piece. *European Journal of Neuroscience 24*(3), 955–958.

Darwin, C. (1871). *The descent of man, and selection in relation to sex.* London: J. Murray.

Darwin, C. (1887). *The life and letters of Charles Darwin.* London: J. Murray.

Dijksterhuis, A. (2005). Why are we social animals: the high road to imitation as social glue. In S. Hurley & N. Chater (Eds.), *Perspectives on imitation: From neuroscience to social science* (Vol. 2, pp. 207–220). Cambridge, MA: MIT Press.

Dijksterhuis, A., Bargh, J. A., & Miedema, J. (2000). Of men and mackerels: Attention, subjective experience, and automatic social behavior. In H. Bless & J. Forgas (Eds.), *The message within: The role of subjective experience in social cognition and behavior* (pp. 37–51). New York: Psychology Press.

Dijksterhuis, A., & van Knippenberg, A. (1998). The relation between perception and behavior, or how to win a game of Trivial Pursuit. *Journal of Personality and Social Psychology, 74*(4), 865–877.

Dolgin, K. G., & Adelson, E. H. (1990). Age changes in the ability to interpret affect in sung and instrumentally presented melodies. *Psychology of Music, 18*(1), 87–98.

Egerton, A., Mehta, M. A., Montgomery, A. J., Lappin, J. M., Howes, O. D., Reeves, S. J., Cunningham, V. J., & Grasby, P. M. (2009). The dopaminergic basis of human behaviors: A review of molecular imaging studies. *Neuroscience and Biobehavioral Reviews, 33*(7), 1109–1132.

Engel, L. R., Frum, C., Puce, A., Walker, N. A., & Lewis, J. W. (2009). Different categories of living and non-living sound-sources activate distinct cortical networks. *NeuroImage, 47*(4), 1778–1791.

Fadiga, L., Craighero, L., & D'Ausilio, A. (2009). Broca's area in language, action, and music. *Annals of the New York Academy of Sciences, 1169*, 448–458.

Fadiga, L., Craighero, L., & Olivier, E. (2005). Human motor cortex excitability during the perception of others' action. *Current Opinion in Neurobiology, 15*(2), 213–218.

Fadiga, L., Fogassi, L., Pavesi, G., & Rizzolatti, G. (1995). Motor facilitation during action observation: A magnetic stimulation study. *Journal of Neurophysiology, 73*(6), 2608–2611.

Fawcett, A. J., & Nicolson, R. I. (1995). Persistent deficits in motor skill of children with dyslexia. *Journal of Motor Behavior, 27*(3), 235–240.

Ferrari, P. F., Bonini, L., & Fogassi, L. (2009). From monkey mirror neurons to primate behaviours: possible 'direct' and 'indirect' pathways. *Philosophical Transactions of the Royal Society of London B: Biological Sciences, 364*(1528), 2311–2323.

Ferrari, P. F., Gallese, V., Rizzolatti, G., & Fogassi, L. (2003). Mirror neurons responding to the observation of ingestive and communicative mouth actions in the monkey ventral premotor cortex. *European Journal of Neuroscience, 17*(8), 1703–1714.

Ferrari, P. F., Rozzi, S., & Fogassi, L. (2005). Mirror neurons responding to observation of actions made with tools in monkey ventral premotor cortex. *Journal of Cognitive Neuroscience, 17*(2), 212–226.

Fitch, W. T., & Martins, M. D. (2014). Hierarchical processing in music, language, and action: Lashley revisited. *Annals of the New York Academy of Sciences, 1316*, 87–104.

Fogassi, L., Ferrari, P. F., Gesierich, B., Rozzi, S., Chersi, F., & Rizzolatti, G. (2005). Parietal lobe: From action organization to intention understanding. *Science, 308*(5722), 662–667.

Fogassi, L., & Luppino, G. (2005). Motor functions of the parietal lobe. *Current Opinion in Neurobiology, 15*(6), 626–631.

Freedberg, D., & Gallese, V. (2007). Motion, emotion and empathy in esthetic experience. *Trends in Cognitive Sciences, 11*(5), 197–203.

Gabrielsson, A. (2001). Emotions in strong experiences with music. In P. Juslin & J. A. Sloboda (Eds.), *Music and emotion: Theory and research* (pp. 431–449). Oxford, UK: Oxford University Press.

Gallese, V. (2001). The 'shared manifold' hypothesis. From mirror neurons to empathy. *Journal of Consciousness Studies, 8*(5–7), 33–50.

Gallese, V. (2003a). The manifold nature of interpersonal relations: the quest for a common mechanism. *Philosophical Transactions of the Royal Society of London B: Biological Sciences, 358*(1431), 517–528.

Gallese, V. (2003b). The roots of empathy: the shared manifold hypothesis and the neural basis of intersubjectivity. *Psychopathology, 36*(4), 171–180.

Gallese, V. (2007). Before and below 'theory of mind': Embodied simulation and the neural correlates of social cognition. *Philosophical Transactions of the Royal Society of London. B, 362*(1480), 659–669.

Gallese, V., Fadiga, L., Fogassi, L., & Rizzolatti, G. (1996). Action recognition in the premotor cortex. *Brain, 119*(Pt 2), 593–609.

Gallese, V., & Goldman, A. (1998). Mirror neurons and the simulation theory of mind-reading. *Trends in Cognitive Sciences, 2*(12), 493–501.

Gallese, V., Keysers, C., & Rizzolatti, G. (2004). A unifying view of the basis of social cognition. *Trends in Cognitive Sciences, 8*(9), 396–403.

Gallese, V., & Sinigaglia, C. (2011). What is so special about embodied simulation? *Trends in Cognitive Sciences, 15*(11), 512–519.

Gamez-Djokic, V., Molnar-Szakacs, I., & Aziz-Zadeh, L. (2015). Embodied simulation: Building meaning through shared neural circuitry. In M. H. Fischer & Y. Coello (Eds.), *Conceptual and interactive embodiment: Foundations of embodied cognition, Volume 2*, (pp. 216–245). London: Psychology Press.

Garrido, S., & Schubert, E. (2011). Individual differences in the enjoyment of negative emotion in music: A literature review and experiment. *Music Perception: An Interdisciplinary Journal, 28*(3), 279–296.

Goldman, A. I. (2006). *Simulating minds: The philosophy, psychology, and neuroscience of mindreading.* New York: Oxford University Press.

Goswami, U., Thomson, J., Richardson, U., Stainthorp, R., Hughes, D., Rosen, S., & Scott, S. K. (2002). Amplitude envelope onsets and developmental dyslexia: A new hypothesis. *Proceedings of the National Academy of Sciences of the United States of America, 99*(16), 10911–10916.

Greenfield, P. (1978). Structural parallels between language and action in development. In A. Lock (Ed.), *Action, gesture and symbol: The emergence of language* (pp. 415–445). London: Academic Press.

Greenfield, P. (1991). Language, tools and brain: The ontogeny and phylogeny of hierarchically organized sequential behavior. *Behavioral and Brain Sciences, 14*(4), 531–595.

Greenfield, P., Maynard, A., Boehm, C., & Schmidtling, E. (2000). Cultural apprenticeship and cultural change: Tool learning and imitation in chimpanzees and humans. In S. T. Parker, J. Langer & M. L. McKinney (Eds.), *Biology, brains & behavior: The evolution in human development* (pp. 237–277). Santa Fe, NM: SAR Press.

Greenfield, P. M., & Dent, C. H. (1982). Pragmatic factors in children's phrasal coordination. *Journal of Child Language, 9*(2), 425–443.

Grezes, J., Armony, J. L., Rowe, J., & Passingham, R. E. (2003). Activations related to 'mirror' and 'canonical' neurones in the human brain: An fMRI study. *Neuroimage, 18*(4), 928–937.

Grossman, M. (1980). A central processor for hierarchically-structured material: Evidence from Broca's aphasia. *Neuropsychologia, 18*(3), 299–308.

Hagen, E. H., & Hammerstein, P. (2009). Did Neanderthals and other early humans sing? Seeking the biological roots of music in the territorial advertisements of primates, lions, hyenas, and wolves. *Musicae Scientiae, 13*(2), 291–320.

Hamzei, F., Rijntjes, M., Dettmers, C., Glauche, V., Weiller, C., & Buchel, C. (2003). The human action recognition system and its relationship to Broca's area: An fMRI study. *Neuroimage, 19*(3), 637–644.

Haslinger, B., Erhard, P., Altenmuller, E., Schroeder, U., Boecker, H., & Ceballos-Baumann, A. O. (2005). Transmodal sensorimotor networks during action observation in professional pianists. *Journal of Cognitive Neuroscience, 17*(2), 282–293.

Haueisen, J., & Knosche, T. R. (2001). Involuntary motor activity in pianists evoked by music perception. *Journal of Cognitive Neuroscience, 13*(6), 786–792.

Hockett, C. D. (1960). The origin of speech. *Scientific American, 203*(3), 89–96.

Huron, D. (2006). *Sweet anticipation: Music and the psychology of expectation.* Cambridge, MA: The MIT Press.

Iacoboni, M., Molnar-Szakacs, I., Gallese, V., Buccino, G., Mazziotta, J. C., & Rizzolatti, G. (2005). Grasping the intentions of others with one's own mirror neuron system. *PLoS Biology, 3*(3), e79.

Iacoboni, M., Woods, R. P., Brass, M., Bekkering, H., Mazziotta, J. C., & Rizzolatti, G. (1999). Cortical mechanisms of human imitation. *Science, 286*(5449), 2526–2528.

Jabbi, M., Bastiaansen, J., & Keysers, C. (2008). A common anterior insula representation of disgust observation, experience and imagination shows divergent functional connectivity pathways. *PLoS ONE, 3*(8), e2939.

Jackson, P. L., Rainville, P., & Decety, J. (2006). To what extent do we share the pain of others? Insight from the neural bases of pain empathy. *Pain, 125*(1–2), 5–9.

Janata, P., & Grafton, S. T. (2003). Swinging in the brain: Shared neural substrates for behaviors related to sequencing and music. *Nature Neuroscience, 6*(7), 682–687.

Johnson-Frey, S. H., Maloof, F. R., Newman-Norlund, R., Farrer, C., Inati, S., & Grafton, S. T. (2003). Actions or hand-object interactions? Human inferior frontal cortex and action observation. *Neuron, 39*(6), 1053–1058.

Juslin, P. N. (2013). From everyday emotions to aesthetic emotions: towards a unified theory of musical emotions. *Physics of Life Reviews, 10*(3), 235–266.

Juslin, P. N. & Västfjäll, D. (2008). Emotional responses to music: The need to consider underlying mechanisms. *Behavioral and Brain Sciences, 31*(5), 559–575.

Keysers, C., & Gazzola, V. (2009). Expanding the mirror: Vicarious activity for actions, emotions, and sensations. *Current Opinion in Neurobiology, 19*(6), 666–671.

Keysers, C., Kaas, J. H., & Gazzola, V. (2010). Somatosensation in social perception. *Nature Reviews Neuroscience, 11*(6), 417–428.

Keysers, C., Kohler, E., Umiltà, M. A., Nanetti, L., Fogassi, L., & Gallese, V. (2003). Audiovisual mirror neurons and action recognition. *Experimental Brain Research, 153*(4), 628–636.

Keysers, C., & Perrett, D. I. (2004). Demystifying social cognition: a Hebbian perspective. *Trends in Cognitive Sciences, 8*(11), 501–507.

Keysers, C., Wicker, B., Gazzola, V., Anton, J. L., Fogassi, L., & Gallese, V. (2004). A touching sight: SII/PV activation during the observation and experience of touch. *Neuron, 42*(2), 335–346.

Kimura, D., & Archibald, Y. (1974). Motor functions of the left hemisphere. *Brain, 97*, 337–350.

Kivy, P. (1980). *The corded shell: Reflections on musical expression.* Princeton, NJ: Princeton University Press.

Koelsch, S. (2010). Towards a neural basis of music-evoked emotions. *Trends in Cognitive Sciences, 14*(3), 131–137.

Koelsch, S., Fritz, T., DY, V. C., Muller, K., & Friederici, A. D. (2006). Investigating emotion with music: An fMRI study. *Human Brain Mapping, 27*(3), 239–250.

Koelsch, S., Maess, B., & Friederici, A. D. (2000). Musical syntax is processed in the area of Broca: An MEG study. *NeuroImage, 11*(56).

Koelsch, S., Rohrmeier, M., Torrecuso, R., & Jentschke, S. (2013). Processing of hierarchical syntactic structure in music. *Proceedings of the National Academy of Sciences of the United States of America, 110*(38), 15443–15448.

Koelsch, S., & Siebel, W. A. (2005). Towards a neural basis of music perception. *Trends in Cognitive Sciences, 9*(12), 578–584.

Kohler, E., Keysers, C., Umilta, M. A., Fogassi, L., Gallese, V., & Rizzolatti, G. (2002). Hearing sounds, understanding actions: Action representation in mirror neurons. *Science, 297*(5582), 846–848.

Koski, L., Wohlschlager, A., Bekkering, H., Woods, R. P., Dubeau, M. C., Mazziotta, J. C., & Iacoboni, M. (2002). Modulation of motor and premotor activity during imitation of target-directed actions. *Cerebral Cortex, 12*(8), 847–855.

Lahav, A., Saltzman, E., & Schlaug, G. (2007). Action representation of sound: Audio-motor recognition network while listening to newly acquired actions. *The Journal of Neuroscience, 27*(2), 308–314.

Langer, S. K. (1954). *Philosophy in a new key: A study in the symbolism of reason, rite, and art* (6th ed.). Cambridge: New American Library.

Launay, J. (2015). Musical sounds, motor resonance, and detectable agency. *Empirical Musicology Review, 10*(1–2), 30–40.

Laurence F. (2008). Music and empathy. In O. Urbain (Ed.), *Music and conflict transformation: Harmonies and dissonances in geopolitics* (pp. 13–25). London: I. B. Tauris.

Leino, S., Brattico, E., Tervaniemi, M., & Vuust, P. (2007). Representation of harmony rules in the human brain: Further evidence from event-related potentials. *Brain Research, 1142,* 169–177.

Lerdahl, F., & Jackendoff, R. (1983). *A generative theory of tonal music.* Cambridge: MIT Press.

Levitin, D. J., & Menon, V. (2003). Musical structure is processed in 'language' areas of the brain: A possible role for Brodmann Area 47 in temporal coherence. *NeuroImage, 20,* 2142–2152.

Lewis, J. W., Brefczynski, J. A., Phinney, R. E., Janik, J. J., & DeYoe, E. A. (2005). Distinct cortical pathways for processing tool versus animal sounds. *The Journal of Neuroscience, 25*(21), 5148–5158.

Leyton, M., Boileau, I., Benkelfat, C., Diksic, M., Baker, G., & Dagher, A. (2002). Amphetamine-induced increases in extracellular dopamine, drug wanting, and novelty seeking: a PET/[11C] raclopride study in healthy men. *Neuropsychopharmacology, 27*(6), 1027–1035.

Lipps, T. (1903). Einfühlung, innere Nachahmung und Organenempfindung. *Archiv für die Gesamte Psychologie* (Vol. I, part 2). Leipzig: W. Engelmann.

Livingstone, R. S., & Thompson, W. F. (2009). The emergence of music from the theory of mind. *Musicae Scientiae, 13*(2 suppl), 83–115.

Lomas, J., & Kimura, D. (1976). Intrahemispheric interaction between speaking and sequential manual activity. *Neuropsychologia, 14*(1), 23–33.

Loui, P., Wu, E. H., Wessel, D. L., & Knight, R. T. (2009). A generalized mechanism for perception of pitch patterns. *The Journal of Neuroscience, 29*(2), 454–459.

Luppino, G., Murata, A., Govoni, P., & Matelli, M. (1999). Largely segregated parietofrontal connections linking rostral intraparietal cortex (areas AIP and VIP) and the ventral premotor cortex (areas F5 and F4). *Experimental Brain Research, 128*(1–2), 181–187.

Maess, B., Koelsch, S., Gunter, T. C., & Friederici, A. D. (2001). Musical syntax is processed in Broca's area: An MEG study. *Nature Neuroscience, 4*(5), 540–545.

Margulis, E. H., Mlsna, L. M., Uppunda, A. K., Parrish, T. B., & Wong, P. C. (2009). Selective neurophysiologic responses to music in instrumentalists with different listening biographies. *Human Brain Mapping, 30*(1), 267–275.

Menon, V., & Levitin, D. J. (2005). The rewards of music listening: Response and physiological connectivity of the mesolimbic system. *Neuroimage, 28*(1), 175–184.

Meyer, L. B. (1967). *Music, the arts, and ideas.* Chicago, IL: University of Chicago Press.

Mitterschiffthaler, M. T., Fu, C. H., Dalton, J. A., Andrew, C. M., & Williams, S. C. (2007). A functional MRI study of happy and sad affective states induced by classical music. *Human Brain Mapping, 28*(11), 1150–1162.

Miu, A. C., & Balteş, F. R. (2012). Empathy manipulation impacts music-induced emotions: A psychophysiological study on opera. *PloS ONE, 7*(1), e30618.

Molnar-Szakacs, I. (2015). Please don't stop the music: Commentary on 'musical sounds, motor resonance, and detectable agency'. *Empirical Musicology Review, 10*(1–2), 46–49.

Molnar-Szakacs, I., Green Assuied, V., & Overy, K. (2012). Shared Affective Motion Experience (SAME) and creative, interactive music therapy. In D. J. Hargreaves, D. E. Miell & R. A. R. MacDonald (Eds.), *Musical imaginations: Multidisciplinary perspectives on creativity, performance and perception* (pp. 313–331). Oxford: Oxford University Press.

Molnar-Szakacs, I., & Heaton, P. (2012). Music: A unique window into the world of autism. *Annals of the New York Academy of Sciences, 1252,* 318–324.

Molnar-Szakacs, I., Iacoboni, M., Koski, L., & Mazziotta, J. C. (2005). Functional segregation within pars opercularis of the inferior frontal gyrus: Evidence from fMRI Studies of imitation and action observation. *Cerebral Cortex, 15*(7), 986–994.

Molnar-Szakacs, I., Kaplan, J., Greenfield, P. M., & Iacoboni, M. (2006). Observing complex action sequences: The role of the fronto-parietal mirror neuron system. *NeuroImage, 33*(3), 923–935.

Molnar-Szakacs, I., & Overy, K. (2006). Music and mirror neurons: From motion to 'e'motion. *Social Cognitive and Affective Neuroscience, 1*(3), 235–241.

Molnar-Szakacs, I., Wu, A. D., Robles, F. J., & Iacoboni, M. (2007). Do you see what I mean? Corticospinal excitability during observation of culture-specific gestures. *PLoS ONE, 2*(7), e626.

Morgane, P. J., Galler, J. R., Mokler, D. J. (2005). A review of systems and networks of the limbic forebrain/limbic midbrain. *Progress in Neurobiology, 75*(2), 143–160.

Newell, A., & Simon, H. (1972). *Human problem solving.* Englewood Cliffs, NJ: Prentice-Hall.

Nishitani, N., & Hari, R. (2000). Temporal dynamics of cortical representation for action. *Proceedings of the National Academy of Sciences of the United States of America, 97*(2), 913–918.

O'Doherty, J. P. (2004). Reward representations and reward-related learning in the human brain: Insights from neuroimaging. *Current Opinion in Neurobiology, 14*(6), 769–776.

Opitz, B., Rinne, T., Mecklinger, A., von Cramon, D. Y., & Schroger, E. (2002). Differential contribution of frontal and temporal cortices to auditory change detection: fMRI and ERP results. *NeuroImage, 15*(1), 167–174.

Overy, K. (2003). Dyslexia and music. From timing deficits to musical intervention. *Annals of the New York Academy of Sciences, 999,* 497–505.

Overy, K., & Molnar-Szakacs, I. (2009). Being together in time: Musical experience and the mirror neuron system. *Music Perception, 26*(5), 489–504.

Overy, K., Nicolson, R. I., Fawcett, A. J., & Clarke, E. F. (2003). Dyslexia and music: measuring musical timing skills. *Dyslexia, 9*(1), 18–36.

Panksepp, J. (1995). The emotional sources of 'chills' induced by music. *Music Perception, 13*(2), 171–207.

Patel, A. D. (2003). Language, music, syntax and the brain. *Nature Neuroscience, 6*(7), 674–681.

Patel, A. D. (2005). The relationship of music to the melody of speech and to syntactic processing disorders in aphasia. *Annals of the New York Academy of Sciences, 1060,* 59–70.

Pizzamiglio, L., Aprile, T., Spitoni, G., Pitzalis, S., Bates, E., D'Amico, S., & di Russo, F. (2005). Separate neural systems for processing action- or non-action-related sounds. *NeuroImage, 24*(3), 852–861.

Preston, S. D., & de Waal, F. B. (2002). Empathy: Its ultimate and proximate bases. *Behavioral and Brain Sciences, 25*(1), 1–20; discussion 20–71.

Preuss, T. M. (1995). *The argument from animals to humans in cognitive neuroscience.* Cambridge, MA: MIT Press.

Rabinowitch, T. C., Cross, I., & Burnard, P. (2013). Long-term musical group interaction has a positive influence on empathy in children. *Psychology of Music, 41*(4), 484–498.

Radford, C. (1989). Emotions and music: a reply to the cognitivists. *The Journal of Aesthetics and Art Criticism, 41*(1), 69–76.

Rizzolatti, G., & Arbib, M. (1998). Language within our grasp. *Trends in Neurosciences, 21*(5), 188–194.

Rizzolatti, G., & Craighero, L. (2004). The mirror-neuron system. *Annual Review of Neuroscience, 27,* 169–192.

Rizzolatti, G., Fadiga, L., Gallese, V., & Fogassi, L. (1996). Premotor cortex and the recognition of motor actions. *Cognitive Brain Research, 3*(2), 131–141.

Rizzolatti, G., Fogassi, L., & Gallese, V. (2001). Neurophysiological mechanisms underlying the understanding and imitation of action. *Nature Reviews Neuroscience, 2*(9), 661–670.

Royet, J. P., Zald, D., Versace, R., Costes, N., Lavenne, F., Koenig, O., & Gervais, R. (2000). Emotional responses to pleasant and unpleasant olfactory, visual, and auditory stimuli: A positron emission tomography study. *The Journal of Neuroscience, 20,* 7752–7759.

Sacks, O. (2007). *Musicophilia: Tales of music and the brain.* London: Picador.

Saffran, J. R. (2003). Musical learning and language development. *Annals of the New York Academy of Sciences, 999,* 397–401.

Salimpoor, V. N., Benovoy, M., Larcher, K., Dagher, A., & Zatorre, R. J. (2011). Anatomically distinct dopamine release during anticipation and experience of peak emotion to music. *Nature Neuroscience, 14*(2), 257–262.

Salimpoor, V. N., van den Bosch, I., Kovacevic, N., McIntosh, A. R., Dagher, A., & Zatorre, R. J. (2013). Interactions between the nucleus accumbens and auditory cortices predict music reward value. *Science, 340*(6129), 216–219.

Scherer, K. S., & Oshinsky, J. S. (1977). Cue utilization in emotion attribution. *Motivation and Emotion, 1*(4), 331–346.

Scherer, K. R., & Zentner, M. R. (2001). Emotional effects of music: Production rules. In P. N. Juslin, & J. A. Sloboda (Eds.), *Music and emotion: Theory and research* (pp. 361–392). Oxford: Oxford University Press.

Schon, D., & Francois, C. (2011). Musical expertise and statistical learning of musical and linguistic structures. *Frontiers in Psychology, 2,* 167.

Schonwiesner, M., Novitski, N., Pakarinen, S., Carlson, S., Tervaniemi, M., & Naatanen, R. (2007). Heschl's gyrus, posterior superior temporal gyrus, and mid-ventrolateral prefrontal cortex have different roles in the detection of acoustic changes. *Journal of Neurophysiology, 97*(3), 2075–2082.

Schott, B. H., Minuzzi, L., Krebs, R. M., Elmenhorst, D., Lang, M., Winz, O. H., Seidenbecher, C. I., Coenen, H. H., Heinze, H. J., Zilles, K., Duzel, E., & Bauer, A. (2008). Mesolimbic functional magnetic resonance imaging activations during reward anticipation correlate with reward-related ventral striatal dopamine release. *The Journal of Neuroscience, 28*(52), 14311–14319.

Singer, T., Seymour, B., O'Doherty, J., Kaube, H., Dolan, R. J., & Frith, C. D. (2004). Empathy for pain involves the affective but not sensory components of pain. *Science, 303*(5661), 1157–1162.

Singer, T., Seymour, B., O'Doherty, J. P., Stephan, K. E., Dolan, R. J., & Frith, C. D. (2006). Empathic neural responses are modulated by the perceived fairness of others. *Nature, 439*(7075), 466–469.

Sloboda, J. A. (1985). *The musical mind.* Oxford: Oxford University Press.

Sloboda, J. A., & Juslin, P. N. (2001). Psychological perspectives on music and emotion. In P. Juslin & J. A. Sloboda (Eds.), *Music and emotion: Theory and research. Series in affective science* (pp. 71–104). New York: Oxford University Press.

Sloboda, J. A., & O'Neill, S. A. (2001). Emotions in everyday listening to music. In P. Juslin & J. A. Sloboda (Eds.), *Music and emotion: Theory and research.* Oxford, UK: Oxford University Press.

Small, D. M., Jones-Gotman, M., & Dagher, A. (2003). Feeding-induced dopamine release in dorsal striatum correlates with meal pleasantness ratings in healthy human volunteers. *Neuroimage, 19*(4), 1709–1715.

Smith, A. (1759). *The theory of moral sentiments.* London: A. Millar.

Tallal, P., Miller, S., & Fitch, R. H. (1993). Neurobiological basis of speech: A case for the preeminence of temporal processing. *Annals of the New York Academy of Sciences, 682*, 27–47.

Tervaniemi, M., Rytkonen, M., Schroger, E., Ilmoniemi, R. J., & Naatanen, R. (2001). Superior formation of cortical memory traces for melodic patterns in musicians. *Learning and Memory, 8*(5), 295–300.

Terwogt, M. M., & Van Grinsven, F. (1988). Recognition of emotions in music by children and adults. *Perceptual and Motor Skills, 67*(3), 697–698.

Tomasello, M., Carpenter, M., Call, J., Behne, T., & Moll, H. (2005). Understanding and sharing intentions: The origins of cultural cognition. *Behavioral and Brain Sciences, 28*(5), 675–691.

Trainor, L. J., McDonald, K. L., & Alain, C. (2002). Automatic and controlled processing of melodic contour and interval information measured by electrical brain activity. *Journal of Cognitive Neuroscience, 14*(3), 430–442.

Trehub, S. E. (2001). Musical predispositions in infancy. *Annals of the New York Academy of Sciences, 930*, 1–16.

Trehub, S. E. (2003). The developmental origins of musicality. *Nature Neuroscience, 6*(7), 669–673.

Trevarthen, C. (1999). Musicality and the intrinsic motive pulse: Evidence from human psychobiology and infant communication. In 'Rhythms, musical narrative, and the origins of human communcation'. *Musicae Scientiae, 1999–2000* (Special Issue), 157–213.

Truslit, A. (1938). *Gestaltung und Bewegung in der Musik.* Berlin: Chr. Friedrich Vieweg.

Valeriani, M., Betti, V., Le Pera, D., De Armas, L., Miliucci, R., Restuccia, D., Avenanti, A., & Aglioti, S. M. (2008). Seeing the pain of others while being in pain: A laser-evoked potentials study. *NeuroImage, 40*(3), 1419–1428.

VanderArk, S. D., & Ely, D. (1992). Biochemical and galvanic skin responses to music stimuli by college students in biology and music. *Perceptual and Motor Skills, 74*(3 Pt 2), 1079–1090.

VanderArk, S. D., & Ely, D. (1993). Cortisol, biochemical, and galvanic skin responses to music stimuli of different preference values by college students in biology and music. *Perceptual and Motor Skills, 77*(1), 227–234.

Vuoskoski, J. K., & Eerola, T. (2011). Measuring music-induced emotion: A comparison of emotion models, personality biases, and intensity of experiences. *Musicae Scientiae, 15*(2), 159–173.

Vuoskoski, J. K., & Eerola, T. (2012). Can sad music really make you sad? Indirect measures of affective states induced by music and autobiographical memories. *Psychology of Aesthetics, Creativity, and the Arts*, 6(3), 204.

Vuoskoski, J. K., Thompson, W. F., McIlwain, D., & Eerola, T. (2012). Who enjoys listening to sad music and why? *Music Perception*, 29(3), 311–317.

Wallin, N., Merker, B., & Brown, S. (2000). *The origins of music*. Cambridge, MA: MIT Press.

Wicker, B., Keysers, C., Plailly, J., Royet, J. P., Gallese, V., & Rizzolatti, G. (2003). Both of us disgusted in my insula: The common neural basis of seeing and feeling disgust. *Neuron*, 40(3), 655–664.

Wise, R. A. (2002). Brain reward circuitry: Insights from unsensed incentives. *Neuron*, 36(2), 229–240.

Wolff, P. H. (2002). Timing precision and rhythm in developmental dyslexia. *Reading and Writing*, 15(1–2), 179–206.

Zatorre, R. J., & Salimpoor, V. N. (2013). From perception to pleasure: music and its neural substrates. *Proceedings of the National Academy of Sciences of the United States of America*, 110(Suppl 2), 10430–10437.

Zentner, M., Grandjean, D., & Scherer, K. R. (2008). Emotions evoked by the sound of music: characterization, classification, and measurement. *Emotion*, 8(4), 494–521.

Zentner, M. R., & Kagan, J. (1996). Perception of music by infants. *Nature*, 383(6595), 29.

4 The social side of music listening

Empathy and contagion in music-induced emotions

Andrei C. Miu and Jonna K. Vuoskoski[1]

Introduction

Music has the ability to evoke powerful emotional responses in listeners. In fact, it has been estimated that we respond emotionally to music more than half of the time we spend listening to it (see, for example, Juslin & Laukka, 2004; Juslin, Liljeström, Västfjäll, Barradas, & Silva, 2008). Why should instrumental music, without explicit semantic meaning, be capable of moving us to tears? Although it is likely that there are multiple mechanisms through which music can induce affective responses in listeners, one compelling account suggests that we might respond to music as we would to the observed experiences of another person – with empathy. In its broadest sense, empathy can be defined as a process by which we can understand and feel what another person is experiencing.

It has been widely documented that music can effectively communicate emotional meaning – through emulating the expressive qualities of human vocal communication and movement (Jackendoff & Lerdahl, 2006; Juslin & Laukka, 2003), as well as through culturally learned cues such as mode (see, for example, Dalla Bella, Peretz, Rousseau, & Gosselin, 2001) and extramusical associations (i.e. evaluative conditioning; Juslin & Västfjäll, 2008). Some researchers have even proposed that we might hear music as the emotional expressions of a virtual person (Levinson, 2006), or as the expressive acts of the performer and/or the composer (Scherer & Zentner, 2001). Thus, as music is imbued with connotations of human emotional expression on multiple levels, it is plausible that listeners might – at least in some occasions – respond to it with empathy.

Recent empirical studies have accumulated compelling evidence to suggest that empathy might actually be more fundamental to our engagement with music than previously thought. Just as people differ in terms of the intensity and type of responses they experience while listening to music, they also differ in terms of how readily they tend to experience empathy in their daily lives. This 'dispositional empathy' can be defined as an individual's general responsiveness to the observed experiences of others, involving both cognitive and affective components such as perspective-taking capabilities and tendencies, and emotional reactivity (for example, Davis, 1980). Although a variety of factors contribute to whether or not we experience empathy in a given situation, those with high dispositional empathy tend to experience empathy more readily across different situations. This inter-individual variability in empathic responsiveness can offer insights into individual differences in emotional responses to music, as a number of studies on music-induced emotions have observed associations between dispositional empathy and emotional responses to music (Balteş & Miu, 2014; Vuoskoski & Eerola, 2011; Vuoskoski & Eerola, 2012).

In this chapter, we will first outline the concepts of empathy and contagion as psychological processes, and discuss current directions in mainstream literature. Next, we will introduce a selection of theories that have proposed some form of empathy as a mechanism of music-induced emotions, and review empirical findings in the light of these theories. We have restricted the empirical studies under consideration to those that have either investigated the contribution of dispositional empathy to individual differences in music-induced emotional responses, or explicitly manipulated empathy in the context of music listening. Finally, we will identify a number of gaps in the current literature on empathy and music-induced emotions, and suggest future directions for empirical explorations.

Empathy and emotional contagion

Imaginatively projecting oneself into another's situation, like artists do when creating their characters, is the process originally referred to as *Einfühlung* by Theodor Lipps (Lipps, 1903) and later coined 'empathy' by Edward Titchener (Titchener, 1909). Due to its fundamental role in social cognition and behaviour, empathy has been a popular topic of investigation in philosophy, psychology and cognitive neuroscience (for a more comprehensive discussion of empathy, see Laurence, this volume). The diversity of theoretical approaches helped uncover many facets and functions of empathy, but also contributed to terminological redundancy and confusion regarding the boundaries of this concept (Batson, 2009; Cuff, Brown, Taylor, & Howat, 2016).

Broad definitions of empathy include processes from perception to behaviour (Decety & Jackson, 2004; Preston & de Waal, 2002), such as taking another's perspective, coming to share his/her state of mind and developing motivation to improve his/her situation (Zaki & Ochsner, 2012). These approaches have been criticised for cancelling the distinction between empathy and related concepts such as theory of mind, defined as the ability to infer what others think or feel (Gallagher & Frith, 2003). Keeping this distinction is important, considering that there are situations in which one seeks to understand another's feelings without actually coming to develop those feelings. Such situations have been viewed either as a cognitive facet of empathy (Shamay-Tsoory, Aharon-Peretz, & Perry, 2009) or an affective facet of theory of mind (Shamay-Tsoory & Aharon-Peretz, 2007). Clearly, empathy and theory of mind are closely related concepts (McCall & Singer, 2013) considering that from an empathy point of view, understanding others' feelings is crucial to coming to feel the same, and from a theory of mind point of view, inferring how others think comes hand in hand with understanding what they feel.

Recent approaches from psychology (Eisenberg, 2000; Hoffman, 2000) and social neuroscience (de Vignemont & Singer, 2006; Hein & Singer, 2008; Singer & Klimecki, 2014) argue that empathy should be defined more narrowly in order to differentiate it from closely related processes. According to one such working definition (de Vignemont & Singer, 2006; Hein & Singer, 2008; Singer & Klimecki, 2014), empathy has three main characteristics. First, empathy involves experiencing an affective state as reaction to another's feelings. By emphasising experience sharing as the specific component of empathy, this approach avoids confusion with theory of mind, which refers to understanding another's state of mind, without necessarily adopting the same thoughts and feelings.

A second characteristic of empathy is the 'isomorphism' between the affective states of protagonists (de Vignemont & Singer, 2006), which means that one reacts with the same emotion as the one perceived or assumed in another (for example, being sad with another who is sad). This characteristic helps distinguish empathy from other forms of emotional responses to others, such as compassion or sympathy in which emotion can differ between protagonists (for example, feeling pity for someone who is sad). Empathy involves affect coupling or 'feeling with the other', whereas compassion refers to caring for another without actually sharing his or her affective state ('feeling for the other') (de Vignemont & Singer, 2006; Singer & Klimecki, 2014). In addition, compassion may also imply motivation to improve others' situations, as illustrated by those in helping professions, such as physicians or psychotherapists, who cannot afford to share the distress of their patients, but often report feelings of warmth, concern or care for them (de Vignemont & Singer, 2006; Singer & Klimecki, 2014).

The third characteristic specifies that in empathy, one is consciously aware that his/her current emotion is related to another's emotion (Decety & Meyer, 2008). This characteristic differentiates empathy from emotional contagion, which refers to processes by which one may 'catch' the affective state of another outside awareness (Hatfield, Cacioppo, & Rapson, 1994). Unlike empathy, emotional contagion does not involve the self–other differentiation or knowing that another person is the source of one's emotion (de Vignemont & Singer, 2006; Decety & Meyer, 2008). Therefore, empathy and contagion both involve affect coupling between protagonists, but through either consciously controlled or automatic mechanisms. While empathy is thought to rely on theory of mind, two mechanisms hypothesised to support contagion are motor mimicry and premotor neural mirroring of emotional expressions.

According to Hatfield *et al.* (1994), one way by which one may 'catch' another's emotion is through reflex mimicry of emotional expressions (for example, facial, vocal, postural) and afferent feedback from activated muscles, which may in turn serve as priming mechanism in emotion generation. A recent critical appraisal of empirical evidence (Hess & Fischer, 2013) suggested that emotional mimicry is selective, and its specificity and role in emotion recognition is more limited than originally thought. There is evidence that automatic mimicry of emotional expressions depends on affiliative intentions, which means that the observer seeks to reinforce a bond with the target (Hess & Fischer, 2013). For instance, people display more emotional mimicry towards friends compared to strangers (Fischer, Becker, & Veenstra, 2012), and positive compared to negative fictional characters (Likowski, Mühlberger, Seibt, Pauli, & Weyers, 2008). These findings are in line with evolutionary thinking which argues that in social species, selection may have favoured responses to conspecifics on which one would rely for help (Preston & de Waal, 2002).

In addition, there is also evidence that automatic facial mimicry may not reflect the specific emotions expressed by others, but only the valence (i.e. positive/negative) of emotional expressions. For instance, people display automatic frowning when observing facial expressions of several different negative emotions, including fear, anger and sadness (Hess & Fischer, 2013). Moreover, it was found that automatic facial mimicry contributes to emotion recognition mostly when expressions are ambiguous, such as in distinguishing true from fake smiles (Maringer, Krumhuber, Fischer, & Niedenthal, 2011). Therefore, it was suggested that: 'emotional mimicry is related to the understanding of emotion in context and is involved in regulating one's relation with the other person, rather than being the synchronization of meaningless individual muscle actions' (Hess & Fischer, 2013, pp. 144, 146).

Recent studies have uncovered a neural mechanism that may contribute to imitation, by matching actions observed in others with one's own actions (Gallese, 2001; Iacoboni, 2009). In other words, observing another's action recruits part of the neural circuits involved in preparing to execute the same action. Therefore, understanding another's action may occur through the internal simulation of those actions in premotor areas of the brain (i.e. responsible for action planning), rather than motor imitation. Studies in primates identified neurons that discharge both when the animal performs an action (for example, grasping an object), and when it observes somebody else performing a similar action (di Pellegrino, Fadiga, Fogassi, Gallese, & Rizzolatti, 1992; Gallese, Fadiga, Fogassi, & Rizzolatti, 1996). These were called 'mirror neurons' because their properties suggest that observing others' actions is, at the neural level, like observing one's own actions in a mirror. Mirror neurons were found in the frontal premotor and posterior parietal cortex of macaque monkeys, but there is evidence that neural circuits with 'mirroring' functions (i.e. mirror neuron system) also exist in similar regions of the human brain (Iacoboni *et al.*, 1999). They seem to code action intention, as the observation of the same action triggers the discharge of different mirror neurons depending on its intention. When monkeys observed a human experimenter grasping for food and intention was cued by the presence of a container (i.e. food was put in the container when it was present, or eaten when it was absent), the neurons that discharged were those active when the monkey performed that action with the same intention (Fogassi *et al.*, 2005). Moreover, two-thirds of mirror neurons fire for observed and executed actions that are not even the same, but achieve the same goal or are related (di Pellegrino *et al.*, 1992; Gallese *et al.*, 1996). Another important finding indicated that mirror neurons are multimodal, which means that they can match one's own actions with others' similar actions both when seeing what others do and hearing the sounds of their actions

(Kohler *et al.*, 2002). Therefore, neural matching between actions observed in others and one's own actions may provide a mechanism for understanding others' intentions, based on visual or auditory observation.

In the case of facial movements, the intention is often to communicate emotion. Therefore, it has been hypothesised that the mirror neuron system may contribute to recognising emotional expressions (i.e. by matching them to one's own expressions) and to developing the corresponding emotion though contagion and empathy (Gallese, 2001; Iacoboni, 2009). There is evidence that activity in frontal premotor areas, which may be part of the human mirror neuron system, is correlated with facial emotion discrimination (Enticott, Johnston, Herring, Hoy, & Fitzgerald, 2008). Although further studies are necessary, the potential role of the mirror neuron system in emotion recognition suggests that this system may also contribute to contagion and empathy. The ability to empathise with others may rely on the interaction between the mirror neuron system involved in the recognition of emotional expressions and the limbic system involved in emotion generation, with the insula playing the mediator role (Carr, Iacoboni, Dubeau, Mazziotta, & Lenzi, 2003). Several studies reported overlapping activity in frontal premotor areas, insula and limbic structures such as the amygdala, during both observation and imitation of facial expressions of emotion (Carr *et al.*, 2003; Pfeifer, Iacoboni, Mazziotta, & Dapretto, 2008). Moreover, activity in this network correlates with dispositional empathy and social skills (Pfeifer *et al.*, 2008). Trait empathy has also been linked to parietal and temporal regions that might be part of the auditory mirror neuron system, being active both during action execution and hearing the sounds of a similar action (Gazzola, Aziz-Zadeh, & Keysers, 2006). For further discussion of mirror neurons, see also Molnar-Szakacs (this volume).

In summary, both empathy and contagion involve affect coupling or developing an affective state seen or assumed in others. This characteristic distinguishes them from theory of mind, which involves understanding another's state of mind without necessarily sharing it. While empathy occurs through consciously controlled processes such as theory of mind, contagion may be supported by automatic processes such as motor mimicry or premotor neural mirroring of emotional expressions. Available evidence shows that affiliative contexts enhance motor mimicry, reflecting the emotional valence of the observed emotional expression and playing a role in emotion recognition when expressions are ambiguous. The mirror neuron system may also contribute to contagion and empathy, by matching emotional expressions observed in others with one's own expressions and spreading activation to the insula and the limbic system.

Empathy, contagion and music-induced emotions

Several theories of music-induced emotions feature empathy and contagion as potential mechanisms through which music might induce emotions in listeners (for example, Davies, 2011, 2013; Juslin & Västfjäll, 2008; Livingstone & Thompson, 2009; Molnar-Szakacs & Overy, 2006; Scherer & Zentner, 2001). The theoretical accounts range from pre-conscious motor simulation (involving the mirror neuron system; Livingstone & Thompson, 2009; Molnar-Szakacs & Overy, 2006) and emotional contagion (Davies, 2011, 2013; Juslin & Västfjäll, 2008; Scherer & Zentner, 2001) to empathising with the imagined emotional experiences of the performer/composer (Scherer & Zentner, 2001) or the music as a 'virtual person' (Levinson, 2006; Watt & Ash, 1998). In this section we will outline some of the main theories that have proposed some form of empathy as a mechanism of music-induced emotions, and review the current empirical evidence in the context of these theories.

Theoretical accounts

Several authors (for example, Davies, 2011; Juslin & Västfjäll, 2008; Scherer & Zentner, 2001) have proposed that emotional contagion might occur between music and the listener. Some of the fundamental ways in which music is able to effectively communicate emotional information include utilising the acoustic code for human vocal expression of emotions (for a review, see Juslin & Laukka, 2003), and emulating the speed, trajectory and smoothness/jerkiness of human movement and gestures (Jackendoff & Lerdahl, 2006). Thus, it is possible that human listeners may respond to emotionally expressive music as they would to the perceived emotional state of a conspecific (for example, Juslin & Västfjäll, 2008; Livingstone & Thompson, 2009). Some authors have argued that the human mirror neuron system might offer a neural mechanism for emotional contagion from music (Livingstone & Thompson, 2009; Molnar-Szakacs & Overy, 2006; Overy & Molnar-Szakacs, 2009). In essence, a listener would engage in a form of pre-conscious 'motor simulation' of those auditory and gestural features that resemble human vocal and motor expression of emotion (Juslin & Västfjäll, 2008; Livingstone & Thompson, 2009; Molnar-Szakacs & Overy, 2006), and/or the intentional motor acts that are carried out to produce the sounds (Overy & Molnar-Szakacs, 2009).

Beyond emotional contagion, it has been postulated that music-induced emotional responses might involve empathy, with underlying theory of mind abilities and awareness that one's emotional responses are related to the observed object. Scherer and Zentner (2001) have proposed that

> there may also be a kind of empathy with the emotion presumed to be felt by the performer that may be construed in our imagination through an underlying "idea" that is seen as responsible for the emotional state that is expressed (for example, the longing of the composer for his homeland, as in Dvoràk's 'New World Symphony').
>
> (Scherer & Zentner, 2001, p. 371)

In other words, it is possible that listeners experience empathy for the performer and/or composer by utilising their imagination and theory of mind abilities. Some authors have even suggested that listeners might experience music as a narrative about a virtual person that they 'hear' as inhabiting it (Lavy, 2001; Levinson, 2006).

According to Matthew Lavy's (2001) account, this 'narrative' is an emergent property of the listening process rather than an object or a property of the music itself, and involves the merging of cues from both sound and context into one, coherent narrative structure. Thus, the listener may – in some instances – experience empathy for the imagined experiences of a virtual person that the music personifies (cf. Levinson, 2006). This tendency to adopt a 'narrative mode of listening' may stem from the frequent pairing of music with narrative content (for example, films, operas, lyrics), and the innate human tendency to make sense of the world and our experiences through the construction of narratives (Lavy, 2001).

Empirical evidence

Brain-imaging studies have shown that music listening is able to activate premotor areas related to vocal sound production (Koelsch, Fritz, Cramon, Muller, & Friederici, 2006) as well as larger-scale motor circuits (Alluri et al., 2012) in the absence of overt singing or movement. Furthermore, studies that have investigated music-induced emotions using facial electromyography have discovered that emotionally expressive music is able to evoke facial muscle activation that is consistent with the emotional expression of the music (Lundqvist, Carlsson, Hilmersson, & Juslin, 2009; Witvliet & Vrana, 1996). Although these findings are consistent with the theoretical predictions related to the role of the mirror neuron system and emotional contagion in music-induced emotions, they do not offer unequivocal evidence. It may be that the activation of motor areas during music listening is related to rhythm and beat perception (cf. Grahn & Brett, 2007) rather than mirroring responses, and that zygomatic (cheek) and corrugator (brow) muscle activations reflect liking and disliking responses rather than emotional contagion, for example. It is also unclear whether emotional contagion in musical contexts might involve actual motor simulation of emotionally expressive acts, or whether the process would be more accurately described as the mirroring of contextualised emotions (cf. Hess & Fischer, 2013). The fact that listening to emotionally expressive music is able to evoke facial muscle activation that is congruent with the emotional expression of the music (for example, Lundqvist et al., 2009; Witvliet & Vrana, 1996) is more consistent with the view that people enact mental representations of emotions (rather than mirroring specific facial muscle activations, for example).

In an experience-sampling study of 32 Swedish college students, Patrick Juslin and colleagues (2008) found that 'emotional contagion' was the most frequently mentioned mechanism of music-induced emotions, occurring in 32 per cent of the episodes. However, the wording that they used in their questionnaire ('the music's emotional expression [caused the feeling]'; Juslin et al., 2008, p. 683) implies that participants must have been consciously aware of their emotional state being a response to the emotional expression observed in the music; a process more consistent with empathy than emotional contagion. Indeed, distinguishing between emotional contagion and empathy has been a serious challenge for empirical investigations of music-induced emotions, and the fact that some researchers have used these terms in a rather inclusive (or even interchangeable) manner has not helped to clarify the potential roles of these two hypothesised mechanisms. However, a rare exception is provided by Hauke Egermann and Stephen McAdams (2013), who attempted to distinguish between the contributions of empathy and emotional contagion to music-induced emotions (valence and arousal, to be specific). They discovered that empathy felt for the musicians performing the music was associated with emotional responses that were congruent with the emotions expressed in the music. Interestingly, they also found an independent effect of emotional expression on felt emotions (i.e. an effect that was not associated with reported levels of empathy), which they interpreted as evidence of emotional contagion. Although there is a possibility that participants may have utilised music's emotionally expressive cues in their responses (especially in the absence of actual felt emotions), this likelihood is rendered small by the fact that participants were very carefully instructed to differentiate between felt and perceived emotions.

One possible approach to gain insight into the potential role of empathy in music-induced emotions is to look at individual differences in empathy, as this might provide indirect evidence for the involvement of empathy in emotional responses to music. Individuals who have a tendency to experience empathy more readily across a range of situations (i.e. high dispositional empathy) tend to be more susceptible to emotional contagion, for example (for example, Doherty, 1997). Neuroimaging studies have shown that individuals who score highly on dispositional empathy measures exhibit stronger mirroring responses to speech prosody and action sounds (Aziz-Zadeh, Sheng, & Gheytanchi, 2010; Gazzola *et al.*, 2006). It might be expected that – if music indeed evoked emotional responses through empathy and emotional contagion – individuals with high dispositional empathy would be more susceptible to the emotional effects of music listening. Indeed, previous studies have found positive associations between dispositional empathy and self-reported responses to music, including the intensity of emotions evoked by sad and tender music (Vuoskoski & Eerola, 2011), music-induced sadness, wonder and transcendence (Miu & Balteş, 2012), and the degree of motor and 'visceral' entrainment experienced while listening to classical music (Labbé & Grandjean, 2014). However, one cannot exclude the possibility that this association only exists on the level of self-report, reflecting participants' response styles rather than their actual reactions.

Jonna Vuoskoski and Tuomas Eerola (2012) set out to clarify this issue by using more objective, indirect measures of experienced emotion, namely emotional judgement and memory biases. They discovered that dispositional empathy was positively associated with a judgement bias towards sadness after listening to unfamiliar sad music, but not after listening to neutral music, and not after sad autobiographical recall. In other words, empathy was associated with the degree of experienced sadness only in the sad music condition. This suggests that dispositional empathy can indeed contribute to emotional responses evoked by unfamiliar sad music. In addition to facilitating emotion induction, dispositional empathy has also been associated with enhanced emotion recognition in the context of musical performance. Another study found that listeners with high dispositional empathy were more accurate at perceiving the expressive intentions of a string quartet, suggesting that listeners may also utilise their 'affective' theory of mind abilities when evaluating musical performances (Wöllner, 2012).

To the best of our knowledge, only one study to date has explicitly manipulated the use of empathy in a musical context. Andrei Miu and Felicia Balteş (2012) investigated emotional responses to a recorded opera performance by giving two groups of participants differing instructions: one group was instructed to 'imagine as vividly as possible how the performer feels about what is described in the music, and try to feel those emotions themselves', while the other group was instructed to 'take an objective perspective toward what is described in the music, and try not to get caught up in how the performer might feel' (Miu & Balteş, 2012, p. 3). These high and low empathy instructions lead to differing psychophysiological responses, and differing ratings of experienced emotion. Specifically, the emotional responses in the high empathy condition were more in line with the emotional expression of the opera performances – a finding consistent with those of Egermann and McAdams (2013). The findings of Miu and Balteş provide the first evidence that adopting an empathic point of view can affect music-induced emotions even at the level of psychophysiology.

Finally, investigations that have collected free descriptions of listeners' thoughts and impressions during music listening have shown that listeners often construct narratives and experience vivid imagery when engaging in focused listening (Vuoskoski & Eerola, 2012; Vuoskoski & Eerola, 2013), but it is still unclear whether these processes could be characterised as forms of empathy, or whether music-induced imagery and empathy are two distinct phenomena. Nevertheless, one study (Vuoskoski & Eerola, 2013) attempted to manipulate music-induced visual and/or narrative imagery by giving two groups of participants differing information regarding the original context of a melancholic-sounding piece of film music. One group received a short, empathy-inducing description of a concentration camp scene, while the other group received a neutral description of a nature documentary. Both descriptions evoked vivid visual and/or narrative imagery (related to their contents) during the music listening, and the empathy-inducing description lead to stronger experienced sadness after the music listening (measured indirectly using a word recall task). These findings are consistent with the view that cues from both sound and context get merged into one, coherent narrative structure in the listener's imagination (cf. Lavy, 2001). Furthermore, the emotions that the listeners experienced were congruent with those cues, as would be expected if empathic processes were involved.

In summary, the empirical studies that have investigated the role of empathy in music-induced emotions have revealed that individuals with high dispositional empathy tend to be more susceptible to the emotional effects of music listening, and that empathy manipulations can intensify the emotional responses evoked by music. Furthermore, when listeners report experiencing empathy, their felt emotions are congruent with the emotional expression of the music. However, the evidence regarding the specific underlying mechanisms and their relative contributions – were it emotional contagion or actual empathy – is far from definitive, as it is possible, or even likely, that multiple different emotion induction mechanisms are at play simultaneously in a given episode of music-induced emotions (for example, Juslin & Västfjäll, 2008).

Conclusions and implications

Stimulated by process theories, which have identified psychological mechanisms underlying emotional responses to music (for example, Juslin & Västfjäll, 2008; Molnar-Szakacs & Overy, 2006; Scherer & Zentner, 2001), a growing number of studies have recently focused on empathy and emotional contagion. The main aim of this chapter has been to put theories and empirical evidence related to music in the context of mainstream research on empathy and emotional contagion, and to derive implications for future research on music.

Drawing from current efforts to reduce conceptual confusion in psychological research on empathy and emotional contagion (for example, de Vignemont & Singer, 2006; Eisenberg, 2000; Hoffman, 2000), this chapter has argued for the need to consistently define these constructs in the music literature. Based on recent work from social neuroscience, empathy and emotional contagion are defined as the processes by which one may consciously or automatically come to share the feelings of another (de Vignemont & Singer, 2006; Singer & Klimecki, 2014). In this framework, theory of mind is distinct from, but crucially supports, empathy. Mechanisms such as automatic motor mimicry (Hatfield *et al.*, 1994) or premotor neural mirroring of emotional expressions (Iacoboni, 2009) are thought to underlie emotional contagion. Understanding that empathy and emotional contagion rely on different mechanisms should limit the use of these concepts as interchangeable in the music literature.

Theories of music-induced emotions have mainly focused on either emotional contagion (Juslin & Västfjäll, 2008; Molnar-Szakacs & Overy, 2006), or empathy (Scherer & Zentner, 2001). The former theories are related to a line of research that argues that music induces emotions based on its similarity with vocal and motor expression of emotion, through automatic mechanisms such as premotor neural mirroring (Juslin & Laukka, 2003). The theories that emphasise the role of empathy in music-induced emotions are based on a different perspective arguing that music listeners seek to understand and share the emotions that the composer or performer strives to express through music (Scherer & Zentner, 2001), or according to another line of argument, empathise with fictional characters evoked by music (Levinson, 2006). It is important to note that while their emphasis is on empathy, Klaus Scherer and Marcel Zentner (2001) also consider the involvement of contagion. These different perspectives are not mutually exclusive and they allow for an integrative theoretical account of both contagion and empathy. Based on current empirical evidence, theories cannot discard the involvement of either contagion or empathy in emotional responses to music.

By comparing evidence on contagion and empathy in relation to music-induced emotions, it seems that there is less evidence on the former mechanism. This is not surprising considering that automatic processes are not accessible through self-report and can only be assessed through objective measures of automatic motor mimicry (for example, behavioural observation, electromyography) and neural measures of mirror neuron system activity during music listening. However, the role of contagion remains theoretically appealing for several reasons. Not only that emotional responses to music have short latency and are non-effortful, but also they emerge early in development (Trehub & Nakata, 2002) and precede the appearance of the self–other distinction (Roth-Hanania, Davidov, & Zahn-Waxler, 2011). Contagion does not involve the self–other distinction and is viewed as a developmental precursor of empathy (Batson, 2009), so it may support emotional processing of music in infants and perhaps continue to play this role in adults, in interaction with complementary mechanisms such as empathy.

The mechanisms underlying emotional contagion are not clear considering that automatic facial mimicry is more limited than once thought (Hess & Fischer, 2013); and there is only correlational evidence on the involvement of premotor neural mirroring in the ability to share others' emotions, particularly in the form of self-reported dispositional empathy rather than active contagion (Carr *et al.*, 2003; Pfeifer *et al.*, 2008). As far as the first mechanism in concerned, an interesting possibility is that music listening may enhance automatic motor mimicry by offering an affiliative context, in which one seeks to share the state of mind that another person expresses through music. Future studies may investigate this hypothesis, as well as provide new evidence linking premotor neural mirroring to music-induced emotions in the absence of empathy. The major challenge of future studies is to disentangle the effects of contagion and empathy. One approach is to focus on affect sharing in early development, before the emergence of empathy. Another ingenious approach illustrated in music research (Egermann & McAdams, 2013) is to use self-report to support the absence of empathy efforts and attribute 'by exclusion' whatever emotions are caught from music to contagion. Furthermore, observing affect coupling under cognitive load, which leaves little resources for empathy, offers another approach to studying contagion. Such approaches to controlling for the effects of empathy could also be used in cognitive neuroscience studies focused on the mirror neuron system and music-induced emotions.

Evidence for the involvement of empathy is currently more compelling and this may be explained by the accessibility of self-report measures focused on dispositional aspects of empathy and the active use of empathy during music listening. Current studies support the view that music is appraised as social stimulus, based on the understanding that it has been created by other people in order to express a state of mind or a situation. Moreover, music listening occurs in social contexts, with other people present with whom one may want to share an emotional bond. Future studies may compare these forms of empathy by distinguishing conditions when the target is absent (for example, the composer, a fictional character) or present (for example, performer, other music listeners). The former type of empathy underscores the interplay between empathy and other psychological mechanisms, including semantic memory for information about the composer or the music, and visual imagery and autobiographical memory as mechanisms by which music may evoke fictional characters or people from one's past. The latter type of empathy draws attention to potential differences between listening music in the form of audio recordings and watching the performer live or on video. It also suggests that empathy might mediate the social facilitation of music-induced emotions under conditions where one listens to music with others (Balteş & Miu, 2014). As a general perspective on current studies on empathy and music, most of the evidence is correlational and refers to dispositional facets of empathy. The causal link between empathy and music-induced emotions (Miu & Balteş, 2012) should be further supported in the future, especially considering that multiple approaches to empathy manipulations are available in the psychological literature.

In conclusion, both contagion and empathy may be involved in the generation of emotional responses to music. Until their effects are disentangled, both processes should be considered in theories on music-induced emotions. In order to support the mediator roles of contagion and empathy, music research should gradually move from correlational to experimental studies in which these psychological mechanisms are manipulated. Future work on music-induced emotions should be synchronised with advances in the general field of contagion and empathy in order to avoid conceptual confusion and draw methodological inspiration. In turn, this work might contribute to uncovering new and fundamental aspects of contagion and empathy considering that music is a socially rich form of emotional expression.

Note

1 Both authors have equal contributions to this chapter and the order of authors is alphabetical.

References

Alluri, V., Toiviainen, P., Jaaskelainen, I. P., Glerean, E., Sams, M., & Brattico, E. (2012). Large-scale brain networks emerge from dynamic processing of musical timbre, key and rhythm. *Neuroimage, 59*(4), 3677–3689.
Aziz-Zadeh, L., Sheng, T., & Gheytanchi, A. (2010). Common premotor regions for the perception and production of prosody and correlations with empathy and prosodic ability. *PLoS One, 5*(1), e8759.
Balteş, F. R., & Miu, A. C. (2014). Emotions during live music performance: Links with individual differences in empathy, visual imagery, and mood. *Psychomusicology: Music, Mind, and Brain, 24*(1), 58–65.
Batson, C. D. (2009). These things called empathy: Eight related but distinct phenomena. In J. Decety & W. Ickes (Eds.), *The social neuroscience of empathy* (pp. 3–15). Cambridge, MA: MIT Press.
Carr, L., Iacoboni, M., Dubeau, M. C., Mazziotta, J. C., & Lenzi, G. L. (2003). Neural mechanisms of empathy in humans: A relay from neural systems for imitation to limbic areas. *Proceedings of the National Academy of Sciences USA, 100*(9), 5497–5502.
Cuff, B. M., Brown, S. J., Taylor, L., & Howat, D. J. (2016). Empathy: A review of the concept. *Emotion Review, 8*(2), 144–153.

Dalla Bella, S., Peretz, I., Rousseau, L., & Gosselin, N. (2001). A developmental study of the affective value of tempo and mode in music. *Cognition, 80*(3), B1–10.

Davies, S. (2011). Infectious music: Music-Listener emotional contagion. In A. Coplan & P. Goldie (Eds.), *Empathy. Philosophical and psychological perspectives* (pp. 134–148). Oxford: Oxford University Press.

Davies, S. (2013). Music-to-Listener emotional contagion. In T. Cochrane, B. Fantini, & K. R. Scherer (Eds.), *The emotional power of music: Multidisciplinary perspectives on musical arousal, expression, and social control* (pp. 169–176). Oxford: Oxford University Press.

Davis, M. H. (1980). A multidimensional approach to individual differences in empathy. *JSAS Catalog of Selected Documents in Psychology, 10*, 85–100.

de Vignemont, F., & Singer, T. (2006). The empathic brain: How, when and why? *Trends in Cognitive Sciences, 10*(10), 435–441.

Decety, J., & Jackson, P. L. (2004). The functional architecture of human empathy. *Behavavioral and Cognitive Neuroscience Reviews, 3*(2), 71–100.

Decety, J., & Meyer, M. (2008). From emotion resonance to empathic understanding: A social developmental neuroscience account. *Development and Psychopathology, 20*(4), 1053–1080.

di Pellegrino, G., Fadiga, L., Fogassi, L., Gallese, V., & Rizzolatti, G. (1992). Understanding motor events: A neurophysiological study. *Experimental Brain Research, 91*(1), 176–180.

Doherty, R. W. (1997). The emotional contagion scale: A measure of individual differences. *Journal of Nonverbal Behavior, 21*(2), 131–154.

Egermann, H., & McAdams, S. (2013). Empathy and emotional contagion as a link between recognized and felt emotions in music listening. *Music Perception, 31*(2), 139–156.

Eisenberg, N. (2000). Emotion, regulation, and moral development. *Annual Review of Psychology, 51*, 665–697.

Enticott, P. G., Johnston, P. J., Herring, S. E., Hoy, K. E., & Fitzgerald, P. B. (2008). Mirror neuron activation is associated with facial emotion processing. *Neuropsychologia, 46*(11), 2851–2854.

Fischer, A. H., Becker, D., & Veenstra, L. (2012). Emotional mimicry in social context: The case of disgust and pride. *Frontiers in Psychology, 3*, 475.

Fogassi, L., Ferrari, P. F., Gesierich, B., Rozzi, S., Chersi, F., & Rizzolatti, G. (2005). Parietal lobe: From action organization to intention understanding. *Science, 308*(5722), 662–667.

Gallagher, H. L., & Frith, C. D. (2003). Functional imaging of 'theory of mind'. *Trends in Cognitive Sciences, 7*(2), 77–83.

Gallese, V. (2001). The 'shared manifold' hypothesis. From mirror neurons to empathy. *Journal of Consciousness Studies, 8*(5–7), 33–50.

Gallese, V., Fadiga, L., Fogassi, L., & Rizzolatti, G. (1996). Action recognition in the premotor cortex. *Brain, 119*(Pt 2), 593–609.

Gazzola, V., Aziz-Zadeh, L., & Keysers, C. (2006). Empathy and the somatotopic auditory mirror system in humans. *Current Biology, 16*(18), 1824–1829.

Grahn, J. A., & Brett, M. (2007). Rhythm and beat perception in motor areas of the brain. *Journal of Cognitive Neuroscience, 19*(5), 893–906.

Hatfield, E., Cacioppo, J. T., & Rapson, R. L. (1994). *Emotional contagion.* Cambridge, UK: Cambridge University Press.

Hein, G., & Singer, T. (2008). I feel how you feel but not always: The empathic brain and its modulation. *Current Opinion in Neurobiology, 18*(2), 153–158.

Hess, U., & Fischer, A. (2013). Emotional mimicry as social regulation. *Personality and Social Psychology Review, 17*(2), 142–157.

Hoffman, M. L. (2000). *Empathy and moral development: Implications for caring and justice.* New York: Cambridge University Press.

Iacoboni, M. (2009). Imitation, empathy, and mirror neurons. *Annual Review of Psychology, 60*, 653–670.

Iacoboni, M., Woods, R. P., Brass, M., Bekkering, H., Mazziotta, J. C., & Rizzolatti, G. (1999). Cortical mechanisms of human imitation. *Science, 286*(5449), 2526–2528.

Jackendoff, R., & Lerdahl, F. (2006). The capacity for music: What is it, and what's special about it? *Cognition, 100*(1), 33–72.

Juslin, P. N., & Laukka, P. (2003). Communication of emotions in vocal expression and music performance: Different channels, same code? *Psychology Bulletin, 129*(5), 770–814.

Juslin, P. N., & Laukka, P. (2004). Expression, perception, and induction of musical emotions: A review and a questionnaire study of everyday listening. *Journal of New Music Research, 33*(3), 217–238.

Juslin, P. N., Liljestrom, S., Vastfjall, D., Barradas, G., & Silva, A. (2008). An experience sampling study of emotional reactions to music: Listener, music, and situation. *Emotion, 8*(5), 668–683.

Juslin, P. N., & Västfjäll, D. (2008). Emotional responses to music: The need to consider underlying mechanisms. *Behavioral and Brain Sciences, 31*(5), 559–621.

Koelsch, S., Fritz, T., v. Cramon, D. Y., Muller, K., & Friederici, A. D. (2006). Investigating emotion with music: An fMRI study. *Human Brain Mapping, 27*(3), 239–250.

Kohler, E., Keysers, C., Umilta, M. A., Fogassi, L., Gallese, V., & Rizzolatti, G. (2002). Hearing sounds, understanding actions: action representation in mirror neurons. *Science, 297*(5582), 846–848.

Labbé, C., & Grandjean, D. (2014). Musical emotions predicted by feelings of entrainment. *Music Perception, 32*(3), 170–185.

Lavy, M. M. (2001). *Emotion and the experience of listening to music: A framework for empirical research* (Unpublished doctoral dissertation). University of Cambridge, UK.

Levinson, J. (2006). Musical expressiveness as hearability-as-expression. In M. Kieran (Ed.), *Contemporary Debates in Aesthetics and the Philosophy of Art* (pp. 192–206). Oxford: Blackwell Publishing.

Likowski, K. U., Mühlberger, A., Seibt, B., Pauli, P., & Weyers, P. (2008). Modulation of facial mimicry by attitudes. *Journal of Experimental Social Psychology, 44*(4), 1065–1072.

Lipps, T. (1903). Einfühlung, inner Nachahmung, und Organ-empfindungen. *Archiv für die gesamte Psychologie, 1*, 185–204.

Livingstone, R. S., & Thompson, W. F. (2009). The emergence of music from the Theory of Mind. *Musicae Scientiae, 13*(2 suppl), 83–115.

Lundqvist, L. O., Carlsson, F., Hilmersson, P., & Juslin, P. N. (2009). Emotional responses to music: Experience, expression, and physiology. *Psychology of Music, 37*(1), 61–90.

Maringer, M., Krumhuber, E. G., Fischer, A. H., & Niedenthal, P. M. (2011). Beyond smile dynamics: Mimicry and beliefs in judgments of smiles. *Emotion, 11*(1), 181–187.

McCall, C., & Singer, T. (2013). Empathy and the brain. In S. Baron-Cohen, H. Tager-Flusberg & M. V. Lombardo (Eds.), *Understanding other minds. Perspectives from developmental social neuroscience* (pp. 195–213). Oxford, UK: Oxford University Press.

Miu, A. C., & Balteş, F. R. (2012). Empathy manipulation impacts music-induced emotions: A psychophysiological study on opera. *PLoS One, 7*(1), e30618.

Molnar-Szakacs, I., & Overy, K. (2006). Music and mirror neurons: From motion to 'e'motion. *Social Cognitive and Affective Neuroscience, 1*(3), 235–241.

Overy, K., & Molnar-Szakacs, I. (2009). Being together in time: Musical experience and the mirror neuron system. *Music Perception, 36*(5), 489–504.

Pfeifer, J. H., Iacoboni, M., Mazziotta, J. C., & Dapretto, M. (2008). Mirroring others' emotions relates to empathy and interpersonal competence in children. *Neuroimage, 39*(4), 2076–2085.

Preston, S. D., & de Waal, F. B. M. (2002). Empathy: Its ultimate and proximate bases. *Behavioral and Brain Sciences, 25*(1), 1–20.

Roth-Hanania, R., Davidov, M., & Zahn-Waxler, C. (2011). Empathy development from 8 to 16 months: Early signs of concern for others. *Infant Behavior and Development, 34*(3), 447–458.

Scherer, K. R., & Zentner, M. R. (2001). Emotional effects of music: Production rules. In P. N. Juslin & J. A. Sloboda (Eds.), *Music and emotion: Theory and research* (pp. 361–392). Oxford: Oxford University Press.

Shamay-Tsoory, S. G., & Aharon-Peretz, J. (2007). Dissociable prefrontal networks for cognitive and affective theory of mind: a lesion study. *Neuropsychologia, 45*(13), 3054–3067.

Shamay-Tsoory, S. G., Aharon-Peretz, J., & Perry, D. (2009). Two systems for empathy: A double dissociation between emotional and cognitive empathy in inferior frontal gyrus versus ventromedial prefrontal lesions. *Brain, 132*(Pt 3), 617–627.

Singer, T., & Klimecki, O. M. (2014). Empathy and compassion. *Current Biology, 24*(18), R875–R878.

Titchener, E. B. (1909). *Lectures on the experimental psychology of the thought processes.* New York: Macmillan.

Trehub, S. E., & Nakata, T. (2002). Emotion and music in infancy. *Musicae Scientiae*(Special Issue 2001–2002), 37–61.

Vuoskoski, J. K., & Eerola, T. (2011). Measuring music-induced emotion: A comparison of emotion models, personality biases, and intensity of experiences. *Musicae Scientiae, 15*(2), 159–173.

Vuoskoski, J. K., & Eerola, T. (2012). Can sad music really make you sad? Indirect measures of affective states induced by music and autobiographical memories. *Psychology of Aesthetics, Creativity, and the Arts, 6*(3), 204–213.

Vuoskoski, J. K., & Eerola, T. (2013). Extramusical information contributes to emotions induced by music. *Psychology of Music. 43*(2), 262–274.

Watt, R. J., & Ash, R. L. (1998). A psychological investigation of meaning in music. *Musicae Scientiae, 2*(1), 33–53.

Witvliet, C., & Vrana, S. (1996). The emotional impact of instrumental music on affect ratings, facial EMG, autonomic response, and the startle reflex: Effects of valence and arousal. *Psychophysiology Supplement, 33*(91).

Wöllner, C. (2012). Is empathy related to the perception of emotional expression in music? A multimodal time-series analysis. *Psychology of Aesthetics, Creativity, and the Arts, 6*(3), 214–233.

Zaki, J., & Ochsner, K. N. (2012). The neuroscience of empathy: Progress, pitfalls and promise. *Nature Neuroscience, 15*(5), 675–680.

5   Audience responses in the light of perception–action theories of empathy

Clemens Wöllner

When attending a musical performance, audience members may feel closely re-lated to the musicians and even collectively related to each other. They may also imagine profound connections to the composer. Some theorists argue that musi-cians should feel what the composer may have felt, and transmit these feelings to the audience. In the third part of his treatise on the *True art of playing keyboard instruments*, C. P. E. Bach (1753) discusses sympathy in musical performance:

> A musician cannot move others if he is not moved himself; therefore he necessarily needs to be able to induce in himself all emotions which he wants to arouse in his audience; he conveys his feelings to them, and thus moves them effectively to experience co-sensations ['Mit-Empfindung'] (p. 122).[1]

As pointed out in this well-known statement, musical performers should re-experience the composer's passions when he/she was writing the music. Accord-ing to Bach, improvisations affect the audience in an even stronger way, since emotions can be transmitted more directly. In doing so, musicians arouse a range of various affects in a 'continuously changing' manner (p. 122). Veridical expe-riences of these emotions, in contrast to Bach's ideas, are an almost impossible goal for musicians to achieve, since they would need to feel the range of affects themselves while at the same time having to concentrate on the more physical and structural components of performing. Therefore, one could argue that musi-cians act *as if* they are experiencing certain emotions, and audience members are moved in ways similar to their emotional involvement when watching actors in a theatre play. Bach further states that in addition to the sound of the music, ex-pressive gestures are useful for conveying a musician's intentions and emotions. The multimodal coupling of body movements and sound is indeed at the core of many present theories of music's emotional impact.

From an audience's perspective, the communicative transmission and reception of emotions has often been equated with musical empathy. Stephen Davies (2011), for example, argues that listeners' empathic responses to music are forms of 'attentional emotional contagion' (p. 144), which are based on mir-roring processes: 'sad music tends to make (some) listeners feel sad' (p. 135). This idea seems somewhat contradictory, given that contagion is usually seen as an automatic, unmediated process, while directing one's attention requires some deliberate, conscious processing (see also Miu & Vuoskoski, this volume). In this regard, Jerrold Levinson (2011) postulates that empathic experiences of musical emotions may lead to forms of 'imagined emotions' which are related to the ones in the experienced 'music's persona' (p. 327). While the potential imaginative nature of some emotions cannot be discussed here, Levinson's concept goes beyond the mere contagiousness in empathic responses to music. By ascribing a 'persona' to music, listeners may rather consciously attempt to take the perspective of this imagined subject – whatever the subject in music is supposed to be.

In this chapter, I will discuss how individual listeners grasp the musical performer's expressive intentions, what role bodily response mechanisms play in these processes, and how empathy may enable and modulate the understanding of what is conveyed in a performance. In particular, I will underline the significance of cognitive facets in the appreciation of music, which are, in turn, regarded as a veridical component of empathic responses that are not limited to emotional contagion. A new model of musical empathic interactions is proposed with perception–action coupling – that is, the idea that perception and action processes are fundamentally interconnected – at its heart. Since there are relatively few existing empirical studies about audience empathy, this chapter will take as a starting point consideration of components of empathy through discussion of original theories and research concepts that underlie empathic interactions in music. It will go on to review perception–action models of empathy prior to the proposal and discussion of a new model in the light of existing empirical findings. This critical and empirical review will inform an understanding of the ways in which audiences interact with music and performers. For the purposes of this chapter, audiences will be regarded in the broadest sense within the Western tradition, referring to one or more listeners in various settings engaging with live or recorded performances, thus accessing sound and/or visual stimuli depending on the context. For example, audiences may include individuals undertaking solitary listening to recorded music, shared listening and/or viewing of recorded performances with friends, or watching live performances in concerts or public venues. Audience members may include individuals with or without specialist training or expertise in music.

Components of empathy

In accordance with the ideas of Davies (2011) and Levinson (2011) as outlined above, most psychological accounts of empathy posit both automatic components of empathy, comprising contagion and mirroring, as well as more conscious components such as taking the perspective of someone else (Bischof-Köhler, 2012; Walter, 2012). In addition to the ability of feeling spontaneously with another individual, there are thus conscious and deliberate facets of empathy. These include trying to understand others by imagining their situation and state of mind, constructing an internal model of their reasoning, and evaluating the various factors that may influence their current behaviour or affect display. A positive consequence of the comprehensive concept of empathy is the possibility for individuals to deliberately try to understand others better and therefore even learn to be more empathic. Music in particular may train listeners 'in social attuning and empathic relationships' (Leman, 2007, p. 126). Contagion, on the other hand, is supposedly more strongly related to personality characteristics that are less susceptible for deliberate changes (for further discussion, see Walter, 2012). Definitions of empathy should thus not be reduced to emotional contagion and mirroring, they should rather integrate the various subcomponents of empathy, including cognitive facets (cf. Bischof-Köhler, 2012; Coplan, 2011). At the same time, definitions need to be adequately specific in order to leave the somewhat slippery terrain of a concept with a rather long history in philosophy and psychology. Only with clear definitions of the subcomponents of empathy, valid hypotheses can be formulated and results be compared across different studies.

In 1980, Mark Davis developed the Interpersonal Reactivity Index (IRI), one of the empathy inventories most widely employed in general psychology and many music-related studies. The first subscale 'Perspective taking' assesses the degree to which individuals 'spontaneously adopt the psychological point of view of others' (Davis, 1983, p. 113). The 'Fantasy' subscale measures the personal transposing into fictitious characters such as those in films or books, and to some degree appears to be related to Levinson's (2011) imagined emotions. The two other subscales, 'Empathic concern' and 'Personal distress' assess emotional components when feeling or interacting with others. In sum, Davis (1983) laid stress on a multifaceted nature of empathy that included both the cognitive component of perspective-taking as well as emotional components. These facets of empathy have ever since been debated and refined in numerous studies across various fields of research (see, for example, Coplan & Goldie, 2011). As a side effect of the definition debates and refinements of components in past decades, researchers may have concentrated less on explaining the underlying psychological processes and behavioural consequences. Early approaches and current theories provide such an explanation, by grounding empathy in bodily response circuits. In the next sections, I will describe early accounts of empathy that influenced more recent theories, albeit some of the original concepts seem not always adequately rendered in some papers (see also Laurence, this volume, for further discussion of early conceptualisations of empathy).

Perception–action models of empathy

The introduction of the concept of empathy, a neologism based on a translation of the term '*Einfühlung*' (feeling-into), dates back to the second half of the nineteenth century. This period was characterised by the so-called psychological turn in aesthetics and the history of arts (cf. Büttner, 2003), in addition to the development of empirical methods in philosophy and early psychological research. Friedrich Theodor Vischer emphasised the importance of the perceiving subject over the discussion of normative qualities of art works that, up to then, rested at the core of academic aesthetics. According to Vischer, individuals attribute psychological qualities to the objects they perceive, which lead to impressions of inner co-experiences. His son, Robert Vischer, developed the theory of an inner 'Me' in his dissertation *On optical feeling of form* (1872). The Me transports itself into an object and empathises with it – a process he termed '*Einfühlung*'. Influenced by Wilhelm Wundt, Vischer argued that the direct sensory and motor impulses evoked by perceptions may in turn cause positive or negative reactions in the observer. It is remarkable that Vischer employed a physiological–psychological evaluation circuit, thus highlighting bodily components in the perception of art, which is also a key principle of feeling-into.

As a psychological explanation for the appreciation of visual art and architecture, the concept of feeling-into inspired many theorists and artists of that epoch, especially those affiliated with expressionism (Wölfflin, 1886; see also Mallgrave & Ikonomou, 1994). Some art historians, on the other hand, criticised the shortcomings of the new psychological explanations, since they would not sufficiently account for the historical context in which art was created and perceived (see Büttner, 2003). Philosophers, including Edmund Husserl (1900/1901) and Edith Stein (1917), employed and developed further the concept of feeling-into, which soon became a key concept in philosophical thinking of that time. It should not be ignored that philosophers of the centuries before had explored facets of empathic behaviour in humans by the related term 'sympathy'. For instance, David Hume (1793), in his *Treatise of human nature*, describes sympathy between people as a type of communication of emotions. The ability to perceive these emotions influences aesthetic responses and ethical behaviour (cf. Coplan & Goldie, 2011).

For current definitions of empathy, however, the work of Theodor Lipps, a philosopher and (theoretical) psychologist around the beginning of the last century, was crucial. His ideas are often presented in a very condensed form and therefore merit detailed attention. Lipps is attributed to first describing the phenomenon of empathy in a systematic way (1903). His attempts to explain the underlying processes show striking parallels to modern theories of empathy (for example, Preston & de Waal, 2002, see below). In short, he proposed that observing someone else results in an inner strive or urge to move, which is particularly pertinent when perceiving affect displays of other people. As a philosopher specialising in aesthetics, Lipps was also influenced by the discoveries made in the first experimental studies of perception carried out by Wundt and Hermann von Helmholtz. Although not employing experimental approaches himself, he attempted to systematise human interactions and emotional responses on the basis of observable perceptual processes.

In the early monograph *Foundations of psychology* ('Grundtatsachen des Seelenlebens', 1883), he laid the foundation for the concept of inner co-sensations when interacting with others. The closer we feel to others, the more 'we mirror and re-experience their life in ours, the more we must feel with and for them...' (p. 687). Understanding other people, according to this view, is deeply grounded in realising the inner sensations that are evoked by perceiving others, and by projecting some of one's own feelings onto other people. Twenty years later, in *Foundations of aesthetics* ('Grundlegung der Ästhetik', 1903) he formulates further that the other is an imagined and 'modified own Me' (p. 106), perceived by visual and auditory gestures and facial expressions. Although this radical approach may resonate with later theories of symbolic interactionism (Mead, 1934) and constructionism, it is the underlying process that is of particular interest here. Lipps suggests that nearly all utterances of life bear some expressive components, either as direct affective utterances or more indirectly in the way people move when being in different moods. In this regard, auditory affective sounds ('Affektlaute', Lipps, 1903, p. 106) may also evoke a feeling with others:

> When I hear a sound that is similar to the one I use for expressing this affect myself, so I find myself – not connected, but directly in this affect. ... I do not merely grasp the concept that the affect has caused the sound, but I *experience* the affect. I co-perform it internally ... I am inclined to jubilate with the jubilating person. We will name this concept ... feeling-into ['*Einfühlung*'].
>
> (Lipps, 1903, pp. 106–107)

According to Lipps, 'feeling-into' someone else is a direct process that is based both on the close perception of other people as well as on own experiences with certain affect displays. People are only able to co-perform affective behaviours internally if this behaviour is grounded in their own nature. The joy of co-performing, without being distracted by any other thoughts or interests, is called 'positive feeling-into' (p. 110), which for Lipps is an explanation for someone's enjoyment of watching other people move. Negative feeling-into may arise when observing, for example, haughty affect displays that resonate with the observer but evoke unpleasant feelings. The positive process of feeling-into, leading to the wish of internally co-performing the movements, is seen as the 'basis for *aesthetic understanding*' (p. 120) of artistic movements such as those of an acrobat dancing on a rope.

Lipps argues that people strive for a 'kinaesthetic image of the movement' (p. 120) that matches the visually perceived optical image. While this kinaesthetic image is based on 'certain processes in our muscles and fibres' (p. 114), Lipps emphasises that 'aesthetic feeling-into' is an inner process that should neither be confounded with conscious acts of imitation nor with direct bodily sensations. Although he repeatedly refers to the resonance in the observer's body, his theory can thus not fully explain the interactions between the physiological and psychological processes of feeling-into. When seeing an acrobat, people do not directly experience any bodily pressures or other physiological reactions but rather feel the urge for 'inner activities' (p. 130). In other words, people do not merely strive for own peripheral sensations but attempt to instinctively grasp another person's state of mind:

> The actual content of my *aesthetic* feeling-into is the entire inner state or manner of the inner behaviour, from which emerge the individual acts of will and action. Or, in short: it is the *personality* that I experience sympathetically in the perceived.
>
> (Lipps, 1903, p. 132)

In this regard, Lipps employs the terms identification and sympathy to illustrate facets of positive 'feeling-into'. These processes are described as instinctive mechanisms that allow people to co-experience the 'inner behaviour' (p. 134) of others. It should be noted that researchers did not follow Lipps in using empathy and sympathy in almost synonymic ways. Empathy is seen as a more comprehensive concept that does not only encompass shared feelings with others (as for sympathy), but also includes taking the perspective of others (see, for example, Coplan, 2011). Lipps noted that familiarity and experiences with a range of different emotions, the corresponding affect displays and emotional movements shape the way people can feel into others. The experience of motion-like qualities is not limited to bodily movements of other people, since even optical 'shapes afford movement *possibilities*' (p. 144). In accordance with earlier ideas formulated by Vischer (1872), Lipps (1903) thus presents an explanation for the aesthetic pleasure that these shapes may offer in a different domain of art.

Taken together, Lipps proposed a theory of inner co-experiences with affect displays of other people that is based on bodily resonance. While the underlying mechanisms are not described in detail and the recurrence to philosophical terms such as 'will' or 'urge' may not offer sufficient psychological explanations, he provided the ground for further efforts to elucidate human interactions and empathic responses. Lipps did not explicitly apply his concept to the experience of musical performances, which is surprising given the high frequency of musical examples he employed in his various other writings, which directly address musical themes, such as harmony (Lipps, 1885). Although he introduces the concept of feeling-into with examples of affective sounds (see above), Lipps primarily refers to visual perception in revisions of his concept. Recently, researchers may have slightly misinterpreted Lipps in overemphasising the direct bodily component in his theory, for instance when stating that his ideas refer to 'inner imitation or inner resonance that is based on a natural instinct and causes us to imitate the movements and expressions we perceive in physical and social objects' (Coplan & Goldie, 2011, p. xii). Instead, Lipps's 'inner activities' do not seem to cause direct movements in observers but rather aim at experiencing facets of someone else's personality. The 'fusion' with another individual or object, nevertheless, has been criticised by Husserl (1900/1901) and Stein (1917), who argued that intersubjective reasoning relies more on conscious self–other distinctions (see Coplan & Goldie, 2011). Indeed, even acts of sympathy with others depend on a clear percept of another person, which helps to explain why more recent accounts of empathy highlight the component of perspective-taking. Lipps, nevertheless, attempted to provide an aesthetic theory of perception, which should primarily explain the aesthetic appreciation of the world rather than explaining ethical behaviour. In the following, I will describe a more recent theory of empathy that partially reflects Lipps's original ideas, and that can be applied to the domain of music performance and appreciation.

Stephanie Preston and Frans B. M. de Waal (2002) refer to Lipps's concept of feeling-into as a bodily response mechanism of empathy in human and non-human primates. Perceiving actions or states of other people should activate representations that correspond with the observed actions or states of others. In turn, these representations may automatically trigger various bodily reactions such as changes in heart rate or other autonomic and somatic responses. By 'representation', Preston and de Waal (p. 54) do not refer to specified cognitive or symbolic contents but simply to general information storage systems. When comparing the proposed mechanism with the original concept of Lipps (1903), it becomes evident that they laid more stress on the body component, since Lipps emphasised the inner strives and urges rather than the direct physiological responses. Given Lipps's focus both on internal, non-physiological processes and on the all-embracing idea of grasping another individual's personality, feeling-into may only partially be regarded as a precursor of perception–action models.

The idea of linking perception and action, on the other hand, can be traced back to early ideomotor accounts of human behaviour (Lotze, 1852; Sperry, 1952). More recently, Wolfgang Prinz and colleagues provided behavioural evidence for perception–action couplings, culminating in the formulation of *Common coding theory* (Prinz, 1997), which postulates that the perception of movements and the potential execution of these movements share mutual representations ('common codes') in the observer's brain. As a consequence, motor familiarity with perceived actions should increase the internal responses and shape subsequent behaviour (cf. Wöllner & Cañal Bruland, 2010). Perception–action coupling is an automatic process that does not depend on conscious processing but requires some degree of attending to another individual's state or actions. The discovery of mirror neurons has been attributed to provide neurophysiological evidence for the link between perception and action (for a review, see Rizzolatti & Sinigaglia, 2010) and for the automatic, unconscious co-experience of others' emotions via internal simulation and imitation (cf. Decety & Ickes, 2009; Iacoboni, 2009).

According to Preston and de Waal's (2002) theory, empathic responses are based on these coupling mechanisms: perceiving someone move in a certain mood should resonate with the observer's own action representations and may lead to physiological responses. It should be noted that the link between perception–action systems and emotional responses remains rather elusive, since the type of physiological arousal is not specified and could be attributed to positive or negative emotions. Other researchers, nevertheless, indicate that internal simulation of others' actions could indeed be related to empathic emotional responses (Gallese, 2007; Gallese, Ferrari, & Umiltà, 2002; Molnar-Szakacs & Overy, 2006). On a neurophysiological level, the insula, connecting the limbic system with cortical areas associated with action representations, may have a fundamental role in this regard (Carr *et al.*, 2003; Preston & Hofelich, 2012; Walter, 2012). A number of studies of empathy provided evidence that familiarity with someone else, as well as perceived similarity and salience of the observed actions or affect displays are likely to increase empathy (see Preston & de Waal, 2002). Furthermore, the higher processing speed of unconscious perception–action coupling facilitates interactions between individuals and may thus have benefits for social interactions in groups, which could be a basic function of empathy.

A perception–action approach to musical empathic interactions

Can musical performances be seen as an arena in which social couplings are exercised, by feeling-into the performers and by sharing mutual feelings with other members of the audience? A model is proposed (see Figure 5.1) to represent the musical empathic interactions between audiences, performers and music. Following embodied cognition approaches (cf. Leman, 2007), perception–action coupling lies at the heart of the model because it is central to (1) the social dimensions of empathy, including the more conscious perspective-taking, established through Audience interactions with Performers, (2) to co-performer empathy and feelings of agency, established through interactions between Performers and Music, as well as (3) attributions of a persona in music (Levinson, 2011), established through Audience interactions with Music. The model therefore reflects the ways in which audiences interact empathically with music (as a subject) and performers (as subjects) alongside the interactions between co-performers themselves.

Discussion about the role of perception–action coupling in musical empathic responses is given below according to a number of existing studies of joint actions between musicians in ensembles as well as between performers and audience members. Further evidence stems from audience research addressing audio–visual 'feeling-into' the performers in the domains of music and dance. Most of these studies correlated subscales or overall scores of empathy inventories with scores in experimental tasks.

In one of these tasks, jazz musicians, as expert listeners, were asked to indicate the perceived spontaneity of piano jazz recordings (Engel & Keller, 2011). Some of the melodies presented to them were improvised, while others were imitated. The overall differentiation accuracy was above chance (55 per cent correct). Individuals scoring higher on perspective-taking were better at differentiating between the two types of recordings. Although the expert

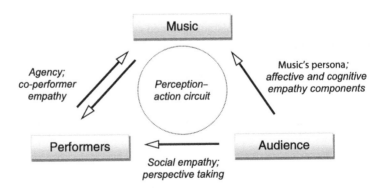

Figure 5.1 Proposed model of musical empathic interactions.

listeners of this study did not perceive the pianists' actions visually, nuances in the sound outcome of the performed actions sufficed for the detection of subtle differences, which was modulated by the cognitive components of empathy. When playing in an ensemble, skilled jazz musicians should also be able to respond to each other's improvisations and changes in timing. In a qualitative observational study, 'empathetic attunement' was seen as being crucial for such successful and spontaneous interactions between jazz musicians (Seddon, 2005, p. 56).

Undoubtedly, these empathic interactions between musicians should be manifest in neural activations of certain brain regions. Evidence for empathic perceptual effects of self-produced actions was provided in an electroencephalogram (EEG) study with jazz ensembles (Babiloni *et al.*, 2012; see also Babiloni *et al.*, this volume). The musicians' brain activation patterns were measured during the actual performance and while they viewed their own performances subsequently. In the observation condition, musicians with higher empathy scores showed activations in a right frontal region (alpha desynchronisation in Brodmann area 44/45). Since these activations were not present in non-musicians, the authors concluded that they are related to the empathetic attunement (to use Seddon's term) of expert musicians when observing their ensemble play and when interacting with others. A further study employed a musical duo paradigm to investigate empathy in relation to action representations of the complementary part of the music. Giacomo Novembre, Luca Ticini, Simone Schütz-Bosbach and Peter Keller (2012) asked amateur pianists to play the melodic lines of several Bach chorales in the right hand. In some conditions, a computer played back the bass line, while in others, no bass line was provided. The pianists were made to believe that the complementary left-hand part, if presented, was played by an actual pianist behind a screen. Transcranial magnetic stimulation (TMS) of the right motor cortex produced motor-evoked potentials for the left hand. These potentials were larger in conditions in which the pianists believed that they played along with another pianist. In addition, the cognitive perspective-taking scale from Davis's (1983) IRI correlated with increased motor-evoked potentials. The authors concluded that the social component of playing together was linked to empathy, which may facilitate action representations of others. Lipps's (1903) idea of feeling-into could thus hold true for cognitive response circuits.

In addition to studies of joint actions, researchers have addressed perception–action couplings that may underlie the emotional and empathic responses of audience members. If aesthetic appreciation of music is modulated by these processes, then empathy may have a role in the perception of a musical performance. The musicians' body movements provide hints about their expressive intentions, which, in turn, should be related to the musical sound outcome and could resonate in the audience members' bodily response systems. In a study based on Preston and de Waal's (2002) perception–action model of empathy, a string quartet was filmed from two perspectives during the performance of

Vaughan Williams's first string quartet in G minor (Wöllner, 2012). A particularly expressive part of the first movement (bars 48–97) was selected for further analysis. This part contained two sections as clearly marked in the original scores, with the second one having homophonic passages and a crescendo over several bars. Videos of the performances were produced under visual-only, auditory-only and audio–visual conditions, showing each member of the quartet individually. Some months after the performance, each member of the quartet judged continuously the level of expressiveness of themselves and their fellow performers. Auditory and visual grand average judgements were correlated, indicating that the musicians perceived strong parallels between their bodily performance movements and the music in terms of expressiveness. Independent observers were then asked to judge the performance under multimodal conditions, and difference values between the quartet's own average ratings and each observer's rating were calculated. For the second section of the music, empathy modulated judgements: that is, observers with higher affective empathy could better decipher the quartet's visual expressive intentions. Similarly, these observers' visual judgements matched the quartet's expressive intentions of the music more closely. In other words, the more empathic the observers were, the better they picked up the musicians' intentions as indicated by themselves in the previous judgements, and empathy did affect the perception of a musical performance.

A further study tackled the question of whether or not empathy is related to judgements of auditory cues derived from social versus non-social situations. In a study with jazz duets, Ana Pesquita, Timothy Corlis and James Enns (2014) asked musically trained participants and novices to indicate whether different jazz standards were recorded in live conditions, meaning that the two musicians played along with each other's performances simultaneously, or in dubbed versions with pre-recorded studio tracks. Participants also filled in Simon Baron-Cohen's (2002) Autism Quotient (AQ), a measure of social aptitude and, indirectly, of empathy. Results show that participants could differentiate between live and dubbed versions, yet differences in sensitivity measures (that is, the differences in ratings between live and dubbed versions) were observed between four ad-hoc groups of participants: musical novices with low social aptitude were not sensitive for the auditory differences between live and dubbed recordings, while novices with high social aptitude as well as musically trained participants (regardless of their aptitude) could successfully discriminate the recordings. This result was generally confirmed in a follow-up experiment that contrasted novices with musical experts from a school of music. For novices, the general AQ showed the highest correlations with judgement sensitivity, so people with high social aptitude could tell more reliably whether the musicians had performed simultaneously or not. Albeit not significant, absolute values in sensitivity measures were highest for 'social novices' and even higher than for the music groups. Musical experts with lower social aptitude, in contrast, did not significantly differ in solving the task than those experts with higher aptitude values. Pesquita, Corlis and Enns (2014) observed that results of the systemising subscale of Baron-Cohen (2002) correlated particularly strongly with musicians' sensitivity to the social recording situation, leading them to conclude that musicians approached the given task differently by paying more attention to musical detail rather than 'using their intuition about social interactions' (p. 182).

While musicians may indeed engage with musical tasks in a different way compared to non-musicians and focus their attention more on technical aspects, it still remains surprising that musical expertise did not influence findings (compared to 'social novices'), in contrast to the social aptitude measures. According to the explanations provided by perception–action accounts of empathy, musicians should be able to internally feel nuances in joint live or dubbed performance situations. In other words, their experience with ensemble situations should allow for higher empathetic attunement. While Pesquita, Corlis and Enns (2014) indicate that only very few musicians had experiences as jazz musicians but all had ensemble experiences, they did not report their respective instruments. It might well be that the perception–action circuits are specific to the musicians' action domains, and that guitarists or clarinettists would have been more sensitive in judging the auditory cues of their own instruments in the duets. Such action-specific effects on perceptual accuracy were shown in a study of string musicians that synchronised better with the entries of a first violinist, compared to musicians of other instruments or non-musicians (Wöllner & Cañal Bruland, 2010).

Further research, on the other hand, suggests that empathy does not increase with musical training *per se*. Gunter Kreutz, Emery Schubert and Laura Mitchell (2008) developed a music-specific empathising–systemising measure based on an earlier inventory by Baron-Cohen (2002). Sample questions included (p. 72): 'I think that I can easily sense how performers feel while playing music' (musical empathising dimension) and 'I especially like the organised way that music is laid out' (musical systematising dimension). Three subgroups established according to musical expertise (professional, amateur or no performance experience) showed consistent differences in the systemising dimension but not in empathising. A follow-up study with a smaller sample and a condensed version of the questionnaire resulted in generally higher systemising as well as empathising scores in relation to musical expertise, although findings were less systematic than in the first study. Taken together, there is evidence that musicians develop specific cognitive styles in relation to their domain of experience that distinguishes them from others with no active experience in music performance. In a recent questionnaire study (Egermann & McAdams, 2013), being musically active was positively related to responses given to the question 'Did you empathise with the musicians you just heard?' (p. 144). Considering the manifold social interactions that playing in musical ensembles typically entail, influences on domain-specific forms of empathy should be further investigated.

Besides potential effects of active musical experience, audience members' empathic responses can to some extent be modulated even on a short-term basis.

Andrei Miu and Felicia Balteş (2012; see also Miu & Vuoskoski, this volume) found out that instructions on empathising with the performer influenced both the type of emotions perceived and the physiological reactions. While watching two commercial video tapes of Cecilia Bartoli, participants were instructed either to imagine 'how the performer feels ... and try to feel those emotions themselves' or to 'take an objective perspective toward what is described in the music, and try not to get caught up in how the performer might feel' (p. 2; instructions adapted by van Lange, 2008). As a result, out of nine music-induced emotions from the *Geneva Emotional Music Scales* (Zentner, Grandjean, & Scherer, 2008), 'feelings of nostalgia' and 'power' were higher in the empathising condition. For one piece of music, skin conductance decreased, while for the other piece, respiration rates increased, suggesting some evidence for relationships with physiological arousal and the experimental instruction conditions. In self-judgements, most participants believed that the music rather than the performer's facial expression or the lyrics were the cause of their attunements. Although the impact of Bartoli's expressive gestures on observers' empathy cannot be ruled out in the experimental design, the main finding suggests that people can indeed consciously direct their levels of empathising with the musician by focusing on different aspects of the performance. In a follow-up study, 'dispositional empathy' – a concept somewhat debated, since empathy is generally not seen as a personality characteristic – was related to feelings of sublimity and unease that was also expressed in a live performance of a Puccini opera (Balteş & Miu, 2014). Empathy may thus enhance the experience of musically expressed emotions. Interestingly, visual imagery skills were related to the feeling of the same emotions, providing some support for the impact of visually perceivable and imaginable movements.

These studies support early theories of feeling-into other people's states when watching them move, or when hearing the corresponding sound outcome of the music they perform. More recent perception–action accounts of empathy further elucidate the advantage musicians may have in observing subtle nuances in performances that resonate with their own action systems. Studies so far used questionnaire approaches or controlled individual experimental sessions. It remains an open question as to whether the listening situation influences empathic responses. Since musical interactions are genuinely social experiences – whether real or with an imagined persona (see Levinson, 2011) – the social situation of listening and the co-presence of other audience members may further influence the ways people react empathically to music.

Aside from the evidence discussed above, music provides auditory and, in live performance contexts, also visual cues for actions that can lead to empathic responses. The perception–action theory of empathy should thus be valid for other performance domains that engender visual perceptions of actions (for a review, see Sevdalis & Raab, 2014). Perceiving a dancer move should resonate in the observers' motor systems, and empathy may modulate responses in relation to the emotional content expressed. Comparable to the field of music, potential links between extensive dance training and enhancements in empathic responses were investigated. In an early study, Kalliopuska (1989) observed that young Finish ballet dancers aged nine to seventeen years had higher empathy scores compared to other students of the same age with no ballet training. She concludes that ballet dancers constantly train to express certain emotions, which would enhance their capacities for empathy.

Using a self–other paradigm, Vassilis Sevdalis and Peter Keller (2011) investigated relations between empathy and accuracy in judging agency and expression. Point-light displays were created from ten individuals dancing to funk music either expressively or with less expression. About half a year later, the same participants watched the point-light videos showing them or other individuals. Participants with higher overall empathy scores (according to the Davis inventory, 1980) were more accurate at indicating whether the point-light dancer had been them or someone else. In addition, participants were more successful at correctly indicating the intended expressiveness when they scored higher on the perspective-taking subscale. Taken together, participants were able to evaluate characteristics of human motion presented to them in very short films and with as little as thirteen body markers, which is in line with previous research showing that self–other distinctions are possible for information-rich motion such as free dancing (cf. Loula *et al.*, 2005).

All participants in Sevdalis and Keller's (2011) study had danced themselves, so one could expect some resonance in their action system when observing the point-light actions. Yet those with higher general empathy scores benefitted more from these coupling processes. This finding raises the question as to whether empathy is indeed mainly grounded in perception–action couplings, or whether components of empathy enhance perceptions of oneself and others in a more abstract way. The first possibility would explain individual differences with regard to the training of these automatic coupling mechanisms. Individuals who are highly experienced in performing certain actions would be more empathic when observing the same actions. The second explanation assumes more indirect empathy effects in action observation of others that may be related to general trait empathy beyond specific domains of expertise. In a related study, even observers not involved in the production of the dance movements were able to judge the level of expressiveness as intended by the dancers, and empathy values correlated again with judgement accuracy (Sevdalis & Keller, 2012). Thus, there is tentative evidence that empathetic attunement to dance is not limited to a repertoire of actions and situations directly experienced by dancers.

Support for this claim stems from studies of individuals taking part in musical activities and tasks involving some form of synchronisation. These activities are supposed to enhance levels of general empathy and socially desirable behaviour beyond the specific domain or situational context. Compared to controls, children with musical training scored higher in an empathy inventory (Hietolahti-Ansten & Kalliopuska, 1990), and show a significant increase in empathy scores after a year of musical training (Rabinowitch, Cross, & Burnard, 2013). Again, these results lead to the question as to whether musicians are indeed more empathic, perhaps by dealing with highly condensed emotions in music, and by synchronising their actions with others for a considerable time of their lives. To my knowledge, no large-scale study has reported higher general empathy scores in professional musicians (cf. Kreutz, Schubert, & Mitchell, 2008). This lack of data is worth considering in terms of what studies of pro-social outcomes share with other research on musical transfer effects, such as those addressing subcomponents of intelligence. One could argue that the effects in question are either rather short term and thus do not profoundly influence an individual's way of responding to other people or objects, or even that the levels of professionalism in musicians may potentially limit pro-social effects in the world of music business.

Conclusions

Investigating empathy in relation to music performance and perception may offer deep insights into fundamental questions of why and how people engage with music. The increased research interest in music and empathy coincides to some extent with what one could call the 'emotional turn' in the psychology of music. A large body of research attributes the significance of music to its emotional impact on many people's lives. For some researchers, feeling-into the perceived subject of the music – whether that is the performer, composer, or some abstract musical persona – and responding emotionally to the music defines the process of empathic behaviour. Those who feel the contagious influence of music more strongly should be particularly empathic.

There are limits to this view. Musicians may not constantly feel the variety of emotions they express musically and, equally, a listener will not necessarily be affected by all emotions a piece of music may embody. Music itself should not be reduced to its emotional impact (Langer, 1941), since it offers a number of important further experiences, among them the structuring of time, enabling perceptions of space and leading to numerous associations, or linking the past with the present. These experiences may coincide with emotions, yet often their experiential significance for a listener may not primarily depend on emotional loadings. Analytic listeners focusing on the musical structure at one extreme, or people hearing music with less attention in the background on the other, typically remain emotionally rather detached. Should they be less empathic than others? My argument here is that responses to music should not be equated with emotional contagion, since such a perspective would limit the plurality of possible aesthetic experiences.

In a similar vein, empathy should not be reduced to emotional contagion. A broader view was expressed in original theorising, philosophical accounts and psychological theory: empathy includes both low-level automatic components, such as contagion, and higher-level conscious processes, such as perspective-taking, the latter showing some similarities to *Theory of Mind* (Walter, 2012; cf. Livingstone & Thompson, 2009), which is also addressed in Baron-Cohen's (2002) Autism Quotient. Only if cognitive elements are involved, then a full understanding of musical interactions and engagement can be reached. In this regard, Martha Nussbaum (2001) distinguishes empathy from 'compassion' by stating that 'empathy is simply an imaginative reconstruction of another person's experience, whether that experience is happy or sad, pleasant or painful or neutral' (p. 302). It should be noted that a number of the studies discussed above resulted in correlations with cognitive perspective-taking (Engel & Keller, 2011; Novembre *et al.*, 2012; Sevdalis & Keller, 2011), thus supporting the argument for comprehensive research on musical empathy. Assuming a perception–action basis for empathy – such as formulated to some extent by Lipps (1903) and more recently by others as discussed above – provides a meaningful and fruitful way to see empathy as an important facet of social experiences, grounded in bodily processes and potentially leading to a deeper understanding of each other.

Do individuals' general levels of empathy explain their responsiveness to music and other forms of art? If so, then listeners who enjoy feeling with other people and taking their views to a greater extent should also appreciate performing arts more than others. Some researchers have recently argued for a genetic component of empathy (for a review, see Walter, 2012), suggesting that individual differences in empathic behaviour are indeed more stable than previously thought. These differences may shape the susceptibility to musical emotions (Vuoskoski *et al.*, 2012). In other studies, researchers suppose that empathy can be enhanced, and call for 'empathy education' (Rabinowitch, Cross, & Burnard, 2013, p. 494; cf. Leman, 2007), which may result in specific music programmes for children. The consistent finding that women appear to be more empathic than men (Egermann & McAdams, 2013; Kreutz, Schubert, & Mitchell, 2008; for a review, see Sevdalis & Raab, 2014) could be both attributed to genetic differences as well as cultural influences. Therefore it is still not clear in what ways empathy may be modulated by musical involvement as a listener or performer. Based on perception–action accounts of empathy, however, there is tentative evidence that sustained training in social interactions – a key component of music performance – should result in fine-tuned skills when responding to others and imagining their thoughts and feelings. If such accounts are based on joint actions, is it also possible that empathy is enhanced in performing musicians, such as pianists, who are practising and performing primarily alone, and audience members who enjoy solitary listening? A potential explanation may lie in the imagination of a person (composer) or a persona in the music (Bach, 1753; Levinson, 2011). In this way, musicians playing solo as well as individual audience members may imagine their activity as being some form of social interaction.

Note

1 Translated by the author, as for all other translations from the German.

References

Babiloni, C., Buffo, P., Vecchio, F., Marzano, N., DelPercio, C., Spada, D., Rossi, S., Bruni, I., Rossini, P. M., & Perani, D. (2012). Brains 'in concert': Frontal oscillatory alpha rhythms and empathy in professional musicians. *Neuroimage, 60*(1), 105–116.

Bach, C. P. E. (1753). *Versuch über die wahre Art, das Clavier zu spielen* (facsimile reprint, ed. L. Hoffmann-Erbrecht, 1969). Leipzig: Breitkopf & Härtel.

Balteş, F. R., & Miu, A. C. (2014). Emotions during live music performance: Links with individual differences in empathy, visual imagery, and mood. *Psychomusicology: Music, Mind, and Brain, 24*(1), 58–65.

Baron-Cohen, S. (2002). The extreme male brain theory of autism. *Trends in Cognitive Sciences, 6*(6), 248–254.

Bischof-Köhler, D. (2012). Empathy and self-recognition in phylogenetic and ontogenetic perspective. *Emotion Review, 4*(1), 40–48.

Büttner, F. (2003). Das Paradigma 'Einfühlung' bei Robert Vischer, Heinrich Wölfflin und Wilhelm Worringer. Die problematische Karriere einer kunsttheoretischen Fragestellung. In C. Drude & H. Kohle (Eds.), *200 Jahre Kunstgeschichte in München. Positionen – Perspektiven – Polemik* (pp. 82–93). Munich: Deutscher Kunstverlag.

Carr, L., Iacoboni, M., Dubeau, M. C., Mazziotta, J. C., & Lenzi, G. L. (2003). Neural mechanisms of empathy in humans: A relay from neural systems for imitation to limbic areas. *Proceedings of the National Academy of Sciences (USA), 100*(9), 5497–5502.

Coplan, A. (2011). Understanding empathy: Its features and effects. In A. Coplan & P. Goldie (Eds.), *Empathy: Philosophical and psychological perspectives* (pp. 3–18). New York: Oxford University Press.

Coplan, A., & Goldie, P. (2011). Introduction. In A. Coplan & P. Goldie (Eds.), *Empathy: Philosophical and psychological perspectives* (pp. ix–xlvii). New York: Oxford University Press.

Davies, S. (2011). Infectious music: Music–listener emotional contagion. In A. Coplan & P. Goldie (Eds.), *Empathy: Philosophical and psychological perspectives* (pp. 134–148). New York: Oxford University Press.

Davis, M. H. (1980). A multidimensional approach to individual differences in empathy. *Journal Supplement Abstract Service Catalogue of Selected Documents in Psychology, 10*(4), 85.

Davis, M. H. (1983). Measuring individual differences in empathy: Evidence for multidimensional approach. *Journal of Personality and Social Psychology, 44*, 113–126.

Decety, J., & Ickes, W. (Eds.) (2009). *The social neuroscience of empathy.* Cambridge, MA: MIT Press.

Egermann, H., & McAdams, S. (2013). Empathy and emotional contagion as a link between recognised and felt emotions in music listening. *Music Perception, 31*(2), 139–156.

Engel, A., & Keller, P. E. (2011). The perception of musical spontaneity in improvised and imitated jazz performances. *Frontiers in Psychology, 2*(83).

Gallese, V. (2007). Empathy, embodied simulation and mirroring mechanisms. Commentary on 'Towards a neuroscience of empathy' by Doug Watt. *Neuropsychoanalysis, 9*(2), 146–151.

Gallese, V., Ferrari, P. F., & Umiltà, M. A. (2002). The mirror matching system: A shared manifold for intersubjectivity. *Behavioral Brain Sciences*, *25*(1), 35–36.

Hietolahti-Ansten, M., & Kalliopuska, M. (1990). Self-esteem and empathy among children actively involved in music. *Perceptual and Motor Skills*, *71*(2), 1364–1366.

Hume, D. (1793). *Treatise of human nature* (Ed. D. F. Norton & M. J. Norton, 2007). Oxford: Clarendon Press.

Husserl, E. G. A. (1900–1901). *Logische Untersuchungen (1. und 2. Teil)*. Halle: Niemeyer.

Iacoboni, M. (2009). Imitation, empathy, and mirror neurons. *Annual Review of Psychology*, *60*, 653–670.

Kalliopuska, M. (1989). Empathy, self-esteem and creativity among junior ballet dancers. *Perceptual and Motor Skills*, *69*(3), 1227–1234.

Kreutz, G., Schubert, E., & Mitchell, L. A. (2008). Cognitive styles of music listening. *Music Perception*, *26*(1), 57–73.

Langer, S. (1941). *Philosophy in a new key* (3rd ed., 1957). Cambridge, MA: Harvard University Press.

Leman, M. (2007). *Embodied music cognition and mediation technology*. Cambridge, MA: The MIT Press.

Levinson, J. (2011). *Music, art, and metaphysics. Essays in philosophical aesthetics*. Oxford: Oxford University Press.

Lipps, T. (1883). *Grundtatsachen des Seelenlebens*. Bonn: Max Cohen & Sohn.

Lipps, T. (1885). *Das Wesen der musikalischen Harmonie und Disharmonie*. Heidelberg: Weiss.

Lipps, T. (1903). *Grundlegung der Ästhetik*. Hamburg and Leipzig: Leopold Voss.

Livingstone, S. R., & Thompson, W. F. (2009). The emergence of music from the Theory of Mind. *Musicae Scientiae, Special Issue 2009–2010*, 83–115.

Lotze, R. H. (1852). *Medizinische Psychologie oder Physiologie der Seele*. Leipzig: Weidmannsche Buchhandlung.

Loula, F., Prasad, S., Harber, K., & Shiffrar, M. (2005). Recognising people from their movement. *Journal of Experimental Psychology: Human Perception and Performance*, *31*(1), 210–220.

Mallgrave, H. F., & Ikonomou, E. (Eds.) (1994). Empathy, form, and space – problems in German aesthetics 1873–1893 [including translated writings by R. Vischer, K. Fiedler, H. Wölfflin, A. Goller, A. von Hildebrand, & A. Schmarsow]. Santa Monica, CA: University of Chicago Press.

Mead, G. H. (1934). *Mind, self, and society* (ed. C. W. Morris). Chicago, IL: University of Chicago Press.

Miu, A. C., & Balteș, F. R. (2012). Empathy manipulation impacts music-induced emotions: a psychophysiological study on opera. *PLoS One*, *7*(1), e30618.

Molnar-Szakacs, I., & Overy, K. (2006). Music and mirror neurons: from motion to 'e'motion. *Social Cognitive and Affective Neuroscience*, *1*(3), 235–241.

Novembre, G., Ticini, L. F., Schütz-Bosbach, S., & Keller, P. E. (2012). Distinguishing self and other in joint action. Evidence from a musical paradigm. *Cerebral Cortex*, *22*(12), 2894–2903.

Nussbaum, M. (2001). *Upheavals of thought. The intelligence of emotions*. Cambridge: Cambridge University Press.

Pesquita, A., Corlis, T., & Enns, J. T. (2014). Perception of musical cooperation in Jazz duets is predicted by social aptitude. *Psychomusicology: Music, Mind, and Brain*, *24*(2), 173–183.

Preston, S. D., & de Waal, F. B. M. (2002). Empathy: Its ultimate and proximate bases. *Behavioral and Brain Sciences, 25*(1), 1–20.

Preston, S. D., & Hofelich, A. J. (2012). The many faces of empathy: Parsing empathic phenomena through a proximate, dynamic-systems view of representing the other in the self. *Emotion Review, 4*(1), 24–33.

Prinz, W. (1997). Perception and action planning. *European Journal of Cognitive Psychology, 9*(2), 129–154.

Rabinowitch, T.-C., Cross, I., & Burnard, P. (2013). Long-term musical group interaction has a positive influence on empathy in children. *Psychology of Music, 41*(4), 484–498.

Rizzolatti, G., & Sinigaglia, C. (2010). The functional role of the parieto-frontal mirror circuit: Interpretations and misinterpretations. *Nature Reviews Neuroscience, 11*(4), 264–274.

Seddon, F. A. (2005). Modes of communication during jazz improvisation. *British Journal of Music Education, 22*(1), 47–61.

Sevdalis, V., & Keller, P. E. (2011). Perceiving performer identity and intended expression intensity in point-light displays of dance. *Psychological Research, 75*(5), 423–434.

Sevdalis, V., & Keller, P. E. (2012). Perceiving bodies in motion: expression intensity, empathy, and experience. *Experimental Brain Research, 222*(4), 447–453.

Sevdalis, V., & Raab, M. (2014). Empathy in sports, exercise, and the performing arts. *Psychology of Sport and Exercise, 15*(2), 173–179.

Sperry, R.W. (1952). Neurology and the mind-body problem. *American Scientist, 40*, 291–312.

Stein, E. (1917). *Das Einfühlungsproblem in seiner historischen Entwicklung und in phänomenologischer Betrachtung* (Unpublished doctoral dissertation). University of Freiburg, Germany.

van Lange, P. A. (2008). Does empathy trigger only altruistic motivation? How about selflessness or justice? *Emotion, 8*(6), 766–774.

Vischer, R. (1872). *Über das optische Formgefühl* [On the optical sense of form: A contribution to aesthetics] (Unpublished doctoral dissertation). University of Tübingen, Germany (cited in Büttner, 2003).

Vuoskoski, J. K., Thompson, W. F., McIlwain, D., & Eerola, T. (2012). Who enjoys listening to sad music and why? *Music Perception, 29*(3), 311–317.

Walter, H. (2012). Social cognitive neuroscience of empathy: Concepts, circuits, and genes. *Emotion Review, 4*(1), 9–17.

Wölfflin, H. (1886). *Prolegomena zu einer Psychologie der Architektur* (Unpublished doctoral dissertation). University of Munich, Germany (cited in Büttner, 2003).

Wöllner, C. (2012). Is empathy related to the perception of emotional expression in music? A multimodal time-series analysis. *Psychology of Aesthetics, Creativity, and the Arts, 6*(3), 214–233.

Wöllner, C., & Cañal-Bruland, R. (2010). Keeping an eye on the violinist: motor experts show superior timing consistency in a visual perception task. *Psychological Research, 74*(6), 579–585.

Zentner, M., Grandjean, D., & Scherer, K. R. (2008). Emotions evoked by the sound of music: Characterisation, classification, and measurement. *Emotion, 8*(4), 494–521.

6 Viewing empathy in jazz performance

Peter Elsdon

While the idea of empathy in music is one that is attracting increasing attention, as this volume testifies to, in many respects empathy can be thought to describe musical values that are age-old. Felicity Laurence, for instance, talks of empathy in terms of 'a musicking based ... upon cooperation, democratic participation, mutual respectful listening' (Laurence, 2008, p. 23; see also Laurence, this volume). These are values that are deeply embedded in music pedagogies, and represent the essence of what I suspect most readers would think of as good music-making. My approach in this chapter is, as my title suggests, premised on the idea of viewing: I am interested in how the empathic comes to play an important role in the way we view performance, and jazz performance in particular. I will first develop an argument about the way in which certain fundamental tropes used to describe jazz coincide with many of the qualities we ascribe to empathy. This argument forms part of the basis for the understanding of empathy that I will explore later in the chapter. Then I will discuss how we view empathy in performance by using a recent example of a filmed performance by the group Snarky Puppy.

Jazz and empathy

Perhaps one of the most pervasive cultural preconceptions about jazz is that it is premised on an aesthetic of individual self-expression. This has sometimes been directly linked to the socio-cultural conditions under which the music emerged, as a means of implying that jazz came into being in order to meet the need for a certain kind of individual expression. Nicholas Gebhardt argues that the way in which this aesthetic has been written into accounts of the music, also plays a part in jazz's commodity value: 'That historians and critics continue to reduce the jazz act to a privileged mode of individual self-expression, however, merely functions to reproduce the *ideological* terms on which the jazz act depends for its economic and historical value *as commodity*' (Gebhardt, 2001, pp. 2–3). Gebhardt also identifies the link between self-expression and facets of authenticity:

> No jazz act is not authentic that does not at the same time express the individual terms of the jazz life ... the jazz life is the very *form* of individual self-expression, of which the musical act is merely its medium' (p. 14).

Thus, the idea of self-expression is, as Gebhardt argues, a constitutive part of the appeal jazz has made, as well as playing a part in a larger political dialogue about democratic expression.

John Corbett suggests that within jazz, the notion of expression is inextricably linked with that of voice – that is, to be individual, to have an identity, one must have a 'voice' and be able to articulate that identity, to express it, musically (Corbett, 1994, p. 80). That aesthetic of individual expression has frequently been used as a guiding principle in historical interpretation, supplying both cause and effect (see, for instance, John Litweiler's (1984) famous study of free jazz, which uses the idea of 'freedom of expression' as a guiding principle). And nowhere has this aesthetic of individual expression been more particularly located than with regard to the practice of improvisation in jazz. At the same time, there is a recognition that in order for individual expression to take place, a collaborative effort is involved. Consider, for instance, how David Borgo writes that successful improvised music 'hinges on one's ability to synchronise intention and action and to maintain a keen awareness of, sensitivity to, and connection with the evolving group dynamics and experiences' (Borgo, 2005, p. 9). What we have, then, is the sense that, in order for individuals to cooperate but also to have the opportunity of free and open expression, there has to be an understanding that might loosely be described as empathic; an ability to acknowledge the contributions of others and to act appropriately, to begin to understand the experiences of others, and feel those experiences for oneself. Thus we find deeply embedded in ideas about jazz, a description that seems to closely parallel the empathic musicking of which Laurence writes (see Laurence, this volume).

A substantial amount of the academic literature on jazz has explored ideas of democracy and cooperation within the jazz ensemble. Consider for instance Ingrid Monson's (1996) landmark study *Saying something: Jazz improvisation and interaction*, which focused attention on the jazz ensemble as a locus of inter-musical and interpersonal exchange. One aspect of Monson's work is the idea of accommodation: that different players have different styles, but in the context of the ensemble those styles must be respected and resolved. She quotes drummer Michael Carvin (Monson, 1996, pp. 64–65) at length in a particular passage, as he talks about fellow drummer Kenny Clarke's description of the drum as a woman. Clarke deploys this metaphor in order to describe the instrument as a matriarchal figure that has to acknowledge the different personalities and moods of the musicians in the ensemble and respond appropriately, what Monson calls the 'nurturing and enabling' elements of this role. The metaphor of performance as conversation that Monson invokes, is premised on seeing ensemble playing in terms of give-and-take, of dialogue, and thus the need for musicians to cultivate empathic understandings of each other. She also concentrates attention on a kind of defining tension within jazz: the need for individual personal expression versus the collective feel of the ensemble. In fact Monson's whole analytical project is based on the idea of using democratic expression as a tool for analysing the functioning of the jazz ensemble, and this approach has opened the way for other scholars concerned with investigating these issues of communication and negotiation within jazz (see, for example, Doffman, 2011; Hodson, 2007).

Viewing empathy in performance

In a recent article, Frederick Seddon suggests that 'empathetic attunement' (Seddon, 2005, p. 49) is critical to jazz improvisation – that is, an ability to 'decentre and see things from other musical perspectives', (p. 50; see also Wöllner, this volume) a view very much in agreement with the work of Monson. Seddon's study took a group of jazz students, and confirmed instances where empathetic or sympathetic attunement was observed, based on gathering responses and confirmation from the individual players who were allowed to review recordings of their performance. For Seddon, the crucial factors which indicate empathetic attunement are, '[w]hen empathetically attuned, the musicians seemed to respond to each other in an atmosphere of risk-taking and challenge … Empathetic attunement was evident in expressions of interest (for example, smiles, collective affirmative nodding and animated body movements)' (p. 55). Without the subsequent confirmation of the participants, interpretation of the performance based solely on viewing can be problematic. But what is crucial in the model outlined by Seddon, is that an outsider must view a performance in order to make an interpretation. Empathy is being ascribed in the interpretative act of viewing.

In her reading of Edith Stein's theorising of empathy, Laurence suggests that empathy can be understood as, 'as a process involving an initial cognitive act of intellectual comprehension of another's feeling and inner state' (Laurence, 2011, p. 17). This is in Stein's view the first empathic act; what follows is 'ensuing reflection leading to one's own feeling in response to the other's experienced feeling' (Laurence, 2011, p. 17). For my purposes, this initial cognitive act is of central importance in developing an understanding of the empathic in viewing performance. So for Gert-Jan Vreeke and Ingrid van der Mark, for instance, empathy is a response to 'perceived feelings' (Vreeke & van der Mark, 2003, pp. 178–179), or a response to signs. For Stephen Darwall, it 'consists in feeling what one imagines he [the other] feels' (Darwall, 1998, p. 261). As summarised by Sandra Garrido and Emery Schubert, '[e]mpathy entails a mirroring of emotion' (Garrido & Schubert, 2011, p. 282). In all of these accounts, that initial act of comprehension is implied even if not made explicit, and thereby necessary for the empathic processes described to take place.

In order to explore empathy through the viewing of performance, I want to develop an understanding of performance based on that espoused by Christopher Small (1998) in his influential book *Musicking*, one also taken up by Laurence (2008). Crucial here is that, in Small's formulation, music is not a thing but an act, and musicking brings into existence a set of relationships between participants. The ritual of performance is thus about affirming and celebrating these relationships. Small's account is premised on the concert hall as an exemplar of a space in which these relationships might be formed, but of course different kinds of relationships will come into existence in different contexts and spaces. It is possible to envisage relationships created across virtual spaces; this is when we consider performances on audio–visual media, such as a commercially produced DVD recording, an internet stream, camera footage taken on a mobile telephone and so on. In such a context social actors most likely play one of three main roles: those of performers on screen, audience members on screen, and viewers of the mediatised performance. In this case, the relationships Small outlines still apply, but with the added complication of the mediating role of technologies.

For participants who view performance on screen, I should like to suggest, via Monson (2008), that this is an act of perceptual agency. This is pertinent to my argument, because it suggests that this cognitive act does not just happen of its own accord, but results from the viewer taking an active position. Monson suggests that perceptual agency is 'the conscious focusing of sensory attention that can yield differing experiences of the same event' (Monson, 2008, s. 37). To take this a little further, we could consider Philip Auslander's (2006) deployment of Erving Goffman's 'frame analysis'. By referencing Goffman, Auslander introduces the idea that we view performance through frames, which are 'socially defined principles of organisation that govern events' (Auslander, 2006, p. 104) Goffman's theory can become slightly unwieldy when applied practically. Auslander suggests, for instance, that experiencing a live recording of music involves three frames: two laminations and one transformation. What is crucial, though, is that 'these frames constitute understandings on which members of a social group can generally agree' (p. 105). Furthermore, Auslander suggests that 'musical genres and subgenres constitute crucial laminations over the basic experience of music' (p. 105). That is, as he suggests, 'to perceive a particular sonic event through the jazz frame is quite different from perceiving it through the classical frame, for example' (p. 106). Thus in qualifying this cognitive act of viewing, which may lead to an empathic response, we need to understand the way in which the shared understanding of what jazz performance means should affect how viewers may respond to viewing a performance. It is here that the kinds of understandings of jazz that I mentioned above come into play. This priming means that we view performance through a lens; as a result of which we are likely to presuppose jazz as a universal musical language transcending race, nationality, sexuality, and regard it as a profoundly democratic art.

If, as I have suggested, the act of viewing is one of perceptual agency, and happens through a series of frames, how can we understand the kinds of relationships that emerge through the musicking that is taking place? Perhaps the most commonplace model of empathy in performance, as I have already alluded to, might reside in that of 'appropriate action'. Daniel Putman's description has it that, empathy is formed from our observations of what we 'think (or feel) other people are experiencing' (Putman, 1994, p. 99). He then suggests that 'we act in a manner that is appropriate'. That is, if two musicians in an ensemble appear to be complementing each other musically, demonstrating good ensemble skills by mirroring each other's phrasing for example, this appropriate action might be a sign of an empathic relationship. This is similar to Seddon's formulation of empathetic attunement. But what about the relationship between viewer and musician? In the discussion which follows, I will present examples where the viewer may identify with something they see on screen, but also instances where that viewer may perceive an empathic response being represented on screen, whether or not that is the case. I am not so much interested here with whether what we are seeing is actually empathic in the strictest sense. Rather, I will argue that we may be seeing the outward gestural signs of what we think of as the empathic, in a context where we are liable to view jazz performance through a set of frames primed with ideas about improvisation, risk-taking, and collective endeavour.

Snarky Puppy, and viewing jazz performance

The analysis I want to present here focuses on some aspects of a recorded performance by the jazz group Snarky Puppy, from their album *We Like It Here*.[1] In doing so I make no claims that this group's performances might be representative or otherwise of empathy in jazz performance. Rather, I will suggest that understanding a little bit about the background to this group and the way that they produce and market their music, reveals something about the frame through which fans of the group are liable to view their performances. It is also important at this point to emphasise the degree to which my analysis engages with the act of viewing. As a result, the examples I present in the following pages do a poor job of standing in for the experience of viewing the performances. I therefore urge the interested reader to seek out these performances on YouTube (which the band make freely available) in order to engage with the interpretative strategy I employ.

As with most of the other albums by the group, this album can be purchased either as a download or in physical form. In physical form it comes as a two-disc set: one disc is an audio CD of the studio performance, the other is a DVD recording of that same performance. Watching the DVD and reading the liner notes reveals that the studio recording took place over a number of nights, with a small audience packed into the large recording space alongside the band.[2] Each night the band performed (presumably) the same set to this audience, and then selected one version of each tune for inclusion on the CD/DVD. Thereby, the DVD allows the consumer to see the performance they hear on CD. The liner notes, authored by leader and bassist Michael League, explain that the performance was recorded without any overdubs, thus making a traditional claim to the idea of the authentic via qualities of liveness and claims of virtuosity.[3]

The idea of recording 'live in the studio' has become quite commonplace in recent years. Even for those consumers who buy a download of this album, Snarky Puppy upload videos from the DVD that fans can watch online through their YouTube channel.[4] Indeed it is this grasp of marketing through new media, including particularly the sites Bandcamp and YouTube, that have enabled Snarky Puppy to come to prominence without the traditional support of a major record label. This use of new media means that the band's fans are very unlikely *not* to have come across footage of them performing online. It is, of course, far from uncommon for fans to be able to watch footage of performers in the studio. But usually that footage merely demonstrates what performers look like in the studio, because very often the actual performances that go on to record are unseen, or are assembled from multiple takes. The live-in-the-studio template that Snarky

Puppy employ is somewhat different, in that the audience is present at the moment of recording, and witness the music being played exactly as it is recorded, without edits or overdubs. This means that in the process of viewing the DVD recording, we see the music being created at the moment of its recording, and the audience reacting to that moment. Because audience members all have headphones on, it is as if they are hearing the mix as it goes direct to 'tape' (computer most likely in this case). It is not just that this is a slightly different paradigm to the concert hall or jazz club, but that it challenges what is meant by 'going into the studio to record'. In addition to ideas of cooperation and self-expression, jazz has often thought to suffer from the confines of the recording studio, with the crafting of performances for recording taking second place to the matter of live performance. The social space of the recording studio is sealed off from the negotiations that happen with an audience in live recording, a fact that has prompted critical reflection on what studio recordings represent (Butterfield, 2001/2002; Elsdon 2010). The recording studio tends to mitigate against risk-taking, in favour of a measured approach that will yield results. Thus, the live-in-the-studio paradigm can be seen as an attempt to redress this balance, to find a middle ground between the fidelity the recording studio offers and the social context of performance provided by the club or concert hall.

As well as the framing of this recording as live in the studio, there is also an important contextual narrative. On the DVD recording, the different pieces are separated by short segments comprising the usual behind-the-scenes 'extras': interviews with band members, footage of the band on tour and shots of them recording in the studio. The narrative this provides is not incidental, but critical in how it positions the viewer. It starts with the dramatic revelation that the group's normal drummer Robert 'Sput' Searight had to pull out at the last minute.[5] A number of the musicians recount their shock on arriving at the studio in The Netherlands to find that he was not present, and explain the trials of having to rehearse new music for four days without a drummer. Bassist Michael League appears on screen confirming that he had been on the telephone to various drummers to see who was available. We later learn that Searight's replacement, Larnell Lewis, travelled on an overnight flight from New York, arrived in a taxi to the studio, and had two hours to learn the music before the first live recording session, having never played most of the music before.[6]

This narrative presents the classic archetype of achieving success under the most trying of performance conditions. The other part of this narrative relates to the album's title, *We Like It Here*. And that is that the band, who started out from scratch in America, playing (as the liner notes explain) for a long time to small, unappreciative audiences, discovered an audience in Europe quite different from what they were used to in America – a quiet audience who listened, and then broke out into huge applause at the end of each number. Thus the very event of the recording is presented as an attempt to document this 'special relationship', to make this music in the presence of, and with the contribution of, European gig-goers. This backstory is important as it helps to position the viewer/listener in certain respects, constructing part of a frame through which we view the performance. I want first of all to look at an example of the way musicians are depicted on screen, in order to investigate how we, as viewers, might be primed to see empathic connections between musicians in the course of performance. It is no coincidence that the examples I use come from improvised solo sections from the Snarky Puppy recording. As I have already suggested, jazz's relationship with improvisation is a prime factor in some of the ways it has and continues to be read as an expression of unsubjective spontaneity.

To begin, it is worth very briefly describing Snarky Puppy's musical style. Their compositions are heavily reliant on riffs, often driven by basslines, and frequently employing odd metres. Rarely, if at all, does any of their music employ standard swing feel, but in sensibility it is far closer to soul, funk and rock. During the improvisation sections, very often the backing instruments have fairly set rhythmic patterns as is typical of funk, rather than the more open approach that jazz musicians can take when 'comping' in straight ahead contexts. Most of the improvised solos in their pieces are arranged in a particular way – the solo will be built over a short riff or chord sequence, and will build gradually as the soloist dictates. On cue from the soloist the band then exit the solo straight into another section. This is slightly different from the standard 'head' arrangements employed in much mainstream jazz. It also has a significant effect on the way the performance is shaped. It requires each soloist to build their solo to the requisite intensity before they can give the cue for the band to move on. In this way, the shape of each solo is predetermined in many respects.

This first example comes from the tune 'Outlier' from *We Like It Here*. The solo on this tune is taken by saxophonist Bob Reynolds, and set against a complex bass riff shown in Example 6.1.[7]

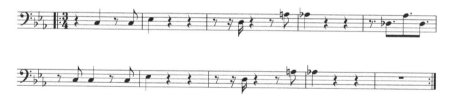

Example 6.1 Bass riff from 'Outlier'.

The solo begins with Reynolds playing over a minimal groove set by bass (here played on a Moog synthesiser) and drums. Over this complicated groove Reynolds plays long phrases that mix standard blues scale tonality with more contemporary angular lines – even hinting at a little 'out' playing. As the solo builds, keyboards enter playing sustained chords over the bass line, and filling out the texture. Then at 4'33" drummer Larnell Lewis plays a complicated passage supporting the increasing intensity Reynolds creates. In doing so he dramatically delays the point of rhythmic resolution. Usually with a complex riff like this, a drummer will always highlight the 'one' at the start of the cycle. Here instead, Lewis plays almost right across the cycle in a very busy manner. This, coupled with Reynolds' solo, has a dramatic effect. Pictured below are keyboardists Cory Henry and Shaun Martin (see Figure 6.1), both reacting to this moment with appreciative and affirmative cries that can be heard on the recording. While the camera is behind Lewis for most of the time so we cannot see his face, other shots from behind him let us see the reaction of other musicians (notice the string players in Figure 6.1).

The sequence of views we are given constitute quite a complicated body of information. There is, first of all, a particular kind of interaction going on between Reynolds and Lewis that creates this peak moment. However that relationship is not itself really framed on screen. As can be seen in Figure 6.1, sometimes we see Reynolds over Lewis's shoulder, and sometimes shots of Lewis and Reynolds independently, but never shots that allow us to see them interacting.[8] What is much more salient are the reactions of others, especially the keyboard players Martin and Henry. But what is it that they are responding to? On the face of it, the answer is simple, that they are responding to a particular peak musical moment. But that moment has come about through the interaction of two musicians within

(a)

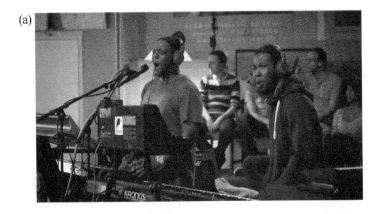

(b)

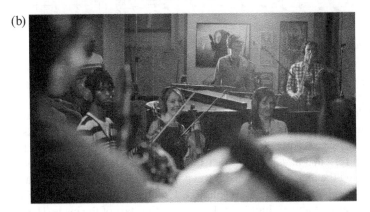

Figure 6.1 Reactions of other musicians during Bob Reynolds's solo on 'Outlier'.

the context of an improvised solo. So the response is actually to the way in which two players are interacting. The response itself also takes the form of affirmation and encouragement. It is an accepted behaviour within the act of musicking in jazz for audience members and musicians to vocalise their approval as an act of encouraging a musician or group of musicians. In some contexts it can even become part of the ritualised behaviour involved in musicking.[9] So vocalising a response here is participation as much as it is reaction, and it is to participate in the relationship being enacted musically between Reynolds and Lewis. To do so is, in the terms I have already described, an empathic act: that is, the response presupposes a certain cognitive act that identifies what is being felt by the musicians playing, and the response itself is appropriate given the circumstances. So where does this place us as viewers? I will return to this a little later following discussion of a second example.

In this second example, I want to explore one of the critical relationships framed on screen, between bassist Michael League, and drummer Larnell Lewis. League is well-known as the leader of Snarky Puppy, a charismatic individual who through sheer force of will managed to bring the band to global prominence without the support of a major record company.[10] In any jazz ensemble, the relationship between bassist and drummer is of particular importance. As the engine that creates the groove or feel, they must find shared musical ground. In other words, the whole feel for an ensemble like this starts and ends with the bassist and drummer. Of course there is a further complicating factor in this case given the scenario I have just explained, one articulated on the DVD recording. That is, that due to the last minute nature of the arrangement, Lewis is seen to be playing some of these pieces for the recording with a matter of hours of rehearsal only.[11] Thus the League–Lewis relationship is central to the kind of narrative the DVD is promoting – one individual is the leader, the driving creative force, attempting to guide the performance from his instrument, the other the musician flown in at the last minute, forced to learn music against the clock. As will become clear, this is not mere background information. Rather, this is critical priming that constructs part of the frame through which we view this performance, and through which we make interpretations about what we are seeing.

Unusually in a context like this, League and Lewis are some physical distance apart. This is likely down to the considerations of recording live in the studio, where 'bleed' from drums into other instrument microphones is a critical factor to be considered. The fact that Lewis is not playing in an isolated drum booth, as is often the practice in recording studios, would only enhance the probability for problems from bleed to occur. There is one particular moment I want to concentrate on. It comes from the end of the second track, 'What About Me'. This is one of the most prominent features for drums from this album for two reasons. While it is built on a funk feel with riff-heavy sections that come close to a rock feel, the drum patterns are particularly busy with lots of snare work, far more than just backbeats. Added to which, the tune ends with a drum solo set against a complex synth bass/bass guitar riff, as seen in Example 6.2.[12]

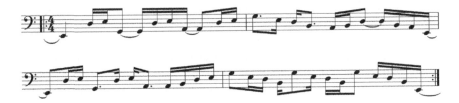

Example 6.2 Bass riff from 'What About Me'.

Lewis's solo must maintain synchronisation against this riff while simultane-ously demonstrating the necessary virtuosity appropriate to the context. This is an extremely common device in contemporary jazz – the drum solo set across a complex riff, and often in unusual time signatures. During Lewis's solo on the recording, there are a few telling camera shots (see Figure 6.2). In this particular instance, these shots demonstrate the framing on screen of relationships between musicians, and the reaction of one musician to another, and also the implication of audience members in this process of participation and attunement.

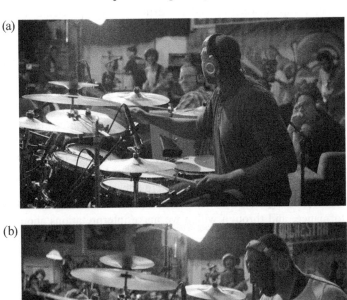

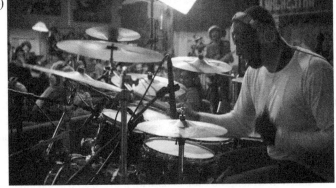

Figure 6.2 Shots framing musicians and audience members during drum solo.

(c)

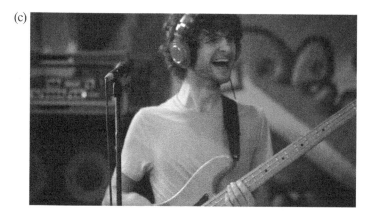

(d)

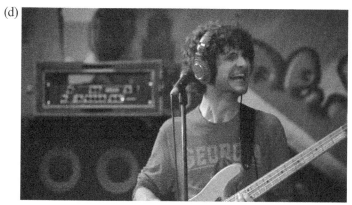

Figure 6.2 Continued

Naturally this sequence does not translate particularly well to still shots, so I would encourage any interested reader to seek it out online. But, as seen in Figure 6.2, Lewis and League are looking at one another during the drum solo. In the second still, taken from one of the extra 'bonus' features on the disc, we see the same tune in a different take, with the same camera shot, this time not demonstrating a direct gaze from one musician to another; but it is obvious that League is keeping his visual attention on Lewis. And in the third and fourth stills, we have reaction shots of League responding to Lewis's solo. In the first still, we can see also an audience member positioned exactly in the sight-line between League and Lewis, also focused on the solo, but oblivious to League's reaction.

In theorising the act of viewing, identification is particularly important. Some-times the camera merely acts as disinterested viewer, but often it encourages us to take a particular position. My suggestion in this case is that we are particularly being encouraged to identify with this audience member, who is party to this moment in the drum solo where League looks on as Lewis solos. The fact that this man is positioned in the shot is important because it is as if he is exactly on the sight-line that connects League directly to Lewis. He is therefore seen to be experiencing the same thing as League and Lewis. This visual trick of foreshortening creates these relationships on screen where they may not have existed in the same way at the actual moment. What is not important here is whether or not this audience member perceived himself to be in this sight-line, but that clearly in the way this shot is framed that is how it appears. Here, then, we have again a relationship between two musicians that displays all the signs of Seddon's empathetic attunement that I have mentioned. But in addition we can see an audience member who, by virtue of their position and facial expression, appears to be empathising with what is going on between bass player and drummer. In this case, not only does the performance on screen seem to enact these empathic relationships, but we are also as viewers encouraged to participate. This happens because we can identify with the experiences of audience members at the recording session, and imagine ourselves in their place.

Concluding remarks

How do we read all the evidence from these performances? For one thing, they certainly speak to all the signs of Seddon's empathetic attunement. There are the expressions of bodily interest – smiles, shouts, animated movements, from both musicians and audience members. These occur particularly at moments of risk-taking, something Seddon sees as key to empathetic attunement in jazz performance. But, what I have presented are outward, gestural signs. As Björn Heile describes, many jazz musicians have cultivated what he calls the performance of spontaneity (Heile, 2016). That is, they have developed ways of presenting and framing performances via repetition, but done in such a way as to promote the idea that the audience are seeing something spontaneous. There is, in other words, a potential gap between what is being gestured at and represented, and the reality of what is actually happening on stage. This is a gap which is far too little acknowledged or understood, and can lead to performances being read literally as direct representations of inner states and feelings. In this case, for instance, one only has to spend a little time watching some of the many videos online of Snarky Puppy performing in a variety of venues in different countries, to find a whole repertoire of gestural behaviours. That these gestures are typical, and repeated, does not in any way necessarily call their truthfulness into question. But it does help to clarify that such gestures are not necessarily the spontaneous indicators of empathetic attunement that they might seem to be. However, if empathy is based on an act of intellectual comprehension, our viewing of empathetic attunement in performance is ultimately unrelated to whether or not certain behaviours are spontaneous or not.

I want to come back at this point to the idea of viewing. Any performance presented to us on screen, whether on television, or via the internet, or from a DVD, has been subject to a range of technological mediations which involve human agency. In viewing a mediatised representation of a performance, we are seeing it through a lens, both literally and figuratively. In all of these cases, we are seeing these gestures and reactions because of human agency – that is, the producers made a conscious decision to choose these shots and these camera angles over others in the process of editing. We are being given a specific point of view of these performances – in other words, we are being shown certain reactions and interactions quite deliberately. So Snarky Puppy's *We Like It Here* presents us with a particular narrative about musical and social relationships, played out on screen, through interviews, and through the notes to the album, and juxtaposed against the wider context of the idea of jazz as a language which crosses divides of race, class, nationality and so on.

I am suggesting that in viewing jazz performance, our idea of empathy emerges from a set of cultural assumptions about jazz as the domain of the democratic, mutually cooperative creative endeavour that rewards risk-taking. When we view what seems to be empathetic attunement in a performance, we are observing outward gestures and behaviours that tally with our cultural assumptions of what we expect. So, the act of viewing is not passive but active or, rather, we construct ideas about empathy in the course of viewing performance.

Acknowledgements

Music examples and illustrations are used by kind permission of GroundUp Music. My thanks to Mike Chadwick for helping arrange this. I am indebted to Paul McIntyre for introducing me to Auslander's use of frame analysis. I also want to acknowledge my fellow collaborators on the Arts and Humanities Research Council (AHRC)-funded project 'The Use of Audiovisual Resources in Jazz Historiography and Scholarship: Performance, Embodiment and Mediatised Representations', Dr Jenny Doctor and Dr Björn Heile. Many of the ideas in this chapter were formed during work on that project. I also want to thank Lewis Kennedy and Sarina Velt for suggestions on a draft version of the chapter, to Alan Drever-Smith for pointing me to the Snarky Puppy transcriptions released by the band, and to the anonymous reviewer who made some helpful suggestions.

Notes

1 Snarky Puppy, *We Like It Here* (Ropeadope, 2013). Much of the background to Snarky Puppy can be found readily available online, not least because they have built their reputation largely through social media and word of mouth, rather than with the support of a record company, as is the traditional model. See, for instance, http://custom. bandframe.com/snarkypuppy/ (accessed 29 August 2014 – 'About' tab) or http:// puregrainaudio.com/interviews/interview-with-snarky-puppy-bassist-guitarist-composer-and-arranger-michael-league (accessed 29 August 2014).

2 It is worth noting that each member of the audience was issued with a pair of headphones precisely because the performance(s) was essentially a recording session.

3 I use the term liveness here as a deliberate reference to Auslander's (1999) important work on this subject.

4 See the band's YouTube channel: www.youtube.com/channel/UColt7ajBc5r44Ejxnod-h7Q (accessed 29 August 2014).

5 The DVD recording does not reveal why, but sources on the internet indicate that an expired passport was the problem.

6 It is not made clear from the DVD, but Lewis had played with the band before. See www.drummerszone.com/news/article/on-stage-6-12488/6/larnell-lewis-takes-care-of-snarky-puppy-dvd-recordings (accessed 29 August 2014). This article also implies that Lewis may have already been familiar with three of the tunes that were being recorded. One of the video interviews on that page subsequently explains that Lewis had MP3s to listen to on his flight, so was in fact learning the music as he was travelling.

7 This notation is drawn from the Snarky Puppy Songbook ebook release. See www. lulu.com/shop/snarky-puppy/the-snarky-puppy-songbook-outlier-we-like-it-here/ ebook/product-21487541.html charts (accessed 6 October 2014). In this case, this is band member and composer Justin Stanton's own notated version.

8 Michael League comments specifically on the interaction between Lewis and Reynolds in his introduction to the Snarky Puppy Songbook version of the tune, noting that the two have an 'incredible' conversation, 'without crossing into kitschy monkey-see-monkey-do territory'.

9 At the same time, there are also jazz contexts where it would be regarded as highly inappropriate behaviour to vocalise encouragement, so generalisation is difficult.

10 The liner notes to *We Like It Here*, authored by League, serve as a prime example of this – recounting the routine of travelling around the US, sleeping on floors, playing to small and/or unappreciative audiences.

11 It is not at all clear from the recording how many of the performances on the CD are actually first takes from the first night of recording. Lewis, therefore, would have had the chance to develop his performance over subsequent nights.

12 As with much of Snarky Puppy's music, the use of notation to represent what is going on is somewhat complex. Most of the music the band play is never notated, and is instead learned by heart by the players. My first attempt at transcribing this passage employed a 15/8 meter to represent what I heard as a quintuple division of the beat. But the ongoing Snarky Puppy Songbook ebook releases present the riff as notated in Example 6.2. www.lulu.com/shop/snarky-puppy/the-snarky-puppy-songbook-what-about-me-we-like-it-here/ebook/product-21486532.html (accessed 6 October 2014). In this case, the ebook presents a transcription of the tune by the band's guitarist Chris McQueen, with notes by Michael League.

References

Auslander, P. (1999). *Liveness: Performance in a mediatized culture*. London: Routledge.

Auslander, P. (2006). Musical personae. *The Drama Review: The Journal of Performance Studies, 50*(1), 100–119.

Borgo, D. (2005). *Sync or swarm: Improvising music in a complex age*. New York: Continuum.

Butterfield, M. (2001/2). Music analysis and the social life of jazz recordings. *Current Musicology, 71–3*, 342–352.

Corbett, J. (1994). *Extended play: Sounding off from John Cage to Dr. Funkenstein*. Durham, NC, London: Duke University Press.

Darwall, S. (1998). Empathy, sympathy, care. *Philosophical Studies, 89*(2–3), 261–282.

Doffman, M. (2011). Jammin' an ending: Creativity, knowledge and conduct amongst jazz musicians. *Twentieth Century Music, 8*(2), 203–225.

Elsdon, P. (2010). Jazz recordings and the capturing of performance. In A. Bayley (Ed.), *Recorded music: Performance, culture and technology* (pp. 146–166) Cambridge: Cambridge University Press.

Garrido, S., & Schubert, E. (2011). Individual differences in the enjoyment of negative emotion in music: A literature review and experiment. *Music Perception, 28*(3), 279–296.

Gebhardt, N. (2001). *Going for jazz: Musical practices and American ideology.* Chicago, IL: University of Chicago Press.

Heile, B. (2016). Play it again Duke: Jazz performance, improvisation, and the construction of spontaneity. In J. Doctor, P. Elsdon & B. Heile (Eds.), *Watching jazz: Encountering jazz performance on film and television* (pp. 238–266). New York: Oxford University Press.

Hodson, R. (2007). *Interaction, improvisation, and interplay in jazz.* New York: Routledge.

Laurence, F. (2008). Music and empathy. In O. Urbain (Ed.), *Music and conflict transformation: Harmonies and dissonances in geopolitics* (pp. 13–25). London: I. B. Tauris.

Litweiler, J. (1984). *The freedom principle: Jazz after 1958.* New York: Da Capo Press.

Monson, I. (1996). *Saying something: Jazz improvisation and interaction.* Chicago, IL: University of Chicago Press.

Monson, I. (2008). Hearing, seeing, and perceptual agency. *Critical Inquiry, 35*(S2), S36–S58.

Putman, D. (1994). Music and empathy. *Journal of Aesthetic Education, 28*(2), 98–102.

Ropeadope (2013). www.ropeadope99.bandcamp.com/album/we-like-it-here (accessed 17 November 2016).

Seddon, F. A. (2005). Modes of communication during jazz improvisation. *British Journal of Music Education, 22*(1), 47–61.

Small, C. (1998). *Musicking: The meanings of performing and listening.* Hanover: Wesleyan University Press.

Vreeke, G. J., & van der Mark, I. L. (2003). Empathy, an integrative model. *New Ideas in Psychology, 21*(3), 177–207.

Part II

Empathy in performing together

7 Otherwise than participation

Unity and alterity in musical encounters

Matthew Rahaim

This chapter considers two distinctive musical orientations: towards unity (communion, empathy, comprehension, participation) and towards alterity (separation, evasion, infinity, striving). This much may sound far removed from playing instruments, singing and dancing. Let's begin, then, from a key practical concern of ethnomusicologists: participatory performance.

Participation

Feeling into a collaborative groove, joining one's voice with others, tuning in to a shared temporality: how could we ever make music together without these powers of participation? A capacity for shared, collective musical feeling allows harmony, unison, polymetre, friction, interlocking rhythm – everyday musical achievements that would be impossible for radically autonomous islands of subjectivity. It's not just that ensemble feels good. A properly well-adjusted modern self would seem to require such participatory capacities in their psychological repertoire alongside self-esteem, coping mechanisms and computer literacy. Think of an otherwise healthy young concert pianist at an American wedding who flatly refuses to join her friends on the dance floor. She is likely to be considered square, or uptight or self-conscious: not just technically lacking, but also, in a crucial sense, morally lacking.

Ethnomusicologists, more than anyone else, have reinforced the sense that participation is a weighty ethical and political matter. We read that 'we need more of this participatory consciousness if we are to get back into ecological synchrony with ourselves and with the natural world' (Keil, 1987, p. 276). We read that the 'feelingful participation' of grooving is a 'positive physical and emotional attachment, a move from being "hip to it" to "getting down" and being "into it"' (Feld, 1988, p. 75). We read that participation allows people to be not just connected, but 'truthfully intimately connected'; that when 'the individual parts create a greater whole … participatory performance is good social life' (Turino, 2008, p. 136). Music educators (for example, Everitt, 1997; Odam, 1995/2001) often proceed with a 'missionary zeal' to encourage musical participation, which is 'essential to our well-being as individuals and social creatures' (Ede, 1997, p. 6). I, too, often find myself zealously insisting that my students get up from their seats in the lecture hall to sing along, dance along and get into the groove. We sweat, we smile, we dance *dabkeh*. At some point in my upbringing, I too was given to understand that this kind of collective participation (social dancing in Eagles halls, community bands, hymn-singing in church) is not just fun, but also *good*.

Lately, though, I have started to wonder about participation. I'm not worrying about fascistic 'rhythmic obedience' here (Adorno, 1941) – advocates of participation are well aware of this danger, and warn us against the evils of statist participatory totalitarianism, highlighting the anarchic and anti-authoritarian potentials of small-scale, egalitarian participatory performance (cf. Feld, 1988, p. 84; Keil, 1987, p. 276; Turino, 2008, pp. 190–210). But the ascription of moral benefits to even non-fascistic participation are nonetheless textured by a distinctive set of economic and political conditions. Thomas Turino (2008) contrasts the virtues of participatory music-making to life 'compartmentalised in private homes, cars, classrooms, and stores' (pp. 156–157). Sian Ede's (1997) plea for participation as a way of nurturing a 'sense of belonging' is made against the backdrop of a 'disconnected society' (p. 6). Charles Keil (1987) presents participation as 'the opposite of alienation from nature, from society, from the body, from labor' (p. 276). This may account for some of the historically specific ways in which, at least for those of us raised among televisions, fast food, and automobiles, participation intuitively 'feels so right' (Feld, 1988, p. 104).

This feeling of rightness is precisely what makes me wonder. The evident powers and pleasures of participation are indeed difficult to untangle from the question of its moral righteousness. We thus might do well to step back for a moment in order to see its metaphysical moorings a bit more clearly.

The metaphysics of unity

Participation, in the technical sense used by ethnographers of performance, does not simply pop out of ethnographic data; it is a concept with a venerable metaphysical pedigree. Its clearest origins are found in the work of anthropologist Lucien Levy-Bruhl and anthroposophist Owen Barfield.[1] Levy-Bruhl used the term to describe a characteristic activity of '*la mentalité primitive*' in which a thing or a person is both itself and something else (for example, both a person *and* a bird) without contradiction (Levy-Bruhl 1910/1926). Barfield went further. In a series of increasingly passionate appeals, he reconstrued participation as a crucial, universal human faculty. Even moderns, according to Barfield (1957/1965), are capable of participation in which 'self and not-self [are] identified in the same moment of experience' (p. 32), so that, rather than standing separate from the world, 'the world itself [is] his self-consciousness displayed before him' (1977, p. 204). Nor, according to Barfield, is this just a momentary failure to distinguish subjectivity and objectivity. The unified, participatory interweave of self and other is a realisation of the universal ground of perception and action, 'built into the structure of the universe' (1977, p. 205). Charles Keil (1995), whose work positively hums with Barfieldian influence, expresses this vision of a unified cosmos in ecstatic musical terms:

> What is beyond our skin is primary reality from the mini-vibes of atomic quarks and mesons up through the molecular vibes of Brownian motion

through the color vibes and life vibes into the James Brown vibes and on out to the galactic rumba but it is also inside us, in our body-minds, and that's why we can participate in it.

(Keil, 1995, p. 3)

Surely, we know where he's coming from. Who has not felt, from time to time, some sort of intuitive musical communion in which we feel ourselves to be part of a grand cosmic Whole? But more is at issue here than a feeling. The metaphysical claims come the next morning, seated at the word processor, in construing such an ecstatic moment as a taste of what is *actually out there*: a primordial unity of vibes, or spirit, or energy, or elementary particles, or what have you. Though this metaphysics has some obvious affinities with certain traditions of practical mysticism, one need not undergo any monastic rigours to become a believer. Timothy Taylor's archive of Electronic Dance Music literature, for example, contains many such unitarian proclamations:

> As we raise our arms with an ecstatic cheer we feel our connection to each other as one tribe united in spirit – the power of the collective. This euphoric dance floor release is…our rite of passage into ecstatic oneness.

(Decker cited in Taylor, 2014, p. 175)

Certainly, many of us can sympathise with a predilection for unity over duality, collectivity over individuality, togetherness over aloneness. But if we turn this into a basic claim about *what is*, if we start from the metaphysical axiom that everything inheres in a single, undivided primary reality, then separation can only appear logically negative (not-one) and morally deviant (alienated.) If face-to-face social life (full of encounters with independent individuals, sovereign interiorities, secrets, separation and duplicity) is taken to be a distortion of a primary unified reality, then the unity produced by participatory music-making would seem to be beckoning us back home. In the starkest metaphysical terms, the 'urge to merge' is calling us to be 'at one with the entire universe' (Keil, 1987, p. 276). Following Jonathan Weidenbaum (2013), I call this orientation the *metaphysics of unity*.

The argument so far is that claims about the moral righteousness of musical participation are grounded in a certain implicit metaphysics.[2] But I am not suggesting that we flee participation and set sail for some non-metaphysical utopia (right next door, perhaps, to that non-political utopia we've heard so much about). Nor am I suggesting that we need to stop dancing, stop singing, or stop participating – far from it. But I am claiming that the metaphysics of unity is a view from somewhere. If we want to reflexively understand the musical implications of this metaphysics, it may be helpful to stand elsewhere for a moment.

The metaphysics of alterity

This chapter focuses on one important *elsewhere*, which (again, following Weidenbaum), I will call the *metaphysics of alterity*.[3] There are numerous precedents for the critique of metaphysical unity from the point of view of alterity,

from many times and places (in the Arabic tradition, Ibn Taymiyyah's rejection
of Ibn Arabi's panentheism in favour of a transcendent Creator absolutely separate from creation; in the Sanskritic tradition, Madhva's insistence on absolute
separation of humanity and divinity as opposed to Shankara's radical *advaita*).
But no one has done it more explicitly, at greater length, or with less confes-
sional specificity than Emmanuel Levinas.[4] Levinas presents a metaphysics[5]
that begins not from primordial unity, but from encountering a separate, never-
fully-comprehensible Other, across a distance. We find ourselves thrown into a
world full of such encounters. Even as I enter into various kinds of relationship,
the Other remains distinct from me (Levinas, 1947/1987, p. 42). Perhaps I may,
at times, join with them as one – through participation, through choreography,
through deep empathy. But upon encountering an Other that I do not grasp, that
I do not control, that I do not understand, joining is by no means the only (or the
best) possibility. A free Other offers me the possibility of open-ended rapport
with someone who is *not* me (in contrast to the autopoetic mutual maintenance of
organs in a cosmic über-organism.) The 'urge to merge', from this point of view,
is an urge to dissolve this separation, so that the face-to-face encounter is assimilated into a larger monad. Levinas points out that the assimilation of separation
into oneness (which, like violence, is often suffused with power and pleasure) has
the same metaphysical form as political domination: it 'establishes an order from
which no one can keep his distance' (Levinas, 1961/1979, p. 21). To participate,
then, requires that the delicate rapport between Self and Other be absorbed into
a single Us: a totality.

   If this account of alterity seems counterintuitive at first, it may be because
the Levinasian Other is not 'the other' that has wide currency in the humanities[6]
and even in everyday speech (for example, marrying someone from an-*other*
race, listening to some *other* kind of music for a change.) This is an important
distinction. Humanists and social scientists have long been concerned with the
processes by which people are represented as 'others' – especially other than
white, other than Christian, other than bourgeois, other than cisgendered, and
so on. This is a matter of difference, of *heteron*. We think of Deep Forest selling
albums with exotic, layered Pygmy voices; we think of Rajasthani folk musicians presented for European audiences in red lighted boxes; we think of white
elementary school students mocking a new Asian–American classmate with
stereotyped pentatonic melodies. Our usual analytic habits direct us to understand these as the results of representation – for example, the results of orientalist
discourse (Said, 1979) or detemporalising ethnographic depiction (Fabian, 1983).
This attention to representation, all the more urgent when illuminating stark
power differentials between ethnographers and ethnographic subjects, continues
to teach us a great deal. But it is an entirely different matter.

   The Other that concerns us here is *not* the qualitatively different figure that
we represent as exotic. We are concerned with the Other whom we meet face-
to-face, who is always escaping representation, by whom we are called to responsibility. This Other certainly may *also* be an ethnographic subject who
speaks another language, but they may just as well be a neighbour, a refugee,

a lover, a teacher, a student. Levinas's phenomenology of encounter is driven by a moral concern about the absorption of the Other into an overarching unity.[7] In this regard, at least, his concerns happen to accord with those of Edward Said and Johannes Fabian. But for Levinas, Otherness itself is not a problem to be solved. To encounter someone face-to-face is already to encounter an Other, in all of their strangeness and vulnerability. Starting from a metaphysics of alterity, the seductive, comforting move highlighted for critical consideration is not *othering*, but *totalising*: grasping the Other, making the Other a mere part of a totality, an appendage of Being, one more thing in our world that we use, know, feel, or encompass. This may, again, seem counterintuitive. It may seem as though our scholarly task is precisely to absorb our baffling musical encounters into ever-more comprehensive totalities. All the more reason, then, that while teaching, writing, and musicking, in distant lands or in our own neighbourhoods, a focus on metaphysical alterity may offer us something of great importance.

The task of this chapter

How might musical life appear to us if we begin from alterity rather than unity, if the formation of a unified totality stands out as a constitutive act rather than as an ontic foundation? This chapter aims to provide just such an account. This is by no means the first attempt at a Levinasian approach to music. Several other musicologists have recently taken up Levinas's ethical challenge – two particularly important examples are Marcel Cobussen and Nanette Nielsen's volume entitled *Music and ethics* (2012) and Jeff Warren's *Music and ethical responsibility* (2014).

Because of the particular arc of my own musical and speculative training, Levinas's account of coming face-to-face with an Other seems to me to *already* be a musical matter in the broadest sense – even if there is no singing or dancing involved. I thus tend to focus especially on the unfolding of rapport in time, and, more generally, on the phenomenological grounding of Levinasian metaphysics, rather than on its ethical and theological implications. This musical bias has led me to some Levinasian considerations of music practice that Levinas himself, for various reasons,[8] never explored. For example, I will attempt to transpose the *visage* (the 'face' of the other) beyond the merely visual, suggesting ways in which it might provide the ground for musical encounters. In the end, we will loop around again to the question of empathetic participation, and what it is that the 'urge to merge' may call us to renounce.

I myself have not signed on once and for all to a metaphysics of alterity. Instead, the line of critique opened by this account is intended to provide a counterpoint to the implicit metaphysics of unity that tends to dominate the human sciences. My aim is not to convert the reader to some kind of 'Levinasianism', or even to produce a prefigured dialectical synthesis between unity and alterity. Rather, I hope to open a speculative path, allowing us to discuss the risks of empathy, participation, and unity alongside their obvious powers and pleasures.

The *chez soi*

Levinasian metaphysics is founded on the radical distance between I and the Other. But this 'I' is no transparent eyeball floating in space. It lives and works in a world of activity, danger and possibility. The world of things and people, which at times can feel so foreign and threatening, is also actively constituted as a place to live, a place for enjoyment, a sensuous and intellectual extension of the Self. In such a world, the I must always exert power in 'recovering its identity throughout all that happens to it' (Levinas, 1961/1979, pp. 36–37). (It is here that the Heideggerian foundation is most obvious.)[9] Levinas often calls this place the *chez soi*, the 'at-home-with-oneself' in the broadest possible sense: the world of power, enjoyment, and comprehension (1961/1979, p. 37).

The *chez soi* is filled with activity: making my coffee, hearing my MP3 player progressing through a playlist, walking to get my daily doughnut around the corner, silently mulling over yesterday's argument with a friend. The *chez soi* is bound together by the constant efforts, big and small, by which I make a place for myself. Though I'm not omniscient, the *chez soi* is still coherent: it is fully available for me to exercise my powers over it. I may not know the exact temperature of my coffee, but I can grasp the handle of my cup; I may not know how this particular MP3 file was encoded, but I can sing along with Nina Simone; I may not know the precise gear ratios on my bike, but I can shift down to ascend a hill. Everything is in play, subject to my powers and my knowledge, so that everything is graspable even if not immediately grasped. I am constantly exerting power to re-organise my world into a totality organised around my needs, my enjoyment, my imagination: the coherence and continuity of my Being.

This is not a world of objects that a transcendental 'I' observes from the outside. Even basic acts of knowing are accomplished *through* it: streetlights, eyeglasses, guitar tuners, the Pythagorean theorem, computer screens, *righty tighty/lefty loosey*, phones, books, eardrums (cf. Levinas, 1961/1979, p. 153). Nor does it simply consist of the things that go as planned. When a guitar string goes slack, I can tune it; when a headphone speaker is crackly, I can solder the loose contact; when I am perplexed by a disagreement with a friend, I can work to assimilate it theoretically (by bolstering or surrendering my position, by caricaturing or empathising with hers.) Even things beyond my immediate control are subject to my powers – when I am trapped by a Minnesota snowstorm, I can survey the situation, I can shovel my way out, I can complain, I can patiently wait for help. Sometimes my efforts fail; always my efforts consist to some degree in passively sojourning in the world I have constituted. But succeeding, failing, abiding in a world subject to my various powers of action and comprehension is what constitutes my *chez soi* – and the 'I' that dwells there.

The *chez soi* reaches far beyond my body. It is a seamless site of personal power, comprehension, and enjoyment ongoingly built by the 'I', a site of an egoism exerting power over a total, coherent lifeworld. When my MP3 player shuffles its way to a recording of Huun-Huur-Tu, I constitute it as 'Tuvan' music, even if I have never been to Tuva myself – even if I am mistaken. As far as my *chez soi* extends its power, 'resistance is futile' – everything and everyone will be assimilated, if I so will it (Berman & Braga, 1995, p. 18). This assimilating power extends far beyond the phenomenal body, far beyond the lived space of a house, to the speculative exploration of distant places I have never been: 'everything is at my disposal, even the stars, if I but reckon them' (Levinas, 1961/1979, p. 37).

Encountering the Other

But this coherent totality is not objectively complete. There is something beyond. Of course there are melodies I have never heard and places I have never heard of, doughnuts I have never eaten and buttons I have never pushed, even in my own apartment; these will offer little resistance to assimilation. But there also are moments when I encounter another person face-to-face who cannot merely be joined with the totality, who remains, for me, utterly Other.

Rushing along a city street, late for a meeting, dodging bodies, I hear a stranger call out to me. I turn to face him and he asks me for directions to the hospital. His confusion, his need, his vulnerability are apparent in his voice and face even if I do not know exactly why he needs to go there. Perhaps later, sitting on the bus, I will stare out of the window, weigh his needs against mine, figure out what a rational being in my position should have done. But right now I am not faced with a call to rational account – *I am faced*, as I might describe it to a friend, *with this guy*. His face and voice reach out to me from beyond the totality of my *chez soi*. Unlike any of the other conditional obstacles in my morning (a late bus, a locked door, a stubbed toe), this man's expression of need is an unconditional demand, utterly incommensurable with my everyday purposes. His call to me demands a response.

If you doubt the force of this demand, try facing someone as they greet you and remaining silent and still. What elaborate psychic feats must you carry out in order to manage *not* to respond? It's not that we must rouse ourselves from a prior unity to convince ourselves to act towards this separate Other. The demand for response – *responsibility* – stands out as quite different from other practical challenges.

But how, we might ask, could this helpless tourist be so strong? Can't I just choose to push him aside and continue on my way? I can. But doing so would be turning away from the encounter, exercising power over his flesh, constituting his body as another element of my world (an intractable algebra problem, a bus to catch, an irritating tourist). In that case I would no longer be faced by an Other. Less obviously violent would be to seal up the hole in my power by absorbing the Other into a theme I already comprehend: 'Ha! You New Yorkers are always getting lost.' This utterance could very well end the encounter; he might turn away in disgust, I might rush on my way.

But suppose the conversation continues; suppose he smiles with me at this unexpected caricature of New Yorkers. Or suppose he contests it, or suppose he points out that he is actually from Philadelphia, or suppose he simply laughs with me, shaking his head: 'you got me there, buddy.' Whatever the theme 'New Yorker' may have been when I said it, no matter how much it may have seemed to account for the figure of this man, my interlocutor now stands outside of it, commenting on it, playing with it, even deliberately using it to grasp his own actions. In doing so, he is now the one deploying the theme rather than the one thematised. He is engaged in what Levinas calls *the saying* (*le dire*) rather than fully grasped in *the said* (*le dit*). This Other 'has quit the theme that encompassed him, and upsurges inevitably behind the said' (1961/1979, p. 195). His response calls for a response in turn. So the rapport continues.

Thus, the simple, everyday sense in which rapport with the Other is *infinite* has nothing to do with large numbers or mind-boggling spans of time or the far reaches of outer space. All of these are totalisable. The infinity at issue can be found in the indeterminate open-endedness of a conversation at the pub: for every n that is *said*, there is always an $n+1$ in the possibility of *saying* (which, in turn, becomes a said). *The saying* is infinite not by virtue of how long we talk or how many topics we cover, but by virtue of always exceeding *the said* that came before. This is not happening through concerted intellectual effort, like a chess game. Inasmuch as we are in rapport, inasmuch as my interlocutor simply continues to be Other, he is constantly evading my grasp, and I his.

This dance by which the Other evades me now begins to appear in its musical dimensions. It has nothing to do with brute force, nothing to do with 'the hardness of the rock [or] the remoteness of a star' (Levinas, 1961/1979, p. 198). He 'opposes to me not a greater force', which would be, by virtue of being relatively *greater than* my own, 'an energy assessable … as though it were part of a whole' (p. 199). His freedom, the unpredictability of his needs, his inevitable upsurge behind any theme in conversation, stands radically outside of the sphere of my ability for power (my *pouvoir de pouvoir*). The Other greets me from the exterior of my *chez soi*, beyond my grasp and thus open to a mode of rapport that preserves the radical separation between the I and the Other. Without any pretense of total comprehension, I am called to responsibility.

It should be clear that such an encounter does not depend on any kind of qualitative difference; it is just as possible between first cousins as between mutual foreigners. The call of the Other demands a response, demands a kind of generosity. Responsibility to the Other 'opens a new dimension' (Levinas, 1961/1979, p. 197) orthogonal to the dimensions of my *chez soi*, orthogonal to my own purposes, enjoyment and comprehension. This, according to Levinas, is the unique dimension in which ethics might occur, prior to my exertions of power to generate and sustain totalities, in which the gentleness of dialogue can occur, in which we are called to ethical account for other people as Others rather than extensions of ourselves.

Totalising

The radical alterity of the Other, however, can be willfully dissolved in a totality. This person who a moment ago spoke to me from across an infinite distance may be reconstituted as one among many items in my total, seamless exercise of power in the world. Physical force, as noted above, is one obvious form of violence. But totalising can take other forms as well: constituting the Other as an attainable object of desire, as a fascinating exotic to be known, as an instrument for my use, as a token of a type, as a theme.

Totalising thus includes not only 'othering' in the familiar representational sense (for example, racialist certainties about 'cunning Arabs' or 'passionate Latinos', saavy disdain for French philosophers or college athletes) but any encompassing comprehension (Levinas, 1961/1979, p. 38). Even the warm embrace of a fellow citizen as *one of us* dissolves the asymmetrical rapport of the I and the Other into an overarching unity. In Levinas's pithy terms, 'the collectivity in which I say "you" or "we" is not a plural of the "I"' (p. 39).

The problem here is not that some particular qualitative distinction between Us and Them is inaccurate or demeaning or politically incorrect (and thus that some other system of difference is accurate or respectful or politically correct). The Levinasian line of critique sees *any* gesture that simultaneously constitutes Them and Us – no matter how empirically accurate or rhetorically convincing or expedient – as a totalising erasure of alterity. This erasure leaves us with a single encompassing totality and forecloses the possibility of rapport with an Other.

Teaching World Music

Shouldn't teaching World Music, then, by highlighting difference, by teaching us about those unlike us, restore the ground of alterity that affords ethical responsibility? Perhaps it should. But again, it is important to distinguish metaphysical alterity (which arises in encounter) from qualitative difference (which is produced in representation). Just as the metaphysics of unity does not require cultural sameness, the metaphysics of alterity does not require cultural difference. Levinas's defence of alterity against the 'imperialism of the Same' (1961/1979, p. 39) should not be confused with the defence of cultural diversity against 'cultural grey-out' that so concerned ethnomusicologists in the 1970s (cf. Lomax, 1972). World Music courses are intended in most institutional curricula to serve something like this latter end. Such courses aim to teach our students to hear and accept difference, to place the musics of colonial subjects on a level playing field with the musics of colonial masters, to provincialise our own listening habits, to teach me that I too, from an alien point of view, am alien too. All worthy goals.

But the Other we are considering here – the other we meet face-to-face – is not Other by virtue of having different traits, playing different music, belonging to a different place. A relationship with an Other that preserves alterity has nothing to do with enumerating her cultural traits ('my scale has twenty-two notes but hers has twenty-four'). Any such distinction, on the contrary, is a way of comprehending the Other in a theme.

Take *culture*, that all-encompassing theoretical recourse of undergraduate World Music textbooks. Leaving aside the question of whether this concept actually accounts for ethnographic data (cf. Gupta & Ferguson, 1991; Laidlaw, 2013, pp. 24–27), what are the implications of teaching our students to hear mbira music as an expression of *Zimbabwean culture*? Why is it such a relief to students to explain away the sting of melodic perplexity by appealing to different *cultural values*? And why does recourse to culture shut down the ongoing, infinite *saying* of face-to-face encounter (in which our interlocutor escapes our every theme) so thoroughly into the seamless totality of the *said* (from which nothing escapes)? When we account for a musicking Other as an economic agent in a market, as an actor in a network, as a member of a society, as a token of a cultural type, we patch up the hole and return to our comfortable sojourn in a world maintained by our own powers.

Again and again, in World Music surveys, we bring students into perplexing encounters with surprising ways of musicking. But this surprise is easily assimilated: neutral thirds, nine-day rituals, asymmetrical metric cycles, feudal patronage. Any such marker of specific difference does its work within a genus: interval, ritual form, metre, patronage structures. Think of the ease and enthusiasm with which a budding jazz musician grasps an unfamiliar groove numerically as 'a seven' or 'an eleven'. Marking difference is not the same as preserving metaphysical alterity; on the contrary, it is a powerful way to render the Other digestible into the Same. As Levinas concisely puts it: 'The alterity of the other does not depend on any quality that would distinguish him from me, for a distinction of this nature would precisely imply between us that community of genus which already nullifies alterity' (1961/1979, p. 194). A Tibetan monk chanting can strike my students as *different* only if they first recognise him empathically as a member of a genus: a man among men, a voice among voices. The off-balance disorientation we feel on hearing the play of two interlocking bell patterns rests on an intuition that there must be a pulse somewhere, feeling our way empathically to where a human might step or play. The sound that I constitute as 'chanting' would not strike me as a different voice, a different subjectivity, were it coming from my furnace; the sound that I constitute as 'bell patterns' would not seem to both invite and frustrate dancing were they coming from a melting glacier. Perhaps the sounds would cause me concern or curiosity (about the workings of my machines or the progress of climate change), perhaps I might even imaginatively constitute them as a kind of cosmic *musica universalis*, but unless I constitute them as a (specific) type of (general) music, they would not arise as exotic, as different, as a 'quality that would distinguish him from me'.

This felt exoticism is a particularly important affective resource in the age of nation-states, in which each person seems to require a nation and each nation seems to require a distinct culture, just as a census form requires each citizen to have unequivocal designations of gender, race and citizenship. When a curious student asks what the music is like in Togo, our answer fills in just such a designative blank (cf. Weiss, 2014). However useful or accurate the answer may be, it also dissolves the student's curiosity within a totality.

For example, a teacher of a World Music class may feel compelled to lead a student from a conception of Asmahan as a *weird singer* to a *singer with an Arab aesthetic sensibility*. To be sure, this is progress along a certain dimension. It moves our students from a concentric view (radiating out from *us* to progressively more exotic *them*-s) to a top-down global map in which each culture – including, necessarily, one's own – is notionally commensurable. It proceeds, in other words, from totalising ethnocentrism to totalising cultural relativism. From this bird's eye view of spatially bounded cultures, a man in Hanoi is *in Vietnamese culture*; any place and person must fall within boundaries, must have a place in a prefigured global totality. This totalising power need not be limited to nation-states; constituting a voice as 'Westernised', or 'working-class', or 'Latin', or 'folk' evokes a prefigured space of exhaustive alternatives, whether empirically accurate or not (for example, 'folk/classical/primitive/pop'). Any such map – oriented around class, gender, region, religion and so on – already comprehends 'us' and 'them'. It locates any musical utterance, any musician, within a prefigured totality from which there is no escape.

But the situation is not so grim as it might seem. Teaching World Music is not simply an exercise in caging alterity within totalities. Just as often, they are occasions for world-shattering musical encounter: with each other, with a teacher, and, perhaps most strikingly, with visiting masters.

Encountering a master

Encounters with such masters[10] have long been a key resource for ethnomusicologists. Many of us were disciples long before we were scholars, returning to our masters as ethnographers only after many years of training. They seem to differ from ordinary interlocutors; they have a special kind of authority quite apart from any *account* of that authority, such as the one I am about to hazard. Here, I will focus here on the master–student[11] relationships I know best, in the Hindustani vocal tradition. Methodological discussions of these relationships often consider ways in which responsibility to a master might skew ethnography or history away from disinterested, objective reportage (see Katz, 2010, p. 34). These concerns parallel the fascinating problematic of charisma and local truths, which has a long tradition in the social sciences (Faubion, 2011; Weber, 1922/1947; Worsley, 1957). Where an acoustician might see the essence of vocal instruction in vibrating air molecules, where a neuroscientist might see the reinforcement of vocal–neural circuitry, a social scientist tends to see various kinds of mutually constitutive structures of truth and power. It is understandable why the idea of writing from within these power structures would be troubling: if our goal is the constitution of an objective-in-principle, universally valid ethnographic account, we need data, not teaching.

For a disciple, the situation is reversed: I need teaching, not data. I am faced with a musical Other who, as a master, stands outside of my preconceived melodic totalities. Listening to a recording of a lesson after the fact, generating data, transcribing our vocal utterances in monochromatic ink as though they were all made of the same stuff: this is an entirely different kind of activity. Surely, at times, a student may step back and question the master, constituting an odd melodic phrase as data subject to dispute. But the moments of most intense instruction, when a lesson is really cooking, are not moments of assimilating data. Likewise, far more is involved in encountering a master than the complex structures of status, semiosis, and authority (enfolded within a totalising cultural system) that are constituted by a social-scientific mode of inquiry. A different understanding of such a relationship is afforded by a metaphysics of alterity; it begins not perched at a distance observing a system, but sitting face-to-face with a teacher, *sina ba sina*.

Sitting face-to-face, my master sings a phrase, and I strive to sing it again. This striving goes beyond mere sonic imitation. I am called to respond. When my rendition falls dramatically short, he corrects me; when it is close enough, we move on to another phrase so the process can begin again. But even as I learn, even as novel phrases are called forth spontaneously from me, I never *become* him. I never accomplish the task of doing what he does or being what he is. Though rituals mark the beginning of the master–disciple relationship, there is no ritual celebration of a final, completed achievement of sameness. The teaching is *never* accomplished in principle, and thus it always generates movement. As one master once said to me, '*Always* I will tell the student to work harder. The guru can never tell you that you have it right.' One singer recently described to me the process of learning from a master like this: 'It's like the horizon. It keeps moving. You keep on going, but the distance is still there.' The distance between the I and the distant Other generates an unending pull.

The metaphysical distance afforded by master–disciple relationships is the inverse of the metaphysical equivalence afforded by participatory performance (Turino, 2008, p. 34). This distance is not merely (or even necessarily) a qualitative difference in ability or in musical wealth. Just as participatory performance does not depend in principle on everyone being equally competent (Turino, 2008, p. 132), rapport with a master does not require a vast difference in technical skill. It is a perfectly common thing for a young student with a brilliant voice to sit before an older master whose voice is ragged and worn. A student may know compositions unknown to the teacher, may have read more books, may even have performed on stage more often. But sitting face-to-face, the master calls to a student from beyond their comprehension and their expectations. It is in this sense – not a difference of any magnitude – that a teacher is infinitely beyond the student. This is no mere matter of technical competence.

Accomplished musicians whose own teachers are physically absent (in another city, in another country, or even long dead) continue to gaze across this musical distance. It is a routine matter to allow the teacher to come to mind before singing. This relation with an infinitely distant master has the same form as a metaphysical relation with an infinite Other that is, for lack of a better word, often called *music* or *sangeet*. When musicians speak of the ocean of music of which they have understood only a drop, they are not referring to some finite corpus of compositions, *raga*-s or techniques. There is no ratio between one's personal understanding and the vast ocean. To claim that music takes many lifetimes to master is not to claim that five or seventeen or a hundred and eight rebirths will be sufficient. Of course, such claims may, from a social-scientific perspective, be construed as functional performances of humility that grant ethical capital

(Laidlaw, 2013, p. 7). But they are also ways of making a key metaphysical distinction: between the totalising achievement of comprehension and an always-deferred, infinite striving. This distinction becomes especially poignant in the age of mass education in raga music, marked by successive examinations, achievements and certificates of completion. To invoke unfathomable oceans or innumerable lifetimes is to invoke a metaphysics of infinite separation, of a distance that *always* exceeds our attempts to span it, and therefore always calls us towards it. Striving, 'a desire that cannot be satisfied' (Levinas, 1961/1979, p. 34), an infinitely deferred comprehension, is the very condition of a musical metaphysics of alterity.

Of course, not all musical encounters, nor even all teaching, requires sitting face-to-face with another person. And even when we do face each other, visual perception itself is neither sufficient nor necessary. It thus will be necessary to develop Levinas's sense of the *visage* beyond its suggestion of visuality.

Improvisation and the Musical *Visage*

Levinas thematises the constant evasion of comprehension in the *visage*, which is ordinarily translated as 'face'. But we should not confuse the *visage* with the visible surface of the nose, mouth, and cheeks. We certainly should not confuse it with a fixed image of another's face as it might be photographed or imagined to be. If we picture a face at all, we might picture someone rolling their eyes, breaking into laughter, raising an eyebrow or smiling warmly. The *visage* is always in motion as expression, always acting and reacting, freely surging beyond what we thought it was a moment ago. It is 'the way in which the other presents himself, exceeding the [totalising] idea of the other in me'. It 'destroys and overflows the plastic image it leaves me' (Levinas, 1961/1979, pp. 50–51). It is the dynamic play of the metaphysically Other, so that the *saying* of each moment exceeds the *said* that came before.

As a practicing musician, this play of theme and evasion feels to me much like improvisation. It seems to me that the dynamics of the *visage* applies not only to face-to-face conversation, but also to a performance of a *taqsim* that playfully affords a glimpse of an unexpected maqam; to a shifting melodic flow that transcends any particular totalisation; to the kind of turbulent rhythmic carriage that one Hindustani vocalist described to me as 'drunken', a gait 'where no one can tell where he will step next'. Though this is clearest when applied to improvisation, it applies equally well to dynamic performances of composed 'pieces' of music that open texts to *saying*. I think of Bootsy Collins playfully mutating a slippery bass line; of Jon Barlow looking over at me and smiling as he finds a new way through a Chopin nocturne; of Essam Rafea taking an unexpected path to the taslim of a classic *semai;* of Padma Talwalkar brilliantly expanding a Hindustani *bandish.* Certainly any of these pieces may also be performed stiffly, so that they arise as a sequence of tones or a reproduction of a style. We may constitute them as mere material to be recorded and played back by a machine in a recognisable way. We may likewise constitute these unexpected moments as tonal or rhythmic deviations, as 'participatory discrepancies' that invite us to join in (Keil, 1995, p. 2). But we may also encounter the musical *visage* of an ungraspable Other who is never quite what we think, with whom we never quite join. We may hear the moment-to-moment musical play between *said* and *saying*, between totality and infinity, between theme and escape.

Improvisation, in this sense, is not a willful expression of pure, active freedom to exert power as one pleases, free from repressive constraints or responsibilities. Even when I am engaging in 'free' improvisation with others, I need not willfully choose which notes to play, move by reasoned move, like playing chess. Nor must I sink into passive entrainment, allowing the 'charm of rhythm' (Levinas, 1961/1979, p. 203) to absorb me into a larger unity. We may instead hearken to a musical call from beyond the *chez soi*. Just as in speech, the *visage* of the Other addresses us from a great distance. Playing in ensemble calls us to respond without fully comprehending what we are hearing. Responsible musical action – even in the midst of a deep groove – may be called forth from us, as when a friend addresses us, or a stranger asks us for directions. Indeed, many of the freest occasions of free improvisation consist in responding to the musical demands of the moment. To respond in this sense is not to obey explicit commands (say, from an orchestral conductor or a square dance caller), nor to meld into a collectivity (where each and all is implicitly understood), but to answer to a call never fully understood, reaching us from outside ourselves.

Powers of empathy, powers of participation

Having outlined a musical metaphysics founded in alterity rather than unity, we can return to our original questions about participation and shared feeling from a different perspective. What do we make of musical empathy, of entrainment, of the realm of *einfühlung* and *einsfühlung*, of *tonglen*, of *hamdardi*, of spontaneously feeling for another as for oneself? Can we encounter another's need as an immediate heartfelt resonance, rather than as some perplexing call from a distant Other? Indeed, *we can* do this – it is very much within our powers. The full accomplishment of musical empathy, whereby we are fully joined together in a single feeling, subsumes the I and the Other. It delivers us from the incomprehensibility of the *visage* to the certainty of connection that 'seems to exclude any possibility of duplicity' (Turino, 2008, p. 136) leaving us instead with a completed unity.

As the other chapters in this volume make clear, the formation of these unities is a perfectly ordinary and widely attested human capacity. From polka parties to the 'muscular bonding' (McNeill, 1995) of military drills, fellow-feeling is all around us. Edith Stein, the phenomenologist of empathy *par excellence*, vividly describes the ways in which a 'we' may emerge as a 'subject of a higher grade [*Stufe*]' than the *I* and the *you*, so that we become suffused with feeling 'as members of a community' [*als Glieder dieser Gemeinschaft*] rather than as separate individuals (Stein, 1917/1964, p. 17). To be sure, this is the mode of feeling that enables musical ensemble. It also is the mode of feeling that enables the solidarities of coordinated violence. There's nothing deviant or fallen or unnatural about it: there is suggestive evidence that empathic action understanding is shared with several species of primates (Iacoboni, 2009) along with fear, pleasure and aggression. The power of a rhythmically flexible orchestra, the power of a tight marching band, the power of a platoon of soldiers in step, the power of thousands of voices chanting slogans in unison – all of these have political and moral implications far beyond their undeniable pleasures.

Surely, we all have felt music taking us 'into deep identification, total participation, and past the logical contradictions of separation of the other' so that 'you now *are* the other, or the other is *in* you' (Keil & Feld, 1994, p. 168). But where a metaphysics of unity sees this identification as a praiseworthy return to a primordial state of oneness, a metaphysics of alterity attends to what is lost when radical separation melts into a comprehensive, finite unity, where 'the subject not only sees the other, but is the other' (Levinas, 1947/1987, p. 43). Fully accomplished, as a form of unifying comprehension, empathy does not hearken beyond the reach of the Same, but extends its dominion. Just as an electronic guitar tuner enables certain kinds of intonation, empathy enables certain kinds of ensemble, pulling individuals into unity, reaffirming the warm embrace of an extended, über-empathetic 'we'. In winking reference to Lucien Levy-Bruhl's account of participatory mentality among 'primitives', Levinas warns, cryptically, that 'a modern consciousness, at least, could not abdicate its secrecy and solitude at so little cost' (Levinas, 1947/1987, p. 43).

But what is this modern consciousness, and what is this solitude that participation calls us to give up? Is it an alienated, egotistical individualism produced by capitalism, propagated by 'power-tripping, control-over people still trapped inside civilization' (Keil, 1995, p. 4), which suppresses an ancient, morally correct regime of fellow-feeling? Is it radical alterity, the necessary condition of ethics, gentleness and responsibility, which hearkens to the call of a free Other outside the totality of the Same? Must feeling-for-others always exclude the possibility of letting others feel for themselves? Might there be modes of empathic striving that proceed through the infinite play of rapport with an unknowable stranger, rather than towards a perfected comprehension? This would seem to be the import of Stein's distinction between *Einfühlen* (empathy) and *Einsfühlen* (a feeling of oneness.) Levinas himself founds his metaphysics on a desire that 'is like goodness – the Desired does not fulfil it, but deepens it', of a mode of encounter that 'is not the disappearance of distance, not a bringing together [*rapprochement*] ... [but] a relationship [*rapport*] whose positivity comes from remoteness, from separation, for it nourishes itself, one might say, with its hunger' (Levinas, 1961/1979, p. 34).

For now, we too remain hungry in the face of these questions. If we have learned anything about alterity, if we have learned anything from the infinite play of musicking, we will be glad to defer the satisfactions of conceptual perfection. Even carving up the world into unity and alterity, after all, is a way of totalising. For my part, I do not intend to renounce the participatory pleasures of dancing *dabke* or singing sacred harp music; I certainly cannot renounce the powers of empathy that make ensemble possible. But a critical consideration of the metaphysics of alterity and unity should help us to feel through these potent musical technologies without conflating power or pleasure with moral righteousness. In this spirit, the questions raised here will be most fruitfully addressed not as problems waiting for solutions to be *said*, but as provocations to *saying*, in the uncertainty of face-to-face conversations and other performances.

Acknowledgements

This chapter has benefitted greatly from critique and inspiration in conversation with colleagues. While taking full responsibility for the shortcomings in this account, I thank the following for their generous provocations: Anaïs Nony, Bruno Chaouat, Michael Gallope, Jonathan Weidenbaum, Jenna Rice and Deniz Peters. I dedicate this chapter to the memory of Jon K. Barlow and Johnny (Way-sa-quo-nabe) Smith, both of whom passed away while it was in preparation.

Notes

1 There are other anthropological precedents as well, as when Alfred Radcliffe-Brown (1922/2013) affirms that 'dancing is a means of uniting individuals into a harmonious whole' (p. 253).
2 The claim here is *not* that Keil, Feld, Turino, or anyone else is explicitly or consistently committed to a metaphysics of unity in all of their work. Rather, I am claiming that this metaphysical orientation (even if adopted provisionally or implicitly) makes the moral stakes of participation appear obvious and closed to critique. For example, Turino's occasional descriptions of 'transcendent' (2014, p. 208, p. 212) experiences of pure Being, analogous to exalted meditative states available to Buddhist adepts (Turino, 2012), are enabled by his creative reorientation of Charles Sanders Peirce's semiotics towards primordial Firstness (pure, unitary Being without a second.) Thus, in such moments, 'the in-and-of-itself character of a First' leads him 'to identify it with "the real"' (Turino, 2014, p. 191). At other moments, however, his nuanced account of the musical 'balancing' of Firstness, Secondness and Thirdness would seem to work against the axiomatic primacy of unity and connection – and therefore participation – at expense of all else (Turino, 2014, p. 213).
3 Alterity and unity are by no means the only possibilities; nor by any means am I suggesting that we swear eternal allegiance to either.
4 Though it's tempting to regard unity and alterity to be characteristic cultural orientations, each bound to a certain time and place (encouraged, perhaps, by Jacques Derrida's construal of Levinas as a Judaic alternative to the Greek tradition (1967/1978), this interpretive habit would obscure more than it would reveal. As noted, representatives of unity and alterity can be found in a range of philosophical and contemplative traditions. I focus here on two of Levinas's early works, *Time and the other* (1947/1987) and *Totality and infinity* (1961/1979), in part because his later works become more closely entangled with his Talmudic readings, and I do not feel I have the spiritual authority to address them fulsomely here. But if the reader is tempted to attribute Levinas's insistence on the primacy of alterity to his Judaic intellectual heritage, one well-known counterexample can be found in the legendary panenthetic mystical tradition of the Baal Shem Tov.
5 I have adopted Jonathan Weidenbaum's handy terms here, in accordance with the loose sense of metaphysics widely used in English – an account of the fundamental conditions of existence prior to (and constitutive of) empirical evidence. Levinas

himself, however, uses the term *métaphysique* with somewhat more specificity: in reference to relation with a transcendental Other, always 'turned toward the "elsewhere" and the "otherwise" and the "other"' (1961/1979, p. 33). Levinas considers what Weidenbaum calls the *metaphysics of unity* (particularly as developed in Heidegger), to be a kind of totalising ontology that privileges Being – but only an orientation to alterity to be worthy of the name *la métaphysique*.

6 Part of why these two concepts are easily confused is that they look identical in print – both take variants of the common word 'other' as a key term, often set apart from its standard meaning with a captial O and the Gallic definite article: '*the* Other'. To make matters more confusing, both traditions were inaugurated in books which had basically the same title: Levinas's *Le temps et l'autre* (1945) and Johannes Fabian's *Time and the other* (1983), though Fabian specifically disavows any connection (2006). A depiction of my *oud*-playing cousin as a token of timeless Oriental culture thus could be critiqued in apparently contradictory terms: (after Fabian) as reducing a co-eval contemporary to a fictional other through representation – *or* (after Levinas) as reducing an Other to a mere object of comprehension.

7 It seems almost certain that Levinas's experiences as a prisoner of the Nazis informed his later philosophical concern with the moral consequences of unfettered totalising. His construal of Martin Heidegger's ontology, in which the assimilating work of Being functions as 'the imperialism of the Same' (not just totalising but totalitarian) might thus appear to require our allegiance in principle. But as illuminating as these biographical considerations might be, they are not sufficient reason to follow (or not follow) his lead. Just as the equation of Heidegger with Nazism fails to account for the divergent paths of thought that emerge from *Sein und Zeit* (including ardent anti-fascists like Hannah Arendt, Jean-Paul Sartre, and Levinas himself), Levinas's own various political commitments (for instance, his struggle against the Nazis in the 1940s, his Zionist apologetics in the 1970s, his 'Third-World decolonialism' in the 1980s) are only a few possible (and by no means necessary) paths to follow from an 'ethics of ethics' founded in alterity (cf. el-Bizri, 2006; Slabodsky, 2010). The sketches of musical alterity I present here should neither be taken as a series of propositions that must follow logically from a set of political axioms (*Alterity is true because not-imperialism!*) nor a system of axioms that must imply certain political imperatives (*Alterity is false because not-Zionism!*) I would hope instead that a careful consideration of alterity and unity might lead us beyond the comforts of slogans, the politics of exclusion, and State-centered political axiomatics.

8 Jeff Warren masterfully addresses Levinas's peculiar ambivalence towards music (2013, pp. 148–157). Levinas himself claimed to be an '*idiot en musique*' (Levinas in Warren, 2013, p. 148), and indeed tended to regard music rather narrowly as a matter of fixed composition, doomed to repetition despite its illusion of novelty, 'covering up the breach of otherness' (p. 150). I add to this Levinas's tendency to consider music categorically as 'art', and thus 'as "devotion" to the Neoplatonic ideal of the One' (1991/1998, p. 184). Despite his support for his son, composer Michaël Levinas (a student of Olivier Messiaen), the elder Levinas nonetheless tended to affect an ignorance of musical *action*. Warren's current work on musical life in the Levinas household should further illuminate these questions.

9 *Totalité et Infini* uses the phenomenological resources of *Sein und Zeit* both to foreground the limits of Being and to point beyond. The *chez soi* is already Being-in-the-World, already involved, already participatory. Levinas's point is that there is something beyond this. Though there is no evidence of Levinas having encountered Owen Barfield's work, Barfield's own account of participation between self and world in *Saving the appearances*– an important part of the ethnomusicological inheritance of 'participation' – bears close comparison to Heidegger's account of *In-der-Welt-sein* (see Terry Hipolito's *Before the new criticism* for more on the connections between Barfield and Heidegger).

10 This account is informed by my relationships with three masters in particular. In Delhi, L. K. Pandit (my music guru); in Minnesota, Johnny (Way-sa-quo-nabe) Smith (Ojibwa keeper of the drum); and in Connecticut, Jon K. Barlow (speculative music theorist).

11 The master–student dyad I am describing here (which typically stretches over many years of intensive training) is variously called *ustad-shagird* or *guru-shishya* in Hindustani languages. The lineage structures thus formed, if not actually congruent with blood relations, often take the form of virtual families. I have not explored here Levinas's subtle consideration of the special forms of alterity that obtains between parents and children (1961/1979, p. 278), though it may be relevant.

References

Adorno, T. W. (1941). On popular music. *Studies in Philosophy and Social Science, 9*(1), 17–48.

Barfield, O. (1957/1965). *Saving the appearances: A study in idolatry*. New York: Harcourt, Brace and World.

Barfield, O. (1977). *The rediscovery of meaning and other essays*. Middletown, CT: Wesleyan University Press.

Berman, R., & Braga, B. (1995). *Star Trek: First contact*. First Draft, September 1995.

el-Bizri, N. (2006). Uneasy interrogations following Levinas. *Studia Phaenomenologica, 6*, 293–315.

Cobussen, M., & Nielsen, N. (2012). *Music and ethics*. Aldershot: Ashgate.

Derrida, J. (1967/1978). Violence and metaphysics: An essay on the thought of Emmanuel Levinas. In his *Writing and Difference* (pp. 97–192) (A. Bass, Trans.). London: Routledge.

Ede, S. (1997). Foreword. In A. Everitt, *Joining in: An investigation into participatory music*. London: Calouste Gulbenkian Foundation.

Fabian, J. (1983). *Time and the other: How anthropology makes its object*. New York: Columbia University Press.

Fabian, J. (2006). The other revisited: Critical afterthoughts. *Anthropological Theory, 6*(2), 139–152.

Faubion, J. (2011). *An anthropology of ethics*. Cambridge: Cambridge University Press.

Feld, S. (1988). Aesthetics as iconicity of style, or 'lift-up-over-sounding': Getting into the Kaluli groove. *Yearbook for Traditional Music, 20*, 74–113.

Gupta, A., & Ferguson, J. (1992). Beyond culture. *Cultural Anthropology, 7*(1), 6–23.

Hipolito, T. (1993). Before the new criticism: Barfield's *Poetic Diction* in context. *Renascence, 46*(1), 3–38.

Iacoboni, M. (2009). Imitation, empathy, and mirror neurons. *Annual Review of Psychology, 60*, 653–70.

Katz, M. (2010). *Hindustani music history and the politics of theory* (Unpublished doctoral dissertation). University of California, Santa Barbara, USA.

Keil, C. (1987). Participatory discrepancies and the power of music. *Cultural Anthropology, 2*(3), 275–283.

Keil, C. (1995). The theory of participatory discrepancies: A progress report. *Ethnomusicology, 39*(1), 1–19.

Keil, C., & Feld, S. (1994). Grooving on participation. In *Music grooves: essays and dialogues* (pp. 151–180). Chicago, IL: University of Chicago Press.

Laidlaw, J. (2013). *The subject of virtue: An anthropology of ethics and freedom*. Cambridge: Cambridge University Press.

Levinas, E. (1945). *Le temps et l'autre.* Paris: Presses Universitaires de France.

Levinas, E. (1947/1987). *Time and the other.* Pittsburgh, PA: Duquesne University Press.

Levinas, E. (1961/1979). *Totality and infinity: An essay on exteriority.* The Hague: Martinus Nijhoff.

Levinas, E. (1991/1998). *Entre nous: On thinking-of-the-other.* New York: Columbia University Press.

Levy-Bruhl, L. (1910/1926). *How natives think.* New York: Washington Square Press.

Lomax, A. (1972). An appeal for cultural equity. *Journal of Communication, 27*(2), 125–138.

McNeill, W. (1995). *Keeping together in time: Dance and drill in human history.* Cambridge, MA: Harvard University Press.

Odam, G. (1995/2001). *The sounding symbol: Music education in action.* Cheltenham: Nelson Thornes, Ltd.

Radcliffe-Brown, A. R. (1922/2013). *The Andaman islanders.* Cambridge: Cambridge University Press.

Said, E. (1979). *Orientalism.* London: Routledge & Keegan Paul.

Slabodsky, S. (2010). Emmanuel Levinas's geopolitics: Overlooked conversations between Rabbinical and third world decolonialisms. *Journal of Jewish Thought and Philosophy, 18*(2), 147–165.

Stein, E. (1917/1964). *On the problem of empathy.* Trans. W. Stein. The Hague: Martinus Nijhoff.

Taylor, N. (2014). Thinking, language and learning in initial teacher education. *Studies in Philosophy and* Education, *25*, 175–190.

Turino, T. (2008). *Music as social life: The politics of participation.* Chicago, IL: University of Chicago Press.

Turino, T. (2012). Peircean phenomenology and musical experience. *Karpa* 5.1–5.2.

Turino, T. (2014). Peircean thought as core theory for a phenomenological ethnomusicology. *Ethnomusicology, 58*(2), 185–221.

Warren, J. (2014). *Music and ethical responsibility.* Cambridge: Cambridge University Press.

Weber, M. (1922/1947). *The theory of social and economic organization.* New York: Simon & Schuster.

Weidenbaum, J. (2013, 28–31 July). The metaphysics of alterity and unity: Levinas and perennialism. Paper presented at the 8th Annual Meeting of the North American Levinas Society, Duquesne University, Pittsburgh, PA.

Weiss, S. (2014). Listening to the world but hearing ourselves: Hybridity and perceptions of authenticity in world music. *Ethnomusicology, 58*(3), 506–525.

Worsley, P. (1957). *The trumpet shall sound: A study of 'cargo' cults in Melanesia.* London: MacGibbon & Kee.

8   In dub conference

Empathy, groove and technology in Jamaican popular music

Rowan Oliver

Groove is usually conceptualised as a phenomenon that arises in the context of musical performance. As such, researchers have primarily examined groove from the perspectives of rhythm and microtiming, typically drawing on examples from jazz and funk as case studies within which to explore the rhythmic interrelationships that exist between instrumentalists.[1] More recently, the role which timbre plays in groove has also begun to be explored, using the interrelationships between timbrally distinct instrumental voices as a focus.[2] Both the temporal and the timbral relationships that contribute to groove rely on a multilayered, shared understanding between musicians, not only in terms of the way that they play together but also how their collective sound fits within – or outside – stylistic conventions.

This chapter will discuss empathic aspects of the way that groove occurs in Jamaican popular music (hereafter 'JPM'), focusing initially on the stylistically specific relationship between the drums and the bass (as well as other instruments in the ensemble). The scope is then broadened to include the ways in which groove changes when a dub mix of a pre-existing recording (known as a 'riddim' in the terminology of JPM) is created. By taking Christopher Small's (1998) ideas around musicking into account, the empathic understanding that exists between instrumentalists can be extended to include the relationship between performers and listeners, whether in the context of live performance or recorded music. This way of thinking is relevant when considering the impact that the dub mixer's subsequent actions have on the original groove that is encapsulated in a given riddim. In dub reggae, the sound engineer who creates the dub mix can thus be seen as a vital musicking participant in the distinctive construction of groove, a participant whose empathic relationships – both with other musicians and also stylistic convention – are akin to those found amongst instrumentalists, but which additionally incorporate a significant technological dimension.

Much of the research that underpins this chapter was carried out at the Center for Black Music Research (CBMR), specifically amidst the wealth of interviews contained in the *Kenneth M. Bilby oral history collection on foundations of Jamaican popular music* that is housed there. Some years ago, Kenneth Bilby – an eminent ethnomusicologist and leading authority on the fruitful intersection between traditional and popular music in Jamaica, amongst other things – realised that not only had the voices of reggae session musicians been conspicuously absent from accounts of the genre, but also that since many of these individuals were growing old there was a consequent risk that their stories may never be recorded for posterity. In response to this scenario, he set about the Herculean task of locating and interviewing as many of these musicians as possible, in order to gather together the first-hand accounts of their crucial involvement in the island's musical development. The collected interviews provide a rich and revealing counter-narrative to the perspectives presented in those more frequently reiterated histories of JPM, which tend to centre around either superstars such as Bob Marley or industry entrepreneurs such as producer Clement 'Sir Coxsone' Dodd.

Feeling in reggae

Before discussing specific recordings as a way to illustrate groove empathy at work in JPM, it is first necessary to consider the extent to which it might be appropriate to characterise the interaction between grooving reggae musicians as having an empathic dimension. Amidst the various (sometimes conflicting) conceptualisations of empathy, there is a broad consensus that it involves the ability to share and understand someone else's feelings while still maintaining a clear sense of self and other.[3] While this can be seen to apply readily to such broad emotional states as sadness, elation or terror, for example, the feeling which reggae musicians have the ability to share with one another is rather less clear-cut and does not even have a name, as such. Nevertheless, 'feeling' and similar, related terms are mentioned or alluded to frequently throughout the interviews conducted by Bilby, as the following extracts illustrate.

Terminologically, the use of the word 'feeling' in this context could be seen to carry associations with the idea of 'feel' in music, a concept that overlaps with, and is sometimes used interchangeably for, 'groove'. 'Feel' is usually used specifically to denote an individual's use of rhythmic nuance in performance though, so a particular instrumentalist's feel results from the characteristic way in which they interpret musical time in their playing. Other musicians participating in the same performance may choose (consciously or otherwise) to align their own timing as closely as possible to this individual's feel via the process of entrainment.[4] As mentioned earlier, however, 'groove' relates to more than simply the temporal aspects of performance, and is more of a multifaceted concept that has been interpreted in numerous, diverse ways by a range of scholars; in effect, feel is one aspect of groove, rather than being an equivalent, interchangeable concept.

Discussing his experience as a session musician in Jamaica, drummer Paul Douglas provides the following point of view: 'Music is a *feeling*. It's like, if I'm playing a groove and you – as the keyboard player – decide to do something else then it's going to influence everyone' (Bilby, 2010). Douglas's statement contains some revealing points; first, he goes beyond the idea that music is an abstract force that either inspires or results from feelings, instead suggesting that music *is* a feeling, and thereby providing a pertinent perspective in the context of this volume. He then draws attention to the multifaceted nature of groove, initially using the term as a noun that describes his individual performance (that is, the drum pattern he has constructed, as it is delivered with personal nuances of timing, dynamics, timbre and so on) but also hinting at the idea of groove as a participatory process that occurs between musicians when they play together. This notion of music as a participatory process is fundamental to Small's writing on the concept of musicking, in which he argues convincingly that 'music is not a thing at all but an activity, something that people do' (Small, 1998, p. 2).

Keyboardist Robert 'Robbie' Lyn describes the typically collaborative approach to composition taken in the recording studio by reggae musicians. He recalls occasions when, for example, the bassist might 'tell the guitarist or keyboard player 'Give me a bassline, because right now I'm not *feeling* this song' or something like that. So it's teamwork' (Bilby, 2010). Lyn alludes, here, to the pressure experienced by musicians working in this context, who were constantly working against the clock, at the behest of the producer, in order to record as much material as possible in the time available. In terms of empathy, however, Lyn's comment reveals an additional empathic dimension to the groove process in a JPM recording session: not only do the musicians need to empathise with one another in order to groove effectively, they must also empathise with the song itself. This idea is explored in more detail later.

In his interview with Cedric Myton, singer with The Congos, Bilby asks whether he has a favourite track on the band's seminal *Heart Of The Congos* (1977) album. The following exchange ensues:

MYTON: The one I would give an edge, really, is 'Congoman'.
BILBY: In terms of the sound?
MYTON: In terms of the *feelings* I get when I'm singing that song.

(Bilby, 2010)

It could be, of course, that Myton's emotional response to the song stems from its lyrical content or, perhaps, from extramusical associations, such as his memories of the context in which it was written, for example. The turn of phrase he uses to describe the response, however, suggests that his empathic link with the music is derived specifically from the process of performing this particular song. This partly echoes the view – as expressed by Lyn in the previous quote – that musicians can empathise with a song and that such empathy simultaneously inspires and results from their performance of the material.

Summing up the connection between feeling and music in JPM in an almost offhand manner, legendary guitarist Ernest Ranglin proposes that 'all this thing is just a *feel*, you know. It's a *feel*. So that's what happens all the time. [The session musicians] come up with their *feel* and it sounds good, so that's it' (Bilby, 2010). As with Douglas's flexible use of the concept of groove to denote both the music performed and the process of performing (discussed above), Ranglin seems here to use the term 'feel' interchangeably, so that it describes not only the characteristic nuances within a musician's performance ('their feel'), but also an underlying feeling associated with either a given song or, perhaps, JPM more broadly ('all this thing is just a feel'). Ultimately, Ranglin implies that by empathising with the song, with the genre and with one another, the musicians are able to spontaneously create a stylistically effective arrangement during the recording session.

By way of an appropriate preamble to the discussion of music examples that follows later (which focuses on the rhythm section's use of empathy and groove), this section concludes with an interview extract that relates specifically to feeling and the role of the bassist. Max Romeo, while a vocalist himself, talks here about working with the eminent bassist Aston 'Family Man' Barrett, underlining the empathic musicking that must initially flow from the rhythm section and then amongst the whole band in order for a JPM recording session to succeed:

BILBY: So you would sit down with Family Man and you would just hum your bassline to him, and then he would develop on it.
[Romeo sings some basslines to illustrate this process in action.]

BILBY: And then would you have to approve what he does before you can go to record it?

ROMEO: Well when you're *vibing* something there is no approval. You just *vibe*, and then at the end of the day you listen to the outcome. It might be perfect or you might have to put it back on the drawing board. But it's different from classical music where you're reading off paper. You're reading the mind. It's a *vibe*. It's coming from within, so you just let it flow.

BILBY: And when you're *vibing* like that, pretty much, at the end of the day if things click, everybody knows it, right?

ROMEO: Everybody knows it. You just *feel* it.

(Bilby, 2010)

Romeo's words here emphasise, once again, the themes that have emerged throughout the preceding interview extracts. His use of the terms 'vibe' and 'vibing' can be added to the list of noun–verb pairings that are relevant to the discussion: feel/feeling, groove/grooving and music/musicking.

Two processes of empathy

The interview extracts above suggest that there may be at least two different – but related – processes of empathy at play simultaneously during a reggae recording session, and that each occurs in relation to a different subject. The first, more abstract process of empathy occurs when the musicians seem to empathise with the song itself; indeed, the interviewed musicians often talk about *feeling* the song, mostly discussing this in terms of whether they do or do not feel it, and what consequent effect this has on their creative approach in the studio. In my previous work on groove, I have noted the significance of a contextual sense of musical time in enabling various musicking participants (instrumentalists, listeners, dancers and so on) to share in grooving (Oliver, 2013). There are various ways that this contextual sense of time can manifest itself – it might be, for example, a stylistically specific timeline such as the Cuban *clave*, an adapted count-in by the bandleader or an isochronous pulse with genre-dependent accents – but the point, throughout all of these examples, is that knowledge of the context informs the way that individuals participate in the groove.

It seems, in reggae, that musicians perceive the song as having its own feeling, and that an understanding of this allows them to perform in ways which are empathically attuned and therefore appropriate. In this context, then, the term 'feeling' does not seem to simply mean the particular emotional state described by the lyrics (although this is likely to be one of several contributing factors), but is, rather, less figurative. Although its effect is not limited to the rhythmic aspects of performance, the way that the song's feeling impacts on the recording session can perhaps be compared to the way that some seemingly more abstract contextual senses of musical time inform groove in performance. The implicit *clave* which Amira and Cornelius (1992) identify in Cuban *batá* drum ensemble performance, for example, can dictate the performance choices made by instrumentalists yet without actually being explicitly sounded by a specific instrument with a time-keeping role; shared knowledge allows the drummers to play in response to the abstract, implicit *clave* and thus its nature is revealed in the sounded, explicit performance. In the case of JPM, the song has an abstract feeling, and the musicians must empathically relate to this feeling in order to perform in ways that will subsequently reveal it to the listener.

This first process of empathy occurs, then, between a musician who is performing and the song that is being performed, but is based on something abstract which exists – at least partly – prior to the performance itself. The second process of empathy, which is the focus of the case studies that follow later in this chapter, occurs between the musicians themselves, dictating and supporting their musical interactions. The two processes of empathy described above therefore enjoy an intriguingly interdependent relationship: the musicians must feel the song in order to perform it, but while revealing this implicit feeling through their performance they must simultaneously empathise with one another's playing, so that 'things click' and 'everybody knows it', to reiterate Max Romeo's summarisation of the processes in action (Bilby, 2010). The combined outworking of these two connected processes of empathy results in the performed version of the song, whose multiple empathic layers are captured via the recording process.

The empathic rhythm section

In his earlier work on the effect of traditional Rastafarian music on the development of popular idioms in Jamaica, Bilby observes that this influence 'helped to promote rhythmic experimentation and led to an expansion of musical space; individual instruments were now free to play a greater variety of rhythmic patterns and began to function more like the interlocking parts of an African drum ensemble' (Bilby, 1995, p. 166).[5] It can, of course, be assumed that when two or more musicians perform simultaneously they will generally strive to create a sense of togetherness and cohesion. Typically, this aim is evident in the extent to which the various parts within an ensemble succeed in achieving rhythmic alignment, but it can also be seen, for example, in the way that a group of singers adapt their vocal production so as to create a timbrally pleasing blend, or in an orchestral violin section's uniformity of phrasing. Bilby's comparison, however, between African musical tendencies and the newfound combination of individual freedom and corporate togetherness which developed in reggae, in response to Rasta influence, seems to have been carefully selected: presumably, this is partly because of the way that some musical developments in the Caribbean inevitably reflect African aspects of the region's cultural heritage, but it also suggests that the degree to which such 'interlocking' is musically significant transcends the standard sense of togetherness to which performance practice elsewhere typically aspires. Michael Veal concurs, noting that reggae 'is a dance music of West African heritage constructed as a web of interlocking parts' (Veal, 2007, p. 70). He goes on to describe the way in which dub mixing subsequently disrupts this interlocking structure by removing its constituent parts at various (often unpredictable) points.

Writing about the *Gahu* drumming tradition in West Africa, David Locke describes the music as 'a beautifully integrated polyphonic whole. Each part asserts its musical character but remains sufficiently stable to be influenced by the others' (Locke, 1987, p. 7). He goes on to describe the percussion ensemble as 'interactive, a feedback network in which instruments 'talk' to each other in all combinations' (Locke, 1987, p. 7). While Locke is specifically describing *Gahu* music, his words also seem highly applicable to the interlocking, interactive approach to ensemble playing found in the JPM tradition, as described in various ways by the reggae musicians interviewed; Bilby's comparison between these traditions is supported by Locke's statements

In his interview, Sly Dunbar underlines the importance of the drummer's role to the grooving process in a JPM recording session: 'Once you [as the drummer] start feeling that groove, *everybody* starts feeling it!' (Bilby, 2010). This viewpoint parallels Lyn's earlier comment about feeling the song, but reframes the idea from the perspective of the rhythm section; here, it is the groove, specifically, which needs to be felt. By working empathically with the groove, Dunbar contributes to the overall feeling that is embodied in the song, which the other musicians will share during the recording, and which the listener will subsequently participate in too.

This idea indicates that there is a causal chain of empathy in some recording session scenarios, in which the drummer (or, potentially, another instrumentalist) feels the song's groove first and then acts as a kind of empathic conduit, an intermediary through whom this groove is communicated to the other musicians. In another extract from the same interview, Dunbar puts forward the idea that the listener should be able to feel the music from the drums alone, without any other instrumentation. While his meaning here relates primarily to the recording session context, he also talks about people being able to dance to the drums alone, suggesting that the listener is another category of musicking participant who might benefit from feeling the music via the drummer's role as an empathic conduit. There is, it seems, a difference between just 'the feel of the music' and being able to 'feel the music'; the latter (as expressed in Dunbar's interview) is more suggestive of empathy at work.[6]

In another section of his interview with Bilby, Robert Lyn talks about the way in which a bassist might then respond to the feeling that the drummer has tapped into, and which is consequently being transmitted to the other musicians:

> Sometimes there's no need for any great bassline, you just need something to ride the rhythm. Sometimes it depends on how the drummer is feeling the song, [or on] where the kick drum is. The bass fills in the space or accentuates how the drummer plays.
>
> (Bilby, 2010)

In this scenario, the bassist responds empathically to the song's groove – as the drummer communicates it in real time – and can choose to either 'fill the space' in it, by playing a line that will interlock with the drum pattern, or to 'accentuate' it, by playing something which aligns with the main drum strokes. (In fact, a bassline is likely to alternate between interlocking and aligning with the drum strokes at various points within a cyclical pattern.)

Aston 'Family Man' Barrett talks about playing melodic basslines which 'let the singer get to swing and flow with the rhythm, and give the drummer that space … to drop. To feel it on the one drop!' (Bilby, 2010). This view highlights the centrality of the bassline to the way that arrangements are structured in JPM: the bass provides a rhythmic springboard for the vocalist while also interlocking with the drummer's playing. The 'one drop' is a distinctive drum pattern associated with much JPM, but reggae in particular, in which the kick drum and snare drum (typically played using a 'side-stick' stroke) are both struck on beat three of the bar. An aesthetically desirable consequence of this approach to patterning is that it creates a considerable amount of space in these drum voices elsewhere in the bar. Such space provides ample opportunity, of course, for the bassist to create lines that will interlock with the drumming. In the following section, I discuss ways that such approaches to patterning, as well as other aspects of performance, are used in groove.

Groove factors

In my research dealing with funk breakbeats (Oliver, 2015) it was necessary to find a way of thinking about groove that could bring together several genres in which breakbeats occur, in order to consider the various ways that musicians (whether instrumentalists or producers) engage with these groovy fragments of drumming. This required a conceptual framework that could accommodate not only the characteristic ways that drummers use nuances of performance in the original funk recordings, but also the range of digital manipulation techniques employed by hip hop and jungle producers when they subsequently sample the breakbeats and recontextualise them into new tracks. Although the practicalities and processes involved in grooving are different for these two groups of musicians, they both, essentially, use techniques that enable them to introduce a range of characteristic nuances to a recorded performance: for drummers, these nuances are introduced primarily by real-time variation in instrumental technique (although instrument design, set-up and tuning, and studio production processes are also contributing factors), whereas, for sampling producers, the nuances are introduced by digital manipulation of the original performance (typically years, or even decades, after the drummer's playing was actually recorded).

I describe this group of variable aspects of performance and production as 'groove factors', and selected inter-onset intervals, patterning, displacement, ghost notes, phrasing/articulation and timbre as the groove factors that seemed most pertinent in my study of breakbeats. In brief, inter-onset intervals are the timespans between the start of each successively sounded note; patterning concerns the grouping of notes within (and between) instrumental voices; displacement occurs when an established pattern is moved to a new beat location in relation to the track's underlying pulse; and ghost notes are light, unaccented notes (typically snare drum strokes) with which funk drummers embellish their drum patterns and whose use, Greenwald notes, 'adds depth to the groove' (2002, p. 261). The remaining groove factors (phrasing/articulation and timbre) are self-explanatory, though their significance in determining groove has sometimes been overlooked by scholars, who have tended to focus primarily on temporal aspects instead.

While these groove factors were initially conceived as a framework within which to assess breakbeats in funk, hip hop and jungle, they can also be usefully applied to the musical context discussed in this chapter; the empathic responses of the rhythm section in a JPM recording session (both to one another and to the song itself) will be manifested in variation of the same groove factors, as will the subsequent actions of the dub mixer. As the track analyses in the following section show, those groove factors that prove most significant differ somewhat in each case.

Empathy and groove in action

The tracks which are analysed in this section are presented in a logical order: in the first, the role of the bass is unchanging, so the focus is on groove factors in the drum voice; in the second, there is variation in both parts; and in the third, it is the dub mixer who uses variation in groove factors to alter aspects of the same track used for the preceding analysis. In the case of all the tracks discussed, various versions of the same original recording have been released, as is common (indeed, fundamental) practice within the Jamaican music industry.[7] This 'versioning' strategy is useful for the purposes of rhythm section analysis, because the detailed nuances in particular instrumental voices which can often be obscured in the full mix are sometimes more clearly revealed in alternative versions, particularly when the deconstructive techniques of dub mixing have been applied. Thus, a single recorded performance of a piece of music has been released by Augustus Pablo – in a range of differently mixed and, therefore, distinct alternative versions – as tracks called 'Rocker's Dub' (1979), 'Frozen Dub' (1976), and 'Hot Dub' (197X).[8,9] While, for the sake of brevity, I simply refer to my first case study as 'Rocker's Dub' for example, the discussion of the rhythm section's performance applies equally to all three of these releases, since they are all mixed from the same master recording.

As Table 8.1 shows, the bassist's performance in 'Rocker's Dub' is very straightforward: only three two-bar patterns are used in total, and these are played as an asymmetrical cyclical sequence across the duration of the track. Rhythmically, all three patterns are identical, as is the phrasing that the bassist employs, so it is only the harmony that shifts from one pattern to the next.

In terms of the other groove factors within the bass part, there is little variation in timbre, no use of ghost notes or the rhythmic displacement technique, and only minimal, stylistically appropriate discrepancies of timing in relation to the tempo (which is 136 beats-per-minute, on average, though some listeners might interpret this as an implied half-time feel of 68 beats-per-minute). In other words, the bassist here provides a solid, virtually unchanging performance as a foundation upon which the drummer can build a series of interlocking variations.

Throughout 'Rocker's Dub', the drum pattern is based on variations of the 'one drop' pattern mentioned in Barrett's interview, as described earlier. Table 8.2 lists the pattern variations found in the first 38-bar section of the track and indicates the frequency with which each occurs. The drummer uses 14 distinct variations during this section alone, which could seem an unusually high number (given the common misconception that this instrument's role tends to vary very little once the main pattern has been established) but is simply the result of his nuanced alteration of the groove factors.

As Table 8.2 shows, the 'one drop' occurs in a range of instrumental voicings, using just a kick drum stroke (Pattern 1), a composite kick-plus-snare drum stroke (Pattern 2) or just a snare drum stroke (Pattern 3). The standard drum kit incorporates instruments whose timbres contrast significantly with one another; by varying the way the 'one drop' is distributed around the drum kit, the drummer here achieves timbrally contrasting iterations of the same basic pattern without needing to alter any other groove factors. Instrumental technique is used

Table 8.1 Bass structure in 'Rocker's Dub'.

Bars	Bass Pattern	Harmony	
1–30	A	D major – E minor	Table 8.2 focuses
31–36	B	B minor – A major	on this 38-bar
37–38	C	F# minor – A major	section
39–58	A	D major – E minor	
59–64	B	B minor – A major	
65–66	C	F# minor – A major	
67–89 (fades out)	A	D major – E minor	

Table 8.2 Drum pattern variations in bars 1–38 of 'Rocker's Dub'.

Pattern		Description	Frequency
1		'One drop' pattern – kick only	13
2	c	'One drop' pattern – kick & snare (centre)	4
	r	'One drop' pattern – kick & snare (rimshot)	2
	s	'One drop' pattern – kick & snare (side-stick)	1
3		'One drop' pattern – snare only (centre)	1
1.1		Pattern 1, plus extra kick on beat 1	1
1.2		Pattern 1, plus open hi-hat on last quaver of bar	4
1.3		Pattern 1, plus extra kick on 4th quaver of bar	1
1 +	Fill 1	The six fills demonstrate the most variation in patterning. Each is unique, but all (except Fill 2) end with a composite stroke consisting of a crash cymbal plus either a kick or snare drum on the last crotchet beat of the fill.	1 (2 bars long)
	Fill 2		1 (2 bars long)
	Fill 3		1 (2 bars long)
Fill 4			1
Fill 5			1
2s + Fill 6			1 (3 bars long)

to further vary the timbral possibilities of the 'one drop', in that the snare drum stroke of Pattern 2 variously uses the centre of the drum head, a rimshot and a side-stick technique; again, the drummer is varying the groove factor of timbre without altering any other aspects of his performance.

Patterns 1.1 and 1.3 incorporate additional kick drum strokes at points in the bar other than beat 3, altering the way that patterning functions within the drum voice yet without destabilising the overall sense that this is still a 'one drop'. Pattern 1.2 adds an open hi-hat stroke on the final quaver beat of the bar, which has the effect of altering the phrasing in this voice as the sound sustains until the cymbals are closed together on the first beat of the following bar. It is common in funk drumming to find similar placement of an open hi-hat stroke at the end of a bar, but in funk the subsequent closing of the hi-hat cymbals typically coincides with a kick drum stroke, whereas in 'Rocker's Dub' there is no kick drum stroke on beat 1, so the closing coincides with the start of the bassist's next phrase instead; thus the same textural pattern occurs in both funk and 'Rocker's Dub' (that is, the sustained high frequency wash of the open hi-hat is terminated by a low frequency sound on the downbeat of the next bar) but in the case of the latter, this textural contour is achieved through an interlocking pattern that emerges from the combined performance of the rhythm section, rather than occurring just within the drums.

By working together as an empathically attuned rhythm section, the bassist and drummer in 'Rocker's Dub' create an interlocking performance in which the varied drum patterns and the unchanging bassline effectively communicate the song's groove to the rest of the ensemble, thereby enabling the other musicians – and, later, the listener – to feel the music. In the next example – Vivian 'Yabby You'

Jackson's 'Love Thy Neighbour' (1977) – both the bass and drums exhibit greater freedom in the way that the instrumentalists alter the groove factors in their performance.[10] As with the preceding example, the use of an alternative version of Yabby You's original recording (released, in this case, as 'Distant Drums' (197X) by Family Man and Knotty Roots) enabled clearer focus on the activity of the rhythm section.

Once again, the 'one drop' pattern forms the basic template for the drumming in 'Love Thy Neighbour', which therefore immediately provides the bassist with some information about what he can expect from the drums (that is, a strong emphasis on the third beat in most bars). When shaping the bassline, he uses this knowledge of how the drummer is feeling the song's groove as a way to inform his own pattern construction, playfully reframing the expected emphasis in a number of different ways. In bars 25–28, for example, there is one bass phrase whose ending coincides with the 'one drop' kick drum stroke, another bass phrase that ends just before the next 'one drop' so that the kick drum stroke is heard in isolation, and a third bass phrase whose beginning coincides with the last 'one drop' before continuing across the following barline. Thus, within a span of four bars, the bassist moves between aligning, interlocking and then aligning (differently) with the groove which the drummer is communicating; in so doing, he exploits the musical space embodied in the 'one drop' pattern.

Rather than passively repeating the 'one drop' pattern throughout this performance however, the drummer instead uses variation in groove factors such as patterning and timbre as he interacts empathically with the bassist. He also toys with the sense of textural expectation created through his use of the 'one drop' pattern, by sometimes omitting the customary emphasis on the third beat. At some of these moments, the bassist still emphasises this point in the bar, creating the impression that the 'one drop' is being passed around the rhythm section. On other occasions, both the kick drum and the bass guitar remain silent on beat three; the 'one drop' is still evident at such points, but through a kind of negative emphasis that is caused by the conspicuous absence of these expected textures. In this way, they not only create rhythmic space within their own patterning, but also textural space within the overall sonic fabric of the track. In dub, Veal notes that 'much of the genre's compositional tension is generated through subversion of the listener's expectations' (Veal, 2007, p. 89); it is interesting to see the rhythm section employing a similarly subversive strategy here, even before any dub mixing has taken place. Such deliberate use of absence accords, again, with Bilby's comments regarding the expansion of musical space in reggae that he attributes to the influence of Rastafarian drumming.

Having explored the instrumentalists' empathic groove interaction, the focus now shifts towards the specific ways in which the dub mixer can become involved in the empathic musicking process by altering groove factors within a previously recorded performance. In order to bring aspects of the dub mixer's role into the discussion at this stage, the final musical example considered here is the 'Frozen Dub' version of Augustus Pablo's 'Rocker's Dub', expertly mixed by Osbourne 'King Tubby' Ruddock.

The technology used to create dub mixes was fairly limited during this era of JPM, so mastery of the form relied on imaginative and resourceful application of the tools at hand. An analogue mixing desk enabled the sound engineer to mute and unmute specific tracks from the multitrack master tape at will, to place sounds at any point in the stereo field, to rebalance the relative volume levels within the ensemble and to alter the timbre of each instrumental voice using an equaliser. Additionally, outboard sound processing equipment made it possible to add artificial reverb, echo, filtering and phasing effects as required, either to individual components within the texture or to the overall mix. Thinking about these capabilities in the context of the groove factors discussed earlier, it is clear that the dub mixer's tools primarily enable variation of timbral aspects of a recorded performance, although selective muting impacts on patterning within and between instrumental voices, echo can add desirable and unpredictable complexity to otherwise simple rhythm patterns, and reverb alters the listener's perception of phrasing and articulation.

In 'Frozen Dub', King Tubby uses his characteristic filter sweeping to achieve a type of timbral variation that could only be the product of studio technology, rather than instrumental technique. He applies reverb to some instrumental voices, but not to others, and so recasts and disrupts the sense of physical space in which the listener perceives the performance as having occurred. Tape echo is used in a number of ways that affect groove factors within the original performance: it adds previously non-existent syncopations by creating rhythmically displaced repetitions of fragments of certain patterns; it sustains some notes and phrases beyond their expected duration; it occasionally foregrounds obscure gestures that had been hidden within the original recording; and, used in conjunction with muting, it imposes deliberately artificial articulation on phrases which had been performed as *legato* in the original recording.

King Tubby's sonic manipulation asserts itself throughout the dub mix, so that at least one technological alteration – and often more – can be heard to affect the instrumentalists' recorded performance at any given moment. As the mix unfolds, a third process of empathy at work in JPM is revealed, one that is specific to the dub mixer's role. Although the sound engineer needs to engage empathically with both the feeling of the song and the recorded groove of the instrumentalists (as is the case with the rhythm section) he also has the potential to extract new, different feelings from the recording, and to communicate these by altering the existing groove factors so that the listener's perception of the performance is changed; sometimes this shift is subtle, but at others it can be more radical.

Conclusions

Both the interviews with Jamaican session musicians and the analyses of relevant music examples indicate that processes of empathy play a significant role in the grooving that occurs during a JPM recording session, and also during the subsequent creation of a dub mix. Two distinct, but related, processes of empathy predominate during the initial recording session: the first exists between each musician and the song itself, while the second enables sharing between the instrumentalists. The bassist's feeling for the song may not be the same as the drummer's, but each needs to share and understand the other's perspective in order to enhance their own performance. This, in turn, will lead to successful grooving within the rhythm section, which will consequently enable the rest of the ensemble, as well as the listener, to participate in this too.

The role of the dub mixer relies on an additional, third process of empathy, in which simple technological manipulation is artfully applied to the groove factors in existing recordings in order to extract alternative or hidden feeling from within a song, and then communicate this to the listener. Although the practicalities of the roles discussed above differ in significant ways, and despite the fact that the dub mixing occurs at a different time (and often in a different place) from the original recording session, it is clear that the various processes of empathy I have described are interconnected, and that they combine to add richness and nuance to groove in JPM.

Acknowledgements

My research visit to Chicago was made possible by a 'Travel to the Collections' grant which CBMR generously provided, thus enabling me to spend a joyful, intense week working with the materials in their archive. I am very grateful to everyone at CBMR for the welcome and support they provided while I was with them. I would also like to offer my heartfelt thanks to Ken Bilby for the illuminating and encouraging conversation we began during my final day in Chicago and have since continued, as well as his efforts in creating the collection of interviews in the first place, of course.

Notes

1 Mark Doffman's (2009) work on jazz trio performance, for example, uses the timing relationship between the playing of the bassist and the drummer as a basis for exploring groove.
2 Drawing on Olly Wilson's (1992) concept of the 'heterogeneous sound ideal', my PhD thesis (Oliver, 2015) discusses the importance of timbre to the way that groove works in breakbeats, for example.
3 Felicity Laurence's work on empathy and musicking presents some less general definitions that are both relevant and illuminating (see, for example, *Music, empathy and intercultural understanding* (2009); and Laurence, this volume).
4 For a detailed discussion of this process (in the context of ethnomusicological research) see Clayton, Sager and Will (2005).
5 It is not my intention to engage in a comparative analysis of composition and performance practice amongst African drum ensembles here; anyone wishing to explore the concept in more detail would benefit from reading the detailed studies of Simha Arom (1991), Kofi Agawu (1995), and John Miller Chernoff (1979), amongst others.
6 The idea of 'feeling the music' also suggests that there is a tactile dimension to the listening experience, which accords with what Julian Henriques (2003) refers to as 'sonic dominance' in his work on reggae sound system performance. In the context that Henriques describes, the physical sensation of bass weight plays an important role and is tied to the audience's perception of musical authenticity.

7 Dick Hebdige (1987) discusses versioning at length, and several commentators link this Jamaican practice to the subsequent emergence of remix culture in popular music more broadly; see, for example, Sullivan (2014).

8 An occasional lack of accurate cataloguing information is one consequence of the sense of immediacy that drove production processes within the Jamaican music industry from the 1960s onwards, where minimising the time that elapsed between recording a song and releasing it on vinyl was seen as a much higher priority than filing precise discographical information. This approach continues to significantly impact the royalty claims of reggae musicians, whose clearly remembered involvement in a given recording session may be difficult to prove in a legal context due to scant or non-existent discographical information. Less significantly (though more pertinently), this approach also impacts on academic referencing. Where it has not been possible to ascertain a record's release date more accurately than by decade, this is indicated in my references with the letter 'X', as in 197X.

9 'Hot Dub', in particular, consists largely of drums and bass, with the majority of the other instrumental voices muted for most of the track, rendering the nuances of the rhythm section's performance exposed for the purpose of closer scrutiny.

10 Given that Yabby You had a strong, if unusual, relationship with Rastafarian culture, it is reasonable to assume that the influence of Rasta drumming (as noted by Bilby) was manifested in his work, giving rise to this greater sense of freedom amongst the instrumentalists.

References

Agawu, K. (1995). *African rhythm: A northern Ewe perspective.* New York: Cambridge University Press.

Amira, J., & Cornelius, S. (1992). *The music of Santería: Traditional rhythms of the batá drums.* Crown Point, IN: White Cliffs Media Co.

Arom, S. (1991). *African polyphony and polyrhythm: Musical structure and methodology.* Cambridge; New York; Paris: Cambridge University Press; Editions de la maison des Sciences de l'homme.

Bilby, K. M. (1995). Jamaica. In P. Manuel (Ed.), *Caribbean currents: Caribbean music from rumba to reggae* (pp. 143–182). Philadelphia, PA: Temple University Press.

Bilby, K. M. (2010). *Kenneth M. Bilby oral history collection on foundations of Jamaican popular music.* Center for Black Music Research, Columbia College Chicago, Chicago, Illinois.

Chernoff, J. M. (1979). *African rhythm and African sensibility: Aesthetics and social action in African musical idioms.* Chicago, IL: University of Chicago Press.

Clayton, M., Sager, R., & Will, U. (2005). In time with the music: The concept of entrainment and its significance for ethnomusicology. *European Meetings in Ethnomusicology, 11*(1), 3–75.

Doffman, M. (2009). *Feeling the groove: Shared time and its meanings for three jazz trios* (Unpublished doctoral dissertation). The Open University, UK.

Family Man & Knotty Roots. (197X). *Distant drums.* Fam's.

Greenwald, J. (2002). Hip-Hop drumming: The rhyme may define, but the groove makes you move. *Black Music Research Journal, 22*(2), 259–271.

Hebdige, D. (1987). *Cut 'n' mix: Culture, identity and Caribbean music.* London: Methuen.

Henriques, J. (2003). Sonic dominance and the reggae sound system session. In M. Bull & L. Back (Eds.), *The auditory culture reader* (pp. 451–480). Oxford, UK; New York: Berg.

Jackson, V. (1977). *Conquering lion.* Prophet Record.

Laurence, F. (2009). *Music, empathy and intercultural understanding.* Retrieved 21 December 2015, from www.slideshare.net/WAAE/music-empathy-and-intercultural-understanding-felicity-laurence.

Locke, D. (1987). *Drum Gahu: The rhythms of West African drumming.* Crown Point, IN: White Cliffs Media Co.

Oliver, R. (2013). Groove as familiarity with time. In E. King & H. M. Prior (Eds.), *Music and familiarity: Listening, musicology and performance* (pp. 239–252). Farnham: Ashgate.

Oliver, R. (2015). *Rebecoming analogue: Groove, breakbeats and sampling* (Unpublished doctoral dissertation). University of Hull, UK.

Pablo, A. (1976). *King Tubby meets rockers uptown.* Yard Music.

Pablo, A. (1979). *Original rockers.* Greensleeves Records.

Pablo, A. (197X). *Hot dub.* Rockers.

Small, C. (1998). *Musicking: The meanings of performing and listening.* Middletown, CT: Wesleyan University Press.

Sullivan, P. (2014). *Remixology: Tracing the dub diaspora.* London: Reaktion Books.

The Congos. (1977). *Heart of the Congos.* Black Art.

Veal, M. E. (2007). *Dub: Soundscapes and shattered songs in Jamaican reggae.* Middletown, CT: Wesleyan University Press.

Wilson, O. (1992). The heterogeneous sound ideal in African American music. In J. Wright, & S. A. Floyd Jr. (Eds.), *New perspectives on music: Essays in honour of Eileen Southern* (pp. 327–340). Michigan, IL: Harmonie Park Press.

9 Empathy of the musical brain in musicians playing in ensemble

Claudio Babiloni, Claudio Del Percio,
Ivo Bruni and Daniela Perani

The musical brain

Measuring the activity of the musical brain

The cognitive neuroscience of music investigates the neurophysiological mechanisms involved in the cognitive processes underlying music listening, mental imagery and auditory–motor interactions, as well as performing, composing, reading, writing and other domains related to musical aesthetics, musical emotion and social cognition in ensemble playing (Leman, 2007; Perani *et al.*, 2011). This discipline is characterised by its reliance on direct observations of brain functioning and the use of functional magnetic resonance imaging (fMRI), positron emission tomography (PET), magnetoencephalography (MEG), electroencephalography (EEG), and others. These techniques complement each other, as they are characterised by different spatial and temporal resolution in the mapping of cortical neural correlates of music experiences. The fMRI and PET allow the highest spatial resolution at the cost of a low temporal resolution (i.e. from a few millimetres and one or more seconds). In contrast, EEG (i.e. centimetres; milliseconds) and MEG (i.e. one or more centimetres; milliseconds) allow a low-moderate spatial resolution with high temporal resolution. This high temporal resolution permits pinpointing of the role of emerging cortical oscillatory activity in the neural processes related to music information processing. Of extreme interest is the modulation of a dominant cortical EEG/MEG oscillatory activity that occurs at about 8–12 Hz (alpha rhythms) in the resting state condition. Amplitude of alpha rhythms decreases as a function of cortical activation during sensorimotor and cognitive events, the so-called desynchronisation of cortical alpha rhythms (Pfurtscheller & Lopes da Silva, 1999). Alpha rhythms have been found to be tightly bound to cortical information processing in music experience (Altenmüller *et al.*, 2002; Schmidt & Trainor, 2001).

The circuits and functions of the musical brain

Neuroimaging techniques such as fMRI and PET have been extensively used to obtain fine spatial details of brain circuits sub-serving music experience (Koelsch, 2010; Koelsch, 2011; Peretz & Zatorre, 2005). Thanks to these techniques, we have the following general picture of these circuits: a circuit including the auditory cortex, intra-parietal, temporal sulcus, ventral frontal gyrus (Brodmann's Area [BA] 44, BA 45 and BA 46), anterior superior insula, and ventral striatum areas (Koelsch, 2010; Koelsch, 2011; Peretz & Zatorre, 2005) appears to sub-serve music perception for the encoding of pitch and spectral features of musical sounds (Foster & Zatorre, 2010a, 2010b; Schönwiesner & Zatorre, 2008; Zatorre & Belin, 2001), melodic information (Foster & Zatorre, 2010a), music categorisation (Klein & Zatorre, 2011; Peretz *et al.*, 2009) and/ or music syntax (Sammler *et al.*, 2009, 2011). In addition, the posterior medial cortex processes melodic and harmonic information in the auditory stream in relation to the cognitive construction of complex multimodal sensory imagery scenes (Spada *et al.*, 2014). Furthermore, a circuit including superior parietal and ventrolateral/dorsolateral frontal areas contributes to the development of music imagery (Zatorre *et al.*, 2010). In this framework, the pre-supplementary motor area and right globus pallidus adapt movements to music imagery, while the left cerebellum adapts the same movements to actual music (Schaefer *et al.*, 2014). Moreover, the left cerebellum, right inferior frontal gyrus and bilateral superior temporal gyri recognise sounds with uneven rhythmical structure (Danielsen *et al.*, 2014). Finally, the anterior part of the left superior frontal gyrus (SFG) sub-serves the execution of movements by musicians according to the rhythm of conductor (Ono *et al.*, 2015).

Compared to fMRI and PET, EEG and MEG have enlightened the fine time course of cortical responses to the execution, imagination and perception of music events (Elbert *et al.*, 1995; Koelsch *et al.*, 2001, 2002; Kristeva *et al.*, 2003; Maess *et al.*, 2001; Petsche *et al.*, 1996). It has been shown that primary and premotor sensorimotor cortical areas are active during both preparation (time preceding the execution) and execution of a music performance (Koelsch *et al.*, 2001, 2002; Kristeva *et al.*, 2003; Maess *et al.*, 2001). Furthermore, they have shown that the imagination, observation and learning of music performances are characterised by peculiar spatio-temporal patterns of cortical activity (Elbert *et al.*, 1995; Kristeva *et al.*, 2003; Petsche *et al.*, 1996).

All of the aforementioned techniques have contributed to modelling the neuro-physiological mechanisms underlying emotional reactions to music listening (Koelsch *et al.*, 2006; Koelsch & Friederici, 2003). Compared to music perception, music production and executive monitoring mainly engage prefrontal, premotor and motor systems (Bangert & Altenmüller, 2003; Kamiyama *et al.*, 2010; Katahira *et al.*, 2008; Maidhof *et al.*, 2009). Expressive music performance evokes emotion and reward-related neural activations, which are conditioned by subjects' musical training (Chapin *et al.*, 2010). Areas associated with emotions and reward are also involved in emotional responding to music (Blood *et al.*, 1999; Chapin *et al.*, 2010; Phan *et al.*, 2002; Royet *et al.*, 2000). More specifically, limbic and paralimbic brain areas responded to the expressive dynamics of human music performance (Chapin *et al.*, 2010). Furthermore, parahippocampus and precuneus activity were found to increase in response to increasing dissonance of short chord sequences (Blood *et al.*, 1999), while increasing consonance was associated with activation of orbitofrontal and frontopolor cortices and sub-callosal cingulate (Phan *et al.*, 2002; Royet *et al.*, 2000). Compared to unpleasant music, listening to pleasant music was associated with activation of the para-hippocampal gyrus, amygdala, temporal poles insula, inferior frontal gyrus (in-cluding BA 44) and ventral striatum (Berridge & Robinson, 2003; Koelsch *et al.*, 2006; Knutson *et al.*, 2001).

The circuits of social cognition of the musical brain: is there a musical empathy?

A bulk of studies has investigated how the brain perceives, learns and produces music, but few have investigated brain activity while music is being generated in the context of playing in ensemble. An fMRI study in jazz pianists revealed an increased activity of the medial prefrontal cortex during music improvisation, which is a brain area linked with self-expression and activities that convey indi-viduality (Limb & Braun, 2008). In parallel, broad areas of the lateral prefrontal cortex, thought to be linked to self-censoring, were deactivated (Limb & Braun, 2008). Furthermore, analysis of listeners' fMRI responses revealed an activation of the amygdala for improvisations, possibly for its role in the detection of be-havioural uncertainty (Engel & Keller, 2011). In addition, a circuit including the medial frontal (premotor) area, frontal operculum and anterior insula was spe-cifically active for melodies judged to be improvised (Engel & Keller, 2011). The frontal lobe is also important in the processes of social cognition-related music experience. Compared to healthy control subjects, patients with lesions of tempo-ral and prefrontal areas due to frontotemporal dementia showed impaired ability to attribute mental states – but not non-mental characteristics – to music excerpts (Downey *et al.*, 2013). Interestingly, this deficit correlated with performance on a standard test of social inference and with career ratings of patients' empathic capacity (Downey *et al.*, 2013).

Another important dimension of the musical brain for playing music in ensem-ble is empathy, one of the main functions of social cognition. This function helps us to understand other people's mental states, such as feelings, emotions, needs and intentions. Empathic abilities can be somewhat measured via standardised questionnaires probing the empathy trait, that is how the person emotionally re-acts to and understands other people's mental states. There is a consensus that the definition of empathy encompasses at least two main dimensions, namely emotional and cognitive empathy. Emotional empathy is defined as the imme-diate affective 'contagion' and understanding of feelings and emotions between the observer and observed person (Shamay-Tsoory, 2011; Shamay-Tsoory *et al.*, 2009). In contrast, cognitive empathy is defined as a process through which the mental states of other people are represented based on mentalisation (i.e. reflec-tions, thinking). It can also be defined as the capacity to adopt the psychological point of view of another person thanks to a perspective-taking ability (Frith & Singer, 2008; Shamay-Tsoory, 2011; Shamay-Tsoory *et al.*, 2009). Such a distinc-tion between these two forms of empathy agrees with phylogenetic/developmental observations and relevant cognitive models (Decety & Jackson, 2004; Leiberg & Anders, 2006; Preston & de Waal, 2002). A form of emotional empathy or conta-gion is found in birds and rodents, while a form of cognitive empathy is observed only in great apes and humans (de Waal, 2008). Furthermore, it becomes observ-able only during childhood and adolescent maturational processes (Decety & Jackson, 2004; Gallese, 2003; Preston & de Waal, 2002).

Two diverse brain circuits may underpin emotional and cognitive empathy (Shamay-Tsoory *et al.*, 2009). Emotional empathy may rely upon ventral-lateral frontal areas (i.e. BA 44/45), as suggested by recent studies probing the recogni-tion of others' emotions (Schulte-Ruther *et al.*, 2007), as well as the experience of empathy with people suffering serious threat or harm (Nummenmaa *et al.*, 2008). Indeed, lesions of ventral-lateral frontal areas are associated with impaired emo-tional contagion and deficits in the recognition of the emotions expressed by other people (Shamay-Tsoory *et al.*, 2009). Interestingly, the BA 44/45 might be part of resonant ventral-lateral frontal and parietal 'mirror' neuron systems sub-serving the understanding of actions and motor intentions performed by others, as well as imitation or observational learning (Gallese *et al.*, 2004; Rizzolatti & Craighero, 2004; Rizzolatti *et al.*, 2006). These frontal areas of 'mirror' neuron systems are active during the observation of musicians playing music as a function of practice (Buccino *et al.*, 2004; Vogt *et al.*, 2007).

In contrast to emotional empathy, cognitive empathy may rely upon the activa-tion of ventromedial prefrontal areas (BA 10/11) when the evaluation of the simi-larities and differences between one's own mental states in relation to those of other individuals is required (Mitchell, 2009). In this line, lesions in the ventro-medial prefrontal cortex result in impaired cognitive empathy (Shamay-Tsoory *et al.*, 2009). Overall, playing music in ensemble is expected to induce substantial empathic feelings in musicians due to several inductors including musical sounds and observations of our own and other bodies in action, as well as the need for the realisation of a common representation and interpretation of the musical piece performed.

A new EEG system to study empathy of the musical brain

The previous section highlighted the importance of empathy for playing music in ensemble and the need for further experiments on brains in concert. However, this scientific endeavour presents a strong methodological challenge. It is hard to record the brain activity of musicians in concert simultaneously. fMRI and PET scanners can be used only on single subjects one-by-one, and the construction of a room for MEG recordings from several scanners would be extremely expen-sive. In addition, the use of metal objects is banned in rooms where MEG and fMRI devices are seated and this is a serious limitation for studies addressing musical performance with real music instruments, although this issue has been successfully dealt with and overcome in some cases (Berkowitz & Ansari, 2008, 2010; Limb & Braun, 2008). Furthermore, slow displacements of a subject's head with respect to the MEG and fMRI sensors may compromise the quality of recordings. In this framework, EEG techniques have the potential to be used for simultaneous recordings in musicians playing in ensemble. Indeed, the tight contact between exploring EEG sensors and subject's head theoretically allows the recording of artefact-free neurophysiological data, provided musicians are trained to minimise head and body movements during their performance.

To overcome the aforementioned barriers to this field research, we have designed and developed a new system allowing the simultaneous EEG recording of four expert musicians playing in ensemble, for the synchronous storage of environmental sounds, digital trigger, and neurophysiological data, including EEG, electrooculographic (EOG) and electromyographic (EMG) signals. In contrast to fMRI, PET and MEG techniques, EEG data can be recorded in an environment allowing the music performance of several musicians, since EEG data can be recorded in very large, unshielded rooms. This approach potentially permits online data acquisition in order to test several hypotheses about particular cortical responses characterising sensorimotor, emotional (including inter-individual empathy) and cognitive processes related to interactions and cooperative behaviour among subjects, including playing music in ensemble.

To test the outcome of the present methodological approach, we simultaneously recorded EEG data from a quartet of professional saxophonists during a music performance executed in ensemble. The quality of the EEG and EMG data was evaluated by several criteria. Full details of this EEG system and validation test can be found in the original study published by our research group (Babiloni *et al.*, 2011).

The design of the new EEG system

The new EEG system was developed by EB-NEURO S.p.A. (www.ebneuro.biz/it). It is formed of several interconnected items. Notably, these items are commercial products whose technical features and quality are well known (they were licensed by European Community regulatory agencies at the time and were approved for commercialisation, and so on). Therefore, the novelty of the EEG system is the design of the interconnection of the existing items for these new scientific purposes.

The EEG system includes four pre-wired EEG caps. Each cap includes 30 electrodes placed according to an augmented 10–20 system (cephalic reference and ground), and is connected to a single multi-channel amplifier box (*Brain Explorer*, EB-Neuro©) that also receives the individual bipolar EOG and EMG signals. Furthermore, this box receives audio signals relative to environmental sounds, which are revealed by two dynamic microphones (*Shure Beta 57©*) placed on proper stands, pre-amplified and mixed by a commercial analogic mixer. The mixer also relays these audio signals in real time to a professional multitrack hard-disk recording system (two channels, 24-bit, sampling rate 48 KHz). The recording of the audio signals allows a descriptive tracking of the music performance synchronised with EEG data and a clear rendering of the music performance.

In the amplifier boxes, analog/digital conversion of EEG–EOG–EMG and audio signals occurs. The four multi-channel amplifier boxes are connected via optical fibres to four *Brain Explorer Net* interfaces (*BE-Net*, EB-Neuro©), which also receive digital trigger signals coming from the experimenter or computer (a trigger represents a common reference signal in the data sets of the four musicians). These four interfaces send (via LAN) all converted signals to a commercial switch. The switch collects and redirects (data transfer rate 100Mb/s) the converted signals from the four musicians towards a single workstation devoted to the data acquisition. Notably, the only possible cause of jitter of the EEG signals recorded from the four musicians was the LAN interconnection inside the switch device, since the delay of these signals was practically equal in the four identical EEG amplifiers and *BE-Net* interface used by the system. The maximum jitter, defined as the maximum variation in the arrival/recording time of the four sets of supposedly synchronous EEG signals, was in the order of hundreds of microseconds (i.e. less than the actual temporal resolution of the present EEG recordings), as reported by the technical report of the commercial switch device used for this study. The operating system of this workstation allows the opening of four sessions of data acquisition software (*GALILEO NT*, EB-Neuro©), for the simultaneous storage of environmental sounds, digital trigger and EEG–EOG–EMG data. A single file is obtained for each individual. Notably, the above system is characterised by the fact that the four subjects were electrically decoupled to satisfy international safety guidelines and to record high-quality EEG–EOG–EMG signals.

The validation of the new EEG system

For the validation of the new system, EEG data were collected simultaneously from the four musicians (bandpass: 0.1–100 Hz, sampling rate: 512 Hz; EB-Neuro Be-family©) by the 30 scalp electrodes of the pre-wired EEG caps. Electrode impedance was kept below 5 KOhm. EEG data were recorded at eyes-open resting state condition (RESTING, duration: 4 minutes) and while the quartet was playing a classical music piece taken from its repertoire (EXECUTION, duration: about 1.5 minutes, with balanced distribution of phrase attacks between subjects). In parallel, we performed the recording of bipolar EOG data (band pass: 0.1–100 Hz; sampling rate: 512 Hz) for the monitoring of blinking and eye movements. Furthermore, EMG activity (band pass: 0.1–100 Hz; sampling rate: 512 Hz) of orbicularis oris, mentalis and right and left extensor digitorum muscles were recorded by bipolar surface electrodes, in order to monitor movements during music performance. For the extensor digitorum communis, bipolar electrodes were placed one-quarter to one-third of the distance of the midpoint between the radial and ulnar styloid processes, as measured from the wrist dorsum and the olecranon process. For the orbicularis oris muscle, the electrodes were positioned on the left side along a medio-lateral axis so that the circular edges of each electrode were aligned with the vermilion border of the upper and the lower lips respectively. For the mentalis muscle, one surface electrode was positioned in the midline above the chin; the other about 1 cm under the chin on a virtual vertical line. Low impedance of the EMG electrodes (<10 KOhm) at the skin–electrode interface was obtained by shaving, abrading and cleaning the skin with alcohol. Special caution was given to the standardisation of the experimental procedure (electrode position), to reduce the susceptibility of EMG to cross-talk.

An additional recording channel was used for triggering the reference instants of the event on the on-going EEG–EOG–EMG data of the four musicians, namely the start and stop instants of the music performance (sampling rate: 512 Hz, no hardware filter). These instants – generally the attacks of musical phrases – could be used to identify the same EEG periods in each of the four musicians.

Recorded EEG data were segmented to single epochs lasting two seconds. The 2-second EEG epochs with ocular, muscular and other types of artefact were preliminarily identified by a computerised automatic procedure (Moretti *et al.*, 2003). The EEG epochs contaminated by ocular artefacts were then corrected by an autoregressive method (Moretti *et al.*, 2003). Finally, two expert electro-encephalographists manually confirmed this automatic selection and correction, with special attention to residual contaminations of the EEG epochs due to head, trunk and eye movements.

The artefact-free EEG data were given as an input to the original standardised low-resolution brain electromagnetic tomography (sLORETA) software for the EEG source analysis (Pascual-Marqui, 2002; www.unizh.ch/keyinst/NewLORETA/LORETA01.htm). sLORETA is a functional imaging technique belonging to a family of standardised linear inverse solution procedures, modelling 3-D distributions of the cortical source patterns generating scalp EEG data (Pascual-Marqui, 2002). sLORETA computes 3-D linear solutions (sLORETA solutions) for the EEG inverse problem standardised with respect to instrumental and biological noise as mathematically defined in the original paper by Pascual-Marqui (2002). sLORETA solutions are computed within a three-shell spherical head model including scalp, skull and brain compartments. The brain compartment is restricted to the cortical grey matter/hippocampus of a head model co-registered to the Talairach probability brain atlas, which has been digitised at the Brain Imaging Center of the Montreal Neurological Institute (Talairach & Tournoux, 1988). This compartment includes 6,239 voxels (5-mm resolution), each voxel containing an equivalent current dipole.

Cortical activation/deactivation was indexed as a task-related power decrease/increase (TRPD/TRPI) of EEG alpha rhythms at about 8–12 Hz, respectively. To this aim, alpha TRPD/TRPI was computed for the EXECUTION condition referenced to the RESTING condition taken as a baseline. Specifically, we used the basic formula used for the computation of event-related desynchronisation/synchronisation (ERD/ERS; Pfurtscheller & Aranibar, 1979; Pfurtscheller & Neuper, 1994; Pfurtscheller *et al.*, 1997; Pfurtscheller & Lopes da Silva, 1999). This formula is as follows:

$$TRPD/TRPI = \left(\frac{event - baseline}{baseline} \times 100 \right)$$

where 'event' refers to the alpha (sLORETA) solutions relative to the EXECUTION condition, while 'baseline' refers to the alpha (sLORETA) solutions relative to the RESTING condition. The procedure was repeated for low- and high-frequency alpha sub-bands. Per cent negative values (i.e. weaker alpha sLORETA solutions during the EXECUTION than during the RESTING condition) represented the alpha TRPD as a reflection of cortical activation (Manganotti *et al.*, 1998). On the contrary, per cent positive values (i.e. stronger alpha sLORETA solutions during the EXECUTION than during the RESTING condition) represented the alpha TRPI as a reflection of cortical deactivation or idling.

The quality of the EOG data was evaluated by a visual inspection of the signals during the EXECUTION. In all subjects, the EOG signal clearly showed quick peaks of voltage due to blinking and slow shift due to saccades. This signal could be used to correct EEG epochs with blinking and saccades and to select artefact-free EEG epochs for further spectral EEG analysis. The EOG data were of good quality for research applications.

The quality of the EMG data was evaluated by a visual inspection of the signals during the EXECUTION. In all subjects, the EMG signal showed low amplitude in the condition of observation of the video of music performance, while it markedly increased in amplitude at a large frequency range during the execution of the music play. The EMG data were of good quality for research applications.

The quality of the EEG data was evaluated by the rate of artefact-free EEG epochs and by the topography and amplitude of EEG rhythms during the RESTING and EXECUTION conditions. This evaluation process showed that about 8 per cent of the recorded 2-second epochs were judged as artefact-free by experts. Furthermore, these epochs revealed typical features of human EEG rhythms. During the resting state condition, alpha rhythms (8–12 Hz) showed dominant amplitude at parietal and occipital electrodes in all subjects, while delta rhythms (<4 Hz) showed dominant amplitude at frontal electrodes. Compared to delta and alpha rhythms, beta (14–30 Hz) and gamma (>30 Hz) rhythms showed lower amplitude at all electrodes in all subjects. During the music performance, the amplitude of posterior and central alpha and beta rhythms decreased, while that of higher frequencies in the beta and gamma range slightly increased in widespread regions of the scalp.

Figure 9.1 maps the grand average (N=4) of sLORETA solutions modelling TRPD/TRPI of distributed EEG sources of low- (about 8–10 Hz) and high-frequency (about 10–12 Hz) alpha rhythms. The maps refer to the TRPD/TRPI in the EXECUTION condition referenced to the RESTING condition. For both sub-bands, there was higher alpha TRPD (i.e. cortical activation) over widely distributed cortical zones. These zones spanned all regions of interest of both hemispheres including BA 3/1/2, BA 4, BA 6 dorsal (6d), BA 6 mesial (6m), BA 6 ventral (6v), BA 17, BA 18, BA 19, BA 40, BA 41, BA 42, BA 44 and BA 45, as expected when playing music. Indeed, this function implies several parallel attentive, perceptive, executive and motor processes impinging upon relative brain circuits. These results were considered as globally satisfying for the validation of the new EEG system.

sLORETA ALPHA TRPD/TRPI

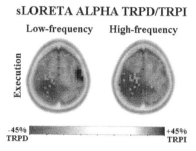

Figure 9.1 Grand average across the saxophonists of 1 quartet (N=4) of sLORETA solutions modelling task-related power decrease/increase (TRPD/TRPI) of distributed EEG sources of low- (about 8–10 Hz) and high-frequency (about 10–12 Hz) alpha rhythms. The TRPD and TRPI index, respectively, cortical activation and inhibition in the EXECUTION condition referenced to the RESTING condition. The modelled cerebral cortex is viewed at top, nose up; left hemisphere is at left side of the brain map. The original colour scale can be appreciated in an electronic version of the figure, available by request from the first author. In this black and white reproduction an intense alpha TRPD is observed as a gray zone distributed in the frontal and parietal regions of the left hemisphere contralateral to the dominant hand.

Testing the experimental hypothesis on the empathy of the musical brain

To test the experimental hypothesis on the empathy of the musical brain, we recorded EEG data from three professional saxophone quartets (i.e. simultaneous recording in each quartet) during the following conditions: music performance in ensemble (EXECUTION); eyes-open resting state condition (RESTING); audio–visual observation of their own music performance of a well-known piece for saxophone quartet played in ensemble (OBSERVATION); and audio–visual observation of themselves turning the pages of a score on a lectern (CONTROL).

General set up, EEG recording parameters, preliminary data analysis, EEG (sLORETA) source estimation and computation of the desynchronisation/synchronisation of alpha rhythms (TRPD/TRPI) were performed as mentioned in the previous section on the validation of the new EEG system. Here, cortical activity was indexed by the percentage reduction (i.e. desynchronisation) of sLORETA alpha sources in the EXECUTION, OBSERVATION and CONTROL conditions with reference to the RESTING condition. Subjects' empathy trait was measured by the Empathy Quotient Test (EQT; Lawrence *et al.*, 2004). The main working hypothesis predicted a correlation across the musicians (Spearman test, $p<0.05$) between EQT score and desynchronisation of alpha sources in BAs typically related to empathy (i.e. 44/45 and 10/11) during the OBSERVATION (when there was no interference of motor activity on the correlates of empathy) but not in the CONTROL (a condition with no empathic contents). All details about this experiment can be found in the original study of our research group (Babiloni *et al.*, 2012).

Figure 9.2 shows the grand average (N=12) of normalised power density spectra of artefact-free EEG data for three representative frontal (Fz), central (Cz) and parietal (Pz) midline electrodes in the RESTING (eyes-open), OBSERVATION and CONTROL conditions. The EXECUTION is omitted here to make it easier to compare the EEG variables between the two conditions in which musicians viewed a video without any movement. The EEG frequencies of interest ranged from 1 to 45 Hz. The normalisation of the EEG power density was obtained by computing the ratio between power density values (frequency bin-by-bin) at each electrode and the power density value averaged across all frequencies (1–45 Hz) and all electrodes. These EEG power spectra revealed the typical features of human cortical EEG rhythms during resting state condition and cognitive–motor events. During the RESTING, power density spectrum showed a dominant peak around 10 Hz at the reference parietal electrode. Furthermore, it showed dominant peak around 1–2 Hz at the reference frontal electrode. In addition, values of EEG power density at higher frequency bands (i.e. beta and gamma) were globally low. During OBSERVATION and CONTROL, the power density spectrum showed a reduced magnitude of the dominant peak around 10 Hz at the reference parietal electrode. Furthermore, it showed an increased magnitude of the dominant peak around 1–2 Hz at the reference frontal electrode. In addition, EEG power density at higher frequency bands (i.e. beta and gamma) was slightly increased in magnitude at the reference frontal electrode. Compared to OBSERVATION and CONTROL, EXECUTION induced similar changes of power density spectrum at reference electrodes. The only difference was that these changes were greater in amplitude in EXECUTION than in OBSERVATION and CONTROL.

For sake of brevity, the following description of the results is focused on the sLORETA solutions of OBSERVATION in comparison to RESTING, since these are the focus of the main working hypothesis of this review. All details of the results can be found in the original paper (Babiloni *et al.*, 2012). Figure 9.3 maps the sLORETA solutions modelling TRPD/TRPI of distributed EEG sources of low- (about 8–10 Hz) and high-frequency (about 10–12 Hz) alpha rhythms in two representative musicians showing a high (EQT=64) and a low (EQT=43) empathy score. The maps refer to the TRPD/TRPI in OBSERVATION referenced to RESTING. The musician with the higher empathy score was characterised by an evident and widespread alpha TRPD (i.e. cortical activity) in OBSERVATION compared to RESTING. In contrast, the musician with the lower empathy score was characterised by an evident and widespread alpha TRPI (i.e. cortical inhibition).

In the OBSERVATION condition, there was a statistically significant negative correlation across all musicians between the EQT score and the alpha TRPD/TRPI in right ventral-lateral BA 44/45 for both high- and low-frequency alpha sub-bands (low-frequency alpha: Spearman $r=-0.75$, $p=0.004$; high-frequency alpha: $r=-0.67$, $p=0.01$). Furthermore, there was a marginal statistical significance between the EQT score values and the low-frequency alpha TRPD/TRPI in ventromedial bilateral BA 10/11 ($r=-0.58$; $p=0.05$). The higher the EQT score, the higher the alpha TRPD (cortical activation). These results suggest that in expert musicians observing their music performance in ensemble, the alpha rhythms

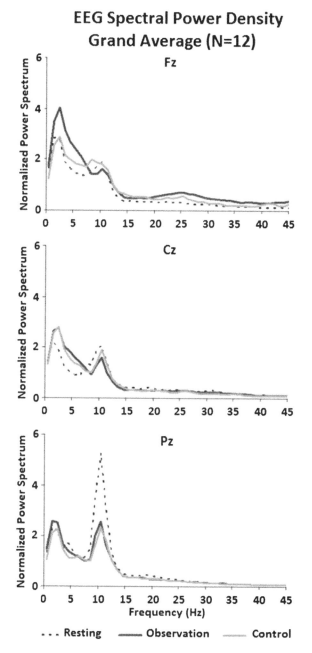

Figure 9.2 Grand average across the saxophonists of three quartets (N=12) of the normalised electroencephalographic (EEG) spectral power density values computed for
three representative electrodes of scalp midline (Fz, Cz and Pz of 10–20 electrode
montage system). These values refer to the EEG frequencies from 1 to 45 Hz and
to three experimental conditions: RESTING, OBSERVATION and CONTROL.

sLORETA MAPS OF ALPHA TRPD/TRPI

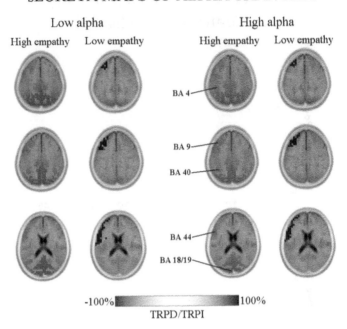

Figure 9.3 sLORETA solutions modelling TRPD/TRPI of distributed EEG sources of low- (about 8–10 Hz) and high-frequency (about 10–12 Hz) alpha rhythms in two representative musicians showing a high (EQT=64) and a low (EQT=43) empathy score. The TRPD and TRPI index, respectively, cortical activation and inhibition in the OBSERVATION condition referenced to the RESTING condition. The three slices of the sLORETA brain model show some BAs of interest of both hemispheres such as BA 4, BA 9, BA 17, BA 18, BA 19, BA 40, BA 44 and BA 45. The modelled cerebral cortex is viewed with nose up; left hemisphere is at left side of the brain map. The original colour scale can be appreciated in an electronic version of the figure, available by request from the first author. In this black and white reproduction an intense alpha TRPD is observed as gray zones distributed in bilateral frontal, parietal, and occipital regions (they are targeted by the BA labels) only in the musician showing the high empathy score.

in the right ventral-lateral frontal regions (BA 44/45) are strictly associated to subjects' global empathy tract.

A control analysis was performed to evaluate whether the main result of the present study was due to emotional empathy, cognitive empathy or both. We divided the 40 empathy items of the EQT in two sub-questionnaires. One questionnaire included 20 items probing emotional empathy, while the other included 20 items probing cognitive empathy. These sub-questionnaires were obtained following the procedures reported in two previous reference studies (Lawrence *et al.*, 2004; Muncer & Ling, 2006). For OBSERVATION, we computed Spearman correlation (two-tailed, N=12, $p < 0.05$) between the cognitive or emotional EQT score and the low- and high-frequency alpha TRPD/TRPI in right

BA 44/45. The results showed only a statistically significant correlation between musicians' emotional EQT score and low-frequency alpha TRPD/TRPI in right BA 44/45 (p<0.05). These control results are in line with the mentioned theory stating that ventral-lateral frontal areas sub-serve emotional but not cognitive empathy (Shamay-Tsoory et al., 2009).

The results of the reviewed experiment extend previous EEG evidence showing a bilateral frontal-parietal alpha desynchronisation during the execution and observation of voluntary movements (Babiloni et al., 1999; Babiloni et al., 2002; Cochin et al., 1998; Pfurtscheller et al. 1997; Ulloa & Pineda, 2007). They also extend previous EEG evidence showing that alpha desynchronisation in bilateral ventral-lateral frontal and parietal areas characterises professional athletes during the judgement of sporting actions performed by others (Babiloni et al., 2009, 2010), as well as dancers during the recognition of dancing performance (Orgs et al., 2008). These results suggest that alpha rhythms (about 8–12 Hz) in the ventral-lateral frontal cortex are a putative physiological mechanism underlying emotional empathy in musicians in concert.

What is the origin and meaning of the cortical alpha rhythms? These rhythms originate from synaptic currents of cortical pyramidal neurons modulated by synchronising/desynchronising signals coming thalamo-cortical and cortico-cortical circuits (Pfurtscheller & Lopes da Silva, 1999). Concerning their neurophysiological meaning, these synchronising/desynchronising signals gate the mentioned circuits, thus facilitating or inhibiting the transmission and retrieval of both sensorimotor and cognitive information (Brunia, 1999; Pfurtscheller & Lopes da Silva, 1999; Steriade & Llinas, 1988). In this framework, alpha rhythms can be distinguished into two frequency sub-bands. Alpha rhythms at low frequencies (about 8–10 Hz) are thought to underlie a subject's global attentive readiness, whereas those at high frequencies (about 10–12 Hz) are thought to underlie synchronising signals of the aforementioned neural loops when they are involved in cognitive–motor tasks (Klimesch, 1996, 1999; Klimesch et al., 1998). Keeping in mind these theoretical considerations, we posit that desynchronisation of low-frequency alpha rhythms in right ventral-lateral frontal cortex represents one of the neurophysiological mechanisms facilitating signal transmission and elaboration in brain circuits sub-serving global cortical arousal related to emotional empathic processes. As a byproduct, this general function would play a relevant role in the experience of cortical arousal and empathy in musicians involved in music experiences.

The results of the reviewed experiment also extend the following bulk of previous fMRI evidence about the role of inferior frontal areas during the observation of motor actions performed by others. During the observation of music performance, lateral frontal areas were active when the observed actions were part of the musicians' motor repertoire (Buccino et al., 2004; Vogt et al., 2007). Furthermore, ventral-lateral frontal areas were also active when expert dancers recognised movements that they had been trained to perform (Calvo-Merino et al., 2005; Cross et al., 2006). Finally, ventral-lateral frontal areas in the right hemisphere were active during pleasant music listening (Koelsch & Friederici, 2003; Koelsch et al., 2006). All these features of the video are common to the video of the present experiment and explain the involvement of ventral-lateral frontal areas.

Keeping in mind these data, it can be speculated that BAs 44 and 45 play a pivotal role in several cognitive–motor functions in humans. They may be part of a resonant frontal-parietal 'mirror' neuron system engaged in the execution of aimed actions, in the understanding of actions performed by others, and in emotional empathy (Gallese *et al.*, 2004; Rizzolatti & Craighero, 2004; Rizzolatti *et al.*, 2006; Shamay-Tsoory *et al.*, 2009). As an original contribution of our experiment, right BAs 44 and 45 may also play a pivotal role in the emotional empathy of musicians engaged in the observation and listening of their own music performance. As mentioned above, emotional empathy of the brain during musicking may be a sub-function of the emotional empathy of the brain.

The results of the reviewed experiment enrich our view of the functions of right hemisphere in humans. It has been previously shown that the human right hemisphere is dominant for the recognition and expression of emotions as well as for related empathic abilities (Leslie *et al.*, 2004; Perry *et al.*, 2001; Rankin *et al.*, 2006; Ruby & Decety, 2003, 2004; Shamay-Tsoory *et al.*, 2003, 2004). Brain activity increased in right frontal areas during the observation of movements having higher group-average aesthetic ratings (Calvo-Merino *et al.*, 2008). Furthermore, right frontal and parietal areas were markedly active during tasks implying the recognition of emotional face expressions (Etcoff, 1984; Gur *et al.*, 1994; Leslie *et al.*, 2004; Rueckert & Pawlak, 2000). A confirmation of this pivotal role also comes from clinical neuropsychology. It has been shown that empathy deficits are correlated to brain atrophy of right hemisphere (Rankin *et al.*, 2006), and that patients with right hemisphere atrophy were characterised by remarkable deficits in empathy when compared to those with left hemisphere atrophy (Perry *et al.*, 2001; Shamay-Tsoory *et al.*, 2003, 2004). Moreover, patients with focal lesions in the right hemisphere experienced difficulties in recognising emotions from facial expressions (Adolphs, 2001; Adolphs *et al.*, 2000) and expressing intense emotions (Borod *et al.*, 1996). In addition, converging data from patients with amusia (Stewart *et al.*, 2006), auditory event-related potentials (Särkämö *et al.*, 2010), structural neuroimaging (Hyde *et al.*, 2006, 2007; Mandell *et al.*, 2007), and functional neuroimaging (Binder *et al.*, 2004) pointed to a critical brain substrate of amusia in right temporal and frontal areas.

One may argue that the human 'mirror' neuron system was proposed as neural basis for language evolution, thus it would be expected that the left BAs 44 and 45, the so-called Broca's area, would play a special role in musical empathy (Corballis, 2002; Iacoboni, 2005; Rizzolatti & Arbib, 1998). In reality, this claim about a dominant role of Broca's area in 'mirror' neuron systems has not been confirmed when properly tested by fMRI (Aziz-Zadeh *et al.*, 2006). Therefore, there is not theoretical bias about a prominent role of right over let BAs 44 and 45 in emotional empathy of musical brain.

Concluding remarks about empathy of the musical brain

This chapter has reviewed the scientific background, the hypotheses and the results of two original studies recently published on the empathy of musical brain in musicians (for details see Babiloni *et al.*, 2011, 2012). In the first study

(Babiloni *et al.*, 2011), we developed and tested a new EEG system to simultaneously record EEG from four musicians playing in ensemble for application to the study of empathy of the musical brain. Results showed that the new EEG system is able to record EEG signals of good quality for that purpose.

In the second study (Babiloni *et al.*, 2012), we used the new EEG system to investigate the neural correlates of empathy in musicians playing in ensemble, with a focus on the mechanism of alpha desynchronisation (cortical activation) of prefrontal areas supposed to sub-serve empathy of the musical brain. Results showed a significant correlation between empathy trait score and low-frequency alpha desynchronisation (indexing cortical activation) estimated in right ventral-lateral frontal gyrus (BAs 44 and 45) in expert musicians involved in the observation of own music performance played in ensemble. The higher the empathy trait score, the higher the low-frequency alpha desynchronisation. The results were confirmed also when only emotional (but not cognitive) items of the empathy trait score were considered for the correlation with alpha desynchronisation in the right BA 44/45. Taken together, these results suggest that low-frequency alpha rhythms of right ventral-lateral frontal regions (BA 44/45) may reflect a neurophysiological mechanism underlying the regulation of general cortical arousal and emotional empathy in musicians engaged in music experiences. It is probable that this is a sub-function of the general neural substrate regulating cortical arousal related to emotional empathy in social interactions. In conclusion, empathy of the musical brain in musicians may be a 'specialisation' of empathy of the human brain.

Acknowledgements

The research was supported by a grant from the EU Project BrainTuning FP6-2004 NEST-PATH-028570 and Association Fatebenefratelli for Research (AFaR). The authors thank all the other co-authors of the two original studies (Babiloni *et al.*, 2011, 2012), which were the basis of the present chapter (i.e. Danilo Spada, Simone Rossi, Fabrizio Vecchio, Francesco Infarinato, Paola Buffo, Nicola Marzano and Paolo M. Rossini).

References

Adolphs, R. (2001). The neurobiology of social cognition. *Current Opinion in Neurobiology, 11*(2), 231–239.

Adolphs, R., Damasio, H., Tranel, D,, Cooper, G., & Damasio, A. R. (2000). A role for somatosensory cortices in the visual recognition of emotion as revealed by three-dimensional lesion mapping. *Journal of Neuroscience, 20*(7), 2683–2690.

Aziz-Zadeh, L., Koski, L., Zaidel, E., Mazziotta, J., & Iacoboni, M. (2006). Lateralization of the human mirror neuron system. *Journal of Neuroscience, 26*(11), 2964–2970.

Babiloni, C., Babiloni, F., Carducci, F., Cincotti, F., Cocozza, G., Del Percio, C., Moretti, D. V., & Rossini, P. M. (2002). Human cortical electroencephalography (EEG) rhythms during the observation of simple aimless movements: A high-resolution EEG study. *NeuroImage, 17*(2), 559–572.

Babiloni, C., Buffo, P., Vecchio, F., Marzano, N., Del Percio, C., Spada, D., Rossi, S., Bruni, I., Rossini, P. M., Perani, D (2012). Brains 'in concert': Frontal oscillatory alpha rhythms and empathy in professional musicians. *NeuroImage, 60*(1), 105–116.

Babiloni, C., Carducci, F., Cincotti, F., Rossini, P. M., Neuper, C., Pfurtscheller, G., & Babiloni, F. (1999). Human movement-related potentials vs desynchronization of EEG alpha rhythm: A high-resolution EEG study. *NeuroImage, 10*(6), 658–665.

Babiloni, C., Del Percio, C., Rossini, P. M., Marzano, N., Iacoboni, M., Infarinato, F., Lizio, R., Piazza, M., Pirritano, M., Berlutti, G., Cibelli, G., & Eusebi, F. (2009). Judgment of actions in experts: A high-resolution EEG study in elite athletes. *NeuroImage, 45*(2), 512–521.

Babiloni, C., Marzano, N., Infarinato, F., Iacoboni, M., Rizza, G., Aschieri, P., Cibelli, G., Soricelli, A., Eusebi, F., & Del Percio, C. (2010) 'Neural efficiency' of experts' brain during judgment of actions: A high-resolution EEG study in elite and amateur karate athletes. *Behavioural Brain Research, 207*(2), 466–475.

Babiloni C., Vecchio, F., Infarinato, F., Buffo, P., Marzano, N., Spada, D., Rossi, S., Bruni, I., Rossini, P. M., & Perani, D. (2011). Simultaneous recording of electroencephalographic data in musicians playing in ensemble. *Cortex, 47*(9), 1082–1090.

Bangert, M., & Altenmüller, E. O. (2003). Mapping perception to action in piano practice: A longitudinal DC-EEG study. *BMC Neuroscience, 4*(1_, 26.

Berkowitz, A. L., & Ansari, D. (2008). Generation of novel motor sequences: the neural correlates of musical improvisation. *NeuroImage, 41*(2), 535–543.

Berkowitz, A. L., & Ansari, D. (2010). Expertise-related deactivation of the right temporoparietal junction during musical improvisation. *NeuroImage, 49*(1), 712–719.

Berridge, K. C., & Robinson, T. E. (2003). Parsing reward. *Trends in Neurosciences, 26*(9), 507–513.

Binder, J. R., Liebenthal, E., Possing, E. T., Medler, D. A., & Ward, B. D. (2004). Neural correlates of sensory and decision processes in auditory object identification. *Nature Neuroscience, 7*(3), 295–301.

Blood, A. J., Zatorre, R. J, Bermudez, P., & Evans, A. C. (1999). Emotional responses to pleasant and unpleasant music correlate with activity in paralimbic brain regions. *Nature Neuroscience, 2*(4), 382–387.

Borod, J. C., Rorie, K. D., Haywood, C. S., Andelman, F., Obler, L. K., Welkowitz, J., Bloom, R. L., & Tweedy, J. R. (1996). Hemispheric specialization for discourse reports of emotional experiences: Relationships to demographic, neurological, and perceptual variables. *Neuropsychologia, 34*(5), 351–359.

Brunia, C. H. (1999). Neural aspects of anticipatory behavior. *Acta Psychologica, 101*(2–3), 213–242.

Buccino, G., Vogt, S., Ritzl, A., Fink, G. R., Zilles, K., Freund, H. J., & Rizzolatti, G. (2004). Neural circuits underlying imitation learning of hand actions: an event-related fMRI study. *Neuron, 42*(2), 323–334.

Calvo-Merino, B., Glaser, D. E., Grèzes, J., Passingham, R. E., & Haggard, P. (2005). Action observation and acquired motor skills: An FMRI study with expert dancers. *Cerebral Cortex, 15*(8), 1243–1249.

Calvo-Merino, B., Jola, C., Glaser, D. E., & Haggard, P. (2008). Towards a sensorimotor aesthetics of performing art. *Conscious and Cognition, 17*(3), 911–922.

Chapin, H., Jantzen, J., Kelso, J. A., Steinberg, F., & Large, E. (2010). Dynamic emotional and neural responses to music depend on performance expression and listener experience. *PLoS One 5*(12), e13812.

Cochin, S., Barthelemy, C., Lejeune, B., Roux, S., & Martineau, J. (1998). Perception of motion and qEEG activity in human adults. *Electroencephalography and Clinical Neurophysiology, 107*(4), 287–295.

Corballis, M. C. (2002). *From hand to mouth: The origins of language.* Princeton, NJ: Princeton University Press.

Cross, E. S., Hamilton, A. F., & Grafton, S. T. (2006). Building a motor simulation de novo: observation of dance by dancers. *NeuroImage, 31*(3), 1257–1267.

Danielsen, A., Otnæss, M. K., Jensen, J., Williams, S. C., & Ostberg, B. C. (2014). Investigating repetition and change in musical rhythm by functional MRI. *Neuroscience, 275*, 469–476.

de Waal, F. B. (2008). Putting the altruism back into altruism: the evolution of empathy. Annual Review of Psychology, *59*(1), 279–300.

Decety, J., & Jackson, P. L. (2004). The functional architecture of human empathy. *Behavioral and Cognitive Neuroscience Reviews, 3*(2), 71–100.

Downey, L. E., Blezat, A., Nicholas, J., Omar, R., Golden, H. L., Mahoney, C. J., Crutch, S. J., & Warren, J. D. (2013). Mentalising music in frontotemporal dementia. *Cortex, 49*(7), 1844–1855.

Elbert, T., Pantev, C., Wienbruch, C., Rockstroh, B., & Taub, E. (1995). Increased cortical representation of the fingers of the left hand in string players. *Science, 270*(5234), 305–307.

Engel, A., & Keller, P. E. (2011). The perception of musical spontaneity in improvised and imitated jazz performances. *Frontiers in Psychology, 2*, 83.

Etcoff, N. L. (1984). Selective attention to facial identity and facial emotion. *Neuropsychologia, 22*(3), 281–295.

Foster, N. E., & Zatorre, R. J. (2010a). Cortical structure predicts success in performing musical transformation judgments. *NeuroImage, 53*(1), 26–36.

Foster, N. E., & Zatorre, R. J. (2010b). A role for the intraparietal sulcus in transforming musical pitch information. *Cerebral Cortex, 20*(6), 1350–1359.

Frith, C. D, & Singer, T. (2008). The role of social cognition in decision making. *Philosophical Transactions of the Royal Society of London. Series B: Biological Sciences, 363*(1511), 3875–3886.

Gallese, V. (2003). The roots of empathy: The shared manifold hypothesis and the neural basis of intersubjectivity. *Psychopathology, 36*(4), 171–80.

Gallese, V., Keysers, C., & Rizzolatti, G. (2004). A unifying view of the basis of social cognition. *Trends in Cognitive Sciences, 8*(9), 396–403.

Gur, R. C., Skolnick, B. E., & Gur, R. E. (1994). Effects of emotional discrimination tasks on cerebral blood flow: Regional activation and its relation to performance. *Brain and Cognition, 25*(2), 271–286.

Hyde, K. L., Lerch, J. P., Zatorre, R. J., Griffiths, T. D., Evans, A. C., & Peretz, I. (2007). Cortical thickness in congenital amusia: When less is better than more. *Journal of Neuroscience, 27*(47), 13028–13032.

Hyde, K. L., Zatorre, R. J., Griffiths, T. D., Lerch, J. P., & Peretz, I. (2006). Morphometry of the amusic brain: A two-site study. *Brain, 129*(10), 2562–2570.

Iacoboni, M. (2005). Understanding others: imitation, language, empathy. In S. Hurley & N. Chater (Eds.), *Perspectives on imitation: Imitation in animals* (pp. 77–99). Cambridge, MA: MIT Press.

Kamiyama, K., Katahira, K., Abla, D., Hori, K., & Okanoya, K. (2010). Music playing and memory trace: Evidence from event-related potentials. *Neuroscience Research, 67*(4), 334–340.

Katahira, K., Abla, D., Masuda, S., & Okanoya, K. (2008). Feedback-based error moni-toring processes during musical performance: An ERP study. *Neuroscience Research, 61*(1), 120–128.

Klein, M. E., & Zatorre, R. J. (2011). A role for the right superior temporal sulcus in cate-gorical perception of musical chords. *Neuropsychologia, 49*(5), 878–887.

Klimesch, W. (1996). Memory processes, brain oscillations and EEG synchronization. *International Journal of Psychophysiology, 24*(1–2), 61–100.

Klimesch, W. (1999). EEG alpha and theta oscillations reflect cognitive and memory per-formance: A review and analysis. *Brain Research Reviews, 29*(2–3), 169–195.

Klimesch, W., Doppelmayr, M., Russegger, H., Pachinger, T., & Schwaiger, J. (1998). Induced alpha band power changes in the human EEG and attention. *Neuroscience Letters, 244*(2), 73–76.

Knutson, B., Adams, C. M., Fong, G. W., & Hommer, D. (2001) Anticipation of increas-ing monetary reward selectively recruits nucleus accumbens. *Journal of Neuroscience, 21*(16), 159.

Koelsch, S. (2010). Towards a neural basis of music-evoked emotions. *Trends in Cognitive Sciences, 14*(3), 131–137.

Koelsch, S. (2011). Toward a neural basis of music perception: A review and updated model. *Frontiers in Psychology, 2*, 110.

Koelsch, S., & Friederici, A. D. (2003). Toward the neural basis of processing structure in music. Comparative results of different neurophysiological investigation methods. *Annals of the New York Academy of Sciences, 999*, 15–28.

Koelsch, S., Fritz, T., V Cramon, D. Y., Müller, K., & Friederici, A. D. (2006). Investi-gating emotion with music: An fMRI study. *Human Brain Mapping, 27*(3), 239–250.

Koelsch, S., Gunter, T. C., v Cramon, D. Y., Zysset, S., Lohmann, G., & Friederici, A. D. (2002). Bach speaks: A cortical 'language-network' serves the processing of music. *NeuroImage. 17*(2), 956–966.

Koelsch, S., Maess, B., Gunter, T. C., & Friederici, A. D. (2001). Neapolitan chords acti-vate the area of Broca. A magnetoencephalographic study. *Annals of the New York Academy of Sciences, 930*, 420–421.

Kristeva, R., Chakarov, V., Schulte-Mönting, J., & Spreer, J. (2003). Activation of cortical areas in music execution and imagining: A high-resolution EEG study. *NeuroImage, 20*(3), 1872–1883.

Lawrence, E. J., Shaw, P., Baker, D., Baron-Cohen, S., & David, A. S. (2004). Measuring empathy: Reliability and validity of the Empathy Quotient. Psychological Medicine, *34*(5), 911–919.

Leiberg, S., & Anders, S. (2006). The multiple facets of empathy: A survey of theory and evidence. *Progress in Brain Research, 156*, 419–440.

Leman, M. (2007). *Embodied music cognition and mediation technology.* Cambridge, MA: MIT Press.

Leslie, K. R., Johnson-Frey, S. H., & Grafton, S. T. (2004). Functional imaging of face and hand imitation: towards a motor theory of empathy. *NeuroImage, 21*(2), 601–607.

Limb, C. J., & Braun, A. R. (2008). Neural substrates of spontaneous musical perfor-mance: An fMRI study of jazz improvisation. *PLoS One, 3*(2), e1679.

Maess, B., Koelsch, S., Gunter, T. C., & Friederici, A. D (2001). Musical syntax is pro-cessed in Broca's area: An MEG study. *Nature Neuroscience, 4*(5), 540–545.

Maidhof, C., Rieger, M., Prinz, W., & Koelsch, S. (2009). Nobody is perfect: ERP effects prior to performance errors in musicians indicate fast monitoring processes. *PLoS One. 4*(4), e5032.

Mandell, J., Schulze, K., & Schlaug, G. (2007). Congenital amusia: An auditory-motor feedback disorder? *Restorative Neurology and Neuroscience, 25*(3–4), 323–334.

Manganotti, P., Gerloff, C., Toro, C., Katsuta, H., Sadato, N., Zhuang, P., Leocani, L., & Hallett, M. (1998). Task-related coherence and task-related spectral power changes during sequential finger movements. *Electroencephalography and Clinical Neurophysiology, 109*(1), 50–62.

Mitchell, J. P. (2009). Inferences about mental states. *Philosophical Transactions of the Royal Society of London. Series B: Biological Sciences, 364*(1521), 1309–1316.

Moretti, D. V., Babiloni, F., Carducci, F., Cincotti, F., Remondini, E., Rossini, P. M., Salinari, S., & Babiloni, C. (2003). Computerized processing of EEG-EOG-EMG artifacts for multi-centric studies in EEG oscillations and event-related potentials. *International Journal of Psychophysiology, 47*(3), 199–216.

Muncer, S. J., & Ling, J. (2006). Psychometric analysis of the Empathy Quotient (EQ) scale. *Personality and Individual Differences, 40*(6), 1111–1119.

Nummenmaa, L., Hirvonen, J., Parkkola, R., & Hietanen, J. K. (2008). Is emotional contagion special? An fMRI study on neural systems for affective and cognitive empathy. *NeuroImage 43*, c571–580.

Ono, K., Nakamura, A., & Maess, B. (2015). Keeping an eye on the conductor: Neural correlates of visuo-motor synchronization and musical experience. *Frontiers in Human Neuroscience, 9*, 154.

Orgs, G., Dombrowski, J. H., Heil, M., & Jansen-Osmann, P. (2008). Expertise in dance modulates alpha/beta event-related desynchronization during action observation. *European Journal of Neuroscience, 27*(12), 3380–3384.

Pascual-Marqui, R. D. (2002). Standardized low-resolution brain electromagnetic tomography (sLORETA): technical details. *Methods and Findings in Experimental Clinical Pharmacology, 24* (Suppl D), 5–12.

Perani, D., Tervaniemi, M., & Toiviainen, P. (2011). Tuning the brain for music. *Cortex, 47*(9), 1023–1025.

Peretz, I., Gosselin, N., Belin, P., Zatorre, R. J., Plailly, J., & Tillmann, B. (2009). Music lexical networks: The cortical organization of music recognition. *Annals of the New York Academy of Sciences, 1169*, 256–265.

Peretz, I., & Zatorre, R. J. (2005). Brain organization for music processing. *Annual Review of Psychology, 56*, 89–114.

Perry, R. J., Rosen, H. R., Kramer, J. H., Beer, J. S., Levenson, R. L., & Miller, B. L. (2001). Hemispheric dominance for emotions, empathy and social behaviour: Evidence from right and left handers with frontotemporal dementia. *Neurocase, 7*(2), 145–160.

Petsche, H., von Stein, A., & Filz, O. (1996). EEG aspects of mentally playing an instrument. *Brain Research and Cognitive Brain Research, 3*(2), 115–123.

Pfurtscheller, G., & Aranibar, A. (1979). Evaluation of event-related desynchronization (ERD) preceding and following voluntary self-paced movement. *Electroencephalography and Clinical Neurophysiology, 46*(2), 138–146.

Pfurtscheller, G., & Lopes da Silva, F. H. (1999). Event-related EEG/MEG synchronization and desynchronization: Basic principles. *Clinical Neurophysiology, 110*(11), 1842–1857.

Pfurtscheller, G., & Neuper, C. (1994). Event-related synchronization of mu rhythm in the EEG over the cortical hand area in man. *Neuroscience Letters, 174*(1), 93–96.

Pfurtscheller, G., Neuper, C., Flotzinger, D., & Pregenzer, M. (1997). EEG-based discrimination between imagination of right and left hand movement. *Electroencephalography and Clinical Neurophysiology, 103*(6), 642–651.

Phan, K. L., Wager, T., Taylor, S. F., & Liberzon, I. (2002) Functional neuroanatomy of emotion: A meta-analysis of emotion activation studies in PET and fMRI. *NeuroImage, 16*(2), 331–348.

Preston, S. D., & de Waal, F. B. (2002). Empathy: Its ultimate and proximate bases. *Behavioral Brain Sciences, 25*(1), 1–20; discussion 20–71.

Rankin, K. P., Gorno-Tempini, M. L., Allison, S. C., Stanley, C. M., Glenn, S., Weiner, M. W., & Miller, B. L. (2006). Structural anatomy of empathy in neurodegenerative disease. *Brain, 129*(11), 2945–2956.

Rizzolatti, G., & Arbib, M. A. (1998). Language within our grasp. *Trends in Neuroscience, 21*(5), 188–194.

Rizzolatti, G., & Craighero, L. (2004). The mirror-neuron system. *Annual Review of Neuroscience, 27*, 169–92.

Rizzolatti, G., Fogassi, L., & Gallese, V. (2006). Mirrors of the mind. *Scientific American, 295*(5), 54–61.

Royet, J. P., Zald, D., Versace, R., Costes, N., Lavenne, F., Koenig, O., & Gervais, R. (2000). Emotional responses to pleasant and unpleasant olfactory, visual, and auditory stimuli: A positron emission tomography study. *Journal of Neuroscience, 20*, 7752–7759.

Ruby, P., & Decety, J. (2003). What you believe versus what you think they believe: A neuroimaging study of conceptual perspective-taking. *European Journal of Neuroscience, 17*(11), 2475–2480.

Ruby, P., & Decety, J. (2004). How would you feel versus how do you think she would feel? A neuroimaging study of perspective-taking with social emotions. *Cognitive Neuroscience, 16*(6), 988–999.

Rueckert, L., & Pawlak, T. (2000). Individual differences in cognitive performance due to right hemisphere arousal. *Laterality, 5*(1), 77–89.

Sammler, D., Koelsch, S., Ball, T., Brandt, A., Elger, C. E., Friederici, A. D., Grigutsch, M., Huppertz, H. J., Knösche, T. R., Wellmer, J., Widman, G., & Schulze-Bonhage, A. (2009). Overlap of musical and linguistic syntax processing: Intracranial ERP evidence. Annals of the New York Academy of Sciences, *1169*, 494–498.

Sammler, D., Koelsch, S., & Friederici, A. D. (2011). Are left fronto-temporal brain areas a prerequisite for normal music-syntactic processing? *Cortex, 47*(6), 659–673.

Särkämö, T., Tervaniemi, M., Soinila, S., Autti, T., Silvennoinen, H. M., Laine, M., Hietanen, M., & Pihko, E. (2010). Auditory and cognitive deficits associated with acquired amusia after stroke: A magnetoencephalography and neuropsychological follow-up study. *PLoS One, 5*(12), e15157.

Schaefer, R. S., Morcom, A. M., Roberts, N., & Overy, K. (2014). Moving to music: Effects of heard and imagined musical cues on movement-related brain activity. *Frontiers of Human Neuroscience, 8*, 774.

Schmidt, L. A., & Trainor, L. J. (2001). Frontal brain electrical activity (EEG) distinguishes *valence* and *intensity* of musical emotions. *Cognition and Emotion, 15*(4), 487–500.

Schönwiesner, M., & Zatorre, R. J. (2008). Depth electrode recordings show double dissociation between pitch processing in lateral Hescl's grus and sound onset processing in medial Hescl's grus. *Experimental Brain Research, 187*(1), 98–105.

Schulte-Ruther, M., Markowitsch, H. J., Fink, G. R., & Piefke, M. (2007). Mirror neuron and theory of mind mechanisms involved in face-to-face interactions: A functional magnetic resonance imaging approach to empathy. *Journal of Cognitive Neuroscience, 19*(8), 1354–1372.

Shamay-Tsoory, S. G. (2011). The neural bases for empathy. *Neuroscientist, 17*(1), 18–24.

Shamay-Tsoory, S. G., Aharon-Peretz, J., & Perry, D. (2009). Two systems for empathy: A double dissociation between emotional and cognitive empathy in inferior frontal gyrus versus ventromedial prefrontal lesions. *Brain, 132*(Pt 3), 617–627.

Shamay-Tsoory, S. G., Tomer, R., Berger, B. D., & Aharon-Peretz, J. (2003). Characterization of empathy deficits following prefrontal brain damage: The role of the right ventromedial prefrontal cortex. *Journal of Cognitive Neuroscience, 15*(3), 324–37.

Shamay-Tsoory, S.G., Tomer, R., Goldsher, D., Berger, B. D., & Aharon-Peretz, J. (2004). Impairment in cognitive and affective empathy in patients with brain lesions: Anatomical and cognitive correlates. *Journal of Clinical and Experimental Neuropsychology, 26*(8), 1113–1127.

Spada, D., Verga, L., Iadanza, A., Tettamanti, M., & Perani, D. (2014). The auditory scene: An fMRI study on melody and accompaniment in professional pianists. *NeuroImage, 102* (Pt 2), 764–775.

Steriade, M., & Llinas, R. R. (1988). The functional states of the thalamus and the associated neuronal interplay. *Physiology Review, 68*(3), 649–742.

Stewart, L., von Kriegstein, K., Warren, J. D., & Griffiths, T. D. (2006). Music and the brain: Disorders of musical listening. *Brain, 129*(10), 2533–2553.

Talairach, J., & Tournoux, P. (1988). *Co-planar stereotaxic atlas of the human brain: 3-Dimensional proportional system – an approach to cerebral imaging.* New York: Thieme Medical Publishers.

Ulloa, E. R., & Pineda, J. A. (2007). Recognition of point-light biological motion: Mu rhythms and mirror neuron activity. *Behavioral Brain Resesarch, 183*(2), 188–194.

Vogt, S., Buccino, G., Wohlschläger, A. M., Canessa, N., Shah, N. J., Zilles, K., Eickhoff, S. B., Freund, H. J., Rizzolatti, G., & Fink, G. R. (2007). Prefrontal involvement in imitation learning of hand actions: Effects of practice and expertise. *NeuroImage, 37*(4), 1371–1383.

Zatorre, R. J, & Belin, P. (2001). Spectral and temporal processing in human auditory cortex. *Cerebral Cortex, 11*(10), 946–953.

Zatorre, R. J., Halpern, A. R., & Bouffard, M. (2010). Mental reversal of imagined melodies: A role for the posterior parietal cortex. *Journal of Cognitive Neuroscience, 22*(4), 775–789.

10 When it clicks

Co-performer empathy in ensemble playing

Caroline Waddington

Ensemble playing is an important area of research in music psychology and education since almost all musicians play, rehearse or perform with others. Small ensembles are not directed by a conductor, and so ensemble playing is a unique social activity in which co-performers interact with one another in a variety of ways. Many researchers have sought to identify and analyse these co-performer interactions (for example, Davidson & Good, 2002; King, 2006; Williamon & Davidson, 2002). Of particular interest to our understanding of co-performer interaction are moments during ensemble performance where players have spoken of achieving a collective state of mind, described variously as being 'in the groove together' (Berliner, 1994), a 'group flow state' (Sawyer, 2006) or 'empathetic attunement' (Seddon, 2005). This collective state of mind seems likely to be related to empathy, a relatively recent intellectual concept (Lipps, 1903; Vischer, 1873/1994) that could be responsible for facilitating co-performer interaction, and may be central to our understanding of group dynamics within small ensembles. The importance of empathy in the rehearsal and performance process has been highlighted by Sharon Myers and Catherine White (2012) in which nine professional musicians described empathy as an essential part of performing well together. More recently, Elizabeth Haddon and Mark Hutchinson (2015) have explored the role and function of empathy in piano duet rehearsal and found that empathy was an important facilitative tool in the construction of shared concerns, reinforcing the duo partnership, pre-emptive conflict resolution and creating a 'safe space'. Empathy has also been identified by Peter Keller (2014) as a likely feature of ensemble playing.

There is much confusion surrounding the conceptualisation of empathy. This is due in no small part to the concept's convoluted research history. Empathy research now spans many disciplines in the arts, humanities and sciences, and each discipline has its own definition, or definitions, of empathy. In addition, the concept of empathy itself seems to overlap with other similar and related concepts, such as sympathy and emotional contagion. There are now many conflicting and overlapping definitions of all three concepts. Amy Coplan (2011) has suggested that rather than trying to find a broad all-encompassing definition for empathy, perhaps the way forward is to adopt specific, narrow definitions of empathy for individual areas of research. Coplan asserts that if all researchers were clear and precise in stating a narrow definition of empathy for their work, then this would lead to greater clarity for the claims they make based on that definition. The present chapter seeks to begin to develop a narrow definition of empathy for the context of ensemble playing. This is achieved through discussion of data obtained from three empirical studies, reported in turn below. The first study investigated expert ensemble musicians' experiences of co-performer empathy via focus group interviews, providing insight into the ways in which they describe and perceive this phenomenon. Following on from this, the second and third studies probed the processes of experiencing and achieving empathy in ensemble performance using observational video-recalls with members of a professional string quartet and string duo respectively. Various models are presented in this account so as to illustrate the process of developing a definition of empathy in ensemble playing.

Study 1: exploring expert ensemble musicians' experiences of co-performer empathy

In order to explore expert ensemble musicians' experiences of co-performer empathy, a focus group study was conducted with five established Western Art ensembles from around the UK (for a full account see Waddington, 2013). The aim of the study was to explore how ensemble musicians themselves describe their experiences of working and performing together, with particular reference to their optimal experiences of performance and co-performer empathy.

A total of 19 participants (ten males and nine females; mean age 37 years) were interviewed in their respective ensembles: a wind quintet, a vocal duo, a contemporary woodwind trio, a mixed piano trio and a string quartet. No brass ensemble was available for a group interview so three members of two brass ensembles were interviewed individually. All participants had been working together in their groups professionally or semi-professionally for a minimum of three years. Interview questions were based, in part, on existing studies on empathy in performance (Myers & White, 2012), peak performance (Privette, 1981) and Strong Experiences with Music (SEM) (Gabrielsson, 2001).

Analysis revealed that co-performer empathy consisted of three main components: a shared approach to interpretation and to working together; an intentional awareness of how colleagues are operating on both a musical and a practical level; and a special connection between players. In addition, it was found that co-performer empathy sometimes led to an ensemble achieving spontaneous interpretative flexibility (SIF) during performance.

Shared approach: a pre-requisite for co-performer empathy

It was found that the ensemble musicians felt that a shared approach to both musical interpretation and to working together was a pre-requisite for co-performer empathy. Regarding interpretation, participants emphasised the importance of a shared approach to expressive detail within the music, as well as an agreement that the music should take priority over all else. One violinist described this second aspect as striving to 'make the whole greater than the sum of the parts'.

There were three distinct aspects of a shared approach to working together. First, it was essential for all players to agree on a style of working. Examples included whether rehearsals should be democratic, whether to work in short bursts or at length, and how blunt players should be. Second, a shared level of commitment to the ensemble was considered vital. If players felt that one colleague was contributing less, then resentment could build. It seems likely, therefore, that an equal commitment is required from all players for an ensemble to function at the highest level. Third, shared goals for the ensemble were essential. This was probably because goals affect an ensemble's approach to rehearsals, the kind of gigs they play, how often they rehearse or how much time they dedicate to the ensemble. Previous research has also shown that shared performance goals are vital for collaborative performance (Keller, 2008; Williamon & Davidson, 2002) and that the interpersonal alignment of fundamental and expressive parameters fosters ensemble cohesion (Keller, 2014). A shared approach both to musical interpretation and to working together was, therefore, a pre-requisite condition for achieving co-performer empathy.

Special connection: 'clicking' together

The second component of co-performer empathy was special connection. A variety of vocabulary was used to express this idea: 'gelling', 'exactly synchronised', 'an intimate connection', 'in harmony', 'eyes', 'ears', 'radar', 'instinctively aware', 'sympathy', 'clicking', 'locking in', 'getting into each other's heads', 'being able to read the other person's mind'. No participants used the word empathy before being asked direct questions about empathy during the interviews, but all agreed either that empathy was a good description of the same phenomenon, or that they understood the term in the same way.

One of the brass players gave an example of a moment of special connection from his ensemble performance experience. His quartet used to perform a particular piece from memory and they would stand in a tight diamond formation, rotating so that whoever was playing the tune was at the front.

> Going back to that 'Air from Suite in D' thing that we as an ensemble worked together. We didn't speak. We couldn't see each other. We used our ears, I guess, or there was something else. And I think there was something else. There was a connection that was made between us as an ensemble that made us all move at the same time, all play at the same time. And that's, I don't think that's an education thing. I think that's something else entirely.
>
> (Tuba player from Tuba Quartet)

A process emerged for forging a special connection between players. It began with an ensemble formed of players with complementary personalities. A socio-emotional connection between players is then consolidated through social bonding experiences, leading to trust between players (see also Gritten, this volume). The connection is developed further through rehearsing together, leading to familiarity between players and a feeling of being able to predict how colleagues are likely to play or respond. Eventually, the process resulted in co-performers experiencing a 'special connection' that is intimate and experienced in varying degrees while playing together. The special connection component characterised almost all of the accounts of optimal performance experiences.

Intentional awareness: perspective-taking

The third component of co-performer empathy was an intentional awareness of how one's colleagues are operating on either a practical or a musical level. This requires a degree of perspective-taking in order to understand the difficulties they may face. On a musical level, players described the importance of an intentional musical awareness of the different expressive ideas and roles embodied by each player at any point within the music. As one flautist explained, being unaware of other parts and retaining only an individual focus results in 'bulldozing through'.

SIF: unplanned moments of ensemble work

SIF was found to be closely related to co-performer empathy. SIF was defined by participants as the spontaneous production of novel expressive variations in performance and was described by all as desirable.

> Changing stuff, changing tempos, changing rits, changing dynamics ... That's part of performing. I mean, if it was the same every time it would be really boring. And that's kind of the joy of working with a group for a long time.
>
> (Flautist from Piano Trio)

All of the ensembles described SIF as something they strived for in performance and it was a feature of almost all of their descriptions of optimal experiences of performance.

Study 2: exploring co-performer empathy and SIF with a string quartet

The production of novel variations in performance has been explored in previous studies. For example, John Sloboda (1985) has suggested that 'expert performance is often characterised by the fresh reconstruction of performance parameters ... on every occasion' (p. 97). Music is a complex-patterned material offering a lot of scope for variability in performance. Variability of musical interpretation in expert performance arises in the moment rather than being pre-planned, and can, therefore, be regarded as 'spontaneous'. An expert performer can approach a performance with a degree of what Sloboda terms 'optionality'. That is, he or she can choose spontaneously during a performance whether to reproduce a previous interpretation, or whether to produce an interpretation that is wholly or partially different in expression. This can be achieved through the spontaneous variation of a number of performance parameters, including dynamics, tempo, articulation, fingering, timbre or intonation. In solo performance, SIF is a relatively simple process involving the soloist spontaneously deviating from an established, practised interpretation and producing some form of novel variation. However, in the context of ensemble playing, the phenomenon becomes more complex by virtue of its becoming a group process involving inter-individual co-variation. SIF in ensemble playing is defined here as the spontaneous production of novel variations differing from an established interpretation, produced by an ensemble while playing together.

All of the professional ensemble players interviewed as part of the Study 1 spoke of SIF as an important and desirable aspect of their performing experiences. These views support evidence from previous research on the production of novel variations in expert performance (for example, Davidson, 1997; Sloboda, 1985). In his book of interviews with the Guarneri String Quartet, David Blum (1986) explored this phenomenon. The players described a sense of spontaneity and a degree of improvisation in their performances as being of crucial importance. Michael Tree described the quartet's approach to performing in terms of flexibility:

> The playing of quartet music is … an organic process. Each of us is influenced by constantly fluctuating circumstances. Each moment of our playing is conditioned by what has just occurred or by what we think is about to occur. It remains creative because just about anything can happen.
>
> (Blum, 1986, p. 20)

Since the results of the focus group analysis revealed SIF to be related to co-performer empathy in some way, an observational study using video-recall was undertaken to examine this relationship more closely. This study was driven by two research questions: what is the process of SIF in expert ensemble playing and how is it related to co-performer empathy?

A rehearsal and a performance of Schubert's *Quartettsatz* were video-recorded within the space of one week by an expert, established string quartet. The quartet had been playing together for over three years, had won several prestigious prizes, and held a fellowship at the European Chamber Music Academy. A code-specific video-recall method was used in which the players were asked to view the video footage individually and identify and comment on examples of three different kinds of moment in the video recordings: intentional awareness, special connection and SIF. For this study it was decided to focus on these three aspects of empathy, assuming that shared approach, the pre-requisite condition, was already in place by virtue of the professional standing of the group. The players were then interviewed individually to discuss their responses, to view and describe in more detail the kind of moments they had identified for each code, and to explain how they thought the codes fitted and related to the workings of their ensemble.

The players' recall logs were read, re-read, explored and compared. Any similarities and differences between participants relating to each code were noted, as well as any overlap between codes. A thematic analysis was then conducted on the interview transcripts to identify any common themes or ideas. The recall logs and interview transcripts were then examined side by side, and considered in relation to the study's research questions.

The relationship between co-performer empathy and SIF

Moments of perceived SIF were coded by all participants in the recall logs. Table 10.1 shows the number of times SIF was coded by each participant.

According to the recall log results, all participants perceived more moments of SIF during performance than during the rehearsal. In addition to supporting evidence in existing literature by John Sloboda (1985) and Jane Davidson (1997), this may also provide some support to the assertion of the players in this study and the focus group that SIF is something that expert ensemble players strive for in performance.

There were a several examples of SIF being coded alongside a component of co-performer empathy by the same performer (see Table 10.2).

There were more examples of SIF being coded alongside intentional awareness in the performance than in the rehearsals. The relatively high incidence of SIF being coded alongside both intentional awareness and special connection in the recall logs, particularly during the performance, suggested that the players perceived there to be a connection between experiencing co-performer empathy and a moment of SIF. In short, there seems to be a relationship between co-performer empathy and SIF, and the nature of this relationship is explored below through discussion of the process of SIF.

Table 10.1 Frequency of SIF coded by each participant during rehearsal and performance.

	Rehearsal (01:31:01)	*Performance (00:09:03)*
Violin 1	0	5
Violin 2	1	1
Viola	1	2
Cello	2	6

Table 10.2 Frequency of SIF coded with components of co-performer empathy.

	Rehearsal (01:30:01)	*Performance (00:09:03)*
Intentional Awareness with SIF	3	7
Special Connection with SIF	1	3

The process of SIF

Figure 10.1 shows a model of the process of SIF in expert ensemble playing, constructed from the analysis of the recall logs and interviews.

The model involves the two components of co-performer empathy (intentional awareness and special connection) and a pre-requisite shared approach, as identified in the focus group study. The central process was determined from the recall logs and interviews in which the players described the way the different components were used in order to achieve SIF. SIF in performance seems to arise as a result of a two-step empathic process involving an intentional awareness of the expressive intentions of one's co-performer(s) followed by an intentional or instinctive response (detailed below). It was often (though not always) characterised by a special connection between players.

The process begins with an intentional awareness, a sort of musical perspective-taking, in which players will shift the focus completely away from their own part and force themselves to listen to another player's part completely. The cellist gave an example of this kind of perspective-taking in a moment of intentional awareness, special connection, and SIF that she had logged during the performance:

> There's a bit just after the double bar, and the first time we play it the first violin goes really quiet and then goes back to … the opening so it kind of just falls into that. But the second time we do it, it goes *subito forte*, and we all come crashing in. And so in those few bars before the crash when [the first violinist] is playing on her own, we all have to be in the zone as they say, and essentially playing her part in our mind so we can all just come in. I don't think you could be sitting there just counting the bars' rest because it wouldn't have the same feeling as if you were actually totally involved, even though you're not playing.
>
> (Cellist from String Quartet)

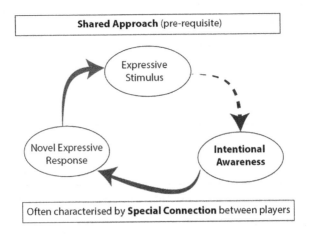

Figure 10.1 Model of the cyclical process of SIF in expert ensemble playing.

The act of musical perspective-taking here is that of the three lower players intentionally imagining playing the leader's part with her. This mental process akin to empathic perspective-taking allows players to identify the musical or expressive intentions of a colleague, through an intentional awareness, and to then respond, creating a moment of SIF. It seems to be similar to Seddon's (2005) notion of 'decentering' in that it requires the players to shift from an individual focus in order to be intentionally aware of the actions of their co-performers.

It is necessary not only that players identify with their colleagues' musical intentions, but that they also respond accordingly – the second step in the process. As the first violinist observed: 'You can't be aware of what someone else is doing on a musical level and then not respond. You wouldn't purposefully not respond would you?' All players agreed that there was a response, but there was no conclusive consensus as to whether the response was intentional or instinctive, with all participants suggesting that perhaps it was a bit of both depending on the circumstances of a particular moment or of a particular performance. Responding in the moment to the novel expressive variation produced by one player completes the process of SIF in ensemble playing.

SIF in performance seems to arise as a result of a two-step empathic process involving an intentional awareness to identify the expressive intentions of one's co-performer(s) and a response. If this is the case, parallels can be drawn with the process of empathic responding more generally. One of the longest-standing debates in the field of empathy research has been over whether empathy is primarily a cognitive or affective phenomenon. More recently a movement has begun towards the wide acceptance of empathy as both a cognitive and affective process. In simple terms, the argument made for empathy as a dual cognitive–affective process is that it is impossible to have an instinctive, affective reaction to an individual's suffering without first having undergone even a subconscious cognitive process to evaluate that individual's state in order to be able to respond appropriately (Baron-Cohen, 2011). Empathy, then, seems to be a two-step process involving cognitive perspective-taking to evaluate an individual's state, followed by an appropriate affective response to that state. Simon Baron-Cohen (2011) has defined empathy as 'our ability to identify what someone else is thinking or feeling, and to respond to their thoughts and feelings with an appropriate emotion'. There are clear similarities between this process of empathy and the process of SIF in ensemble playing.

Just as in the process of empathy, the results of this study suggested that it is impossible to respond to a co-performer's expressive stimulus without first having some kind of intentional awareness of how that co-performer is operating on a musical level. Intentional awareness allows players to identify or anticipate their co-performer's expressive intention and respond to it, to create a moment of SIF. The parallels that can be drawn between the process of SIF and the process of empathy more broadly, further suggest a close relationship between SIF and co-performer empathy. Figures 10.2 and 10.3 show the similarities between the two processes.

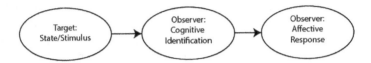

Figure 10.2 The process of empathy (Baron-Cohen, 2011).

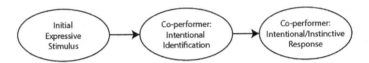

Figure 10.3 The process of SIF in ensemble playing.

SIF as a case of intense co-performer empathy

It seems likely from the analysis of the players' recall interviews and logs that even when players were not producing moments of SIF while playing together, there was an ongoing, cyclical process of co-performer empathy underpinning their collaborative musical interactions. Figure 10.4 shows the initial model developed from the observational study using video-recall with the string quartet and shows that responses to an expressive stimulus may be novel or expected.

Expert ensemble performance seems to involve a continuous, cyclical process of co-performer empathy. At the end of a single cycle, a player's response becomes the new expressive stimulus and the process is repeated. Whether or not

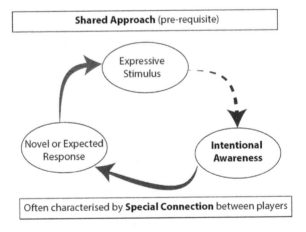

Figure 10.4 Initial model of the cyclical process of co-performer empathy/SIF in ensemble playing.

a cycle results in a moment of SIF depends on whether the response stage is expected or novel.

SIF may be considered to be a type of intense co-performer empathy. When an ensemble strives for SIF, both the shared approach pre-requisite condition and the intentional awareness component of co-performer empathy take on a greater importance. The production of novel expressive variations in the moment require greater intentional awareness since actions are not pre-planned, and the response to a player's expressive variation (stimulus) by other players has to be based on a shared approach to musical interpretation.

As indicated in the focus group study, a shared approach is an essential pre-requisite for both co-performer empathy and the more intense case of SIF. It is imperative that players share the same vision of musical interpretation, because a disagreement over how the music should be interpreted could ruin a performance. The cyclical process of co-performer empathy should occur throughout a performance. Players must constantly be intentionally aware of the expressive actions or intentions of their colleagues in order to be able to respond appropriately to them throughout the performance. If the expressive actions are pre-planned, then the response is more predictable. However, if one player produces a novel expressive variation in the moment, other players must be aware that this has occurred, and adjust their response accordingly. In this way, ensemble performance is a constantly evolving process of empathic responding through which there is the optionality for a piece to be performed differently every time. Players may choose to adhere strictly to a pre-planned interpretation, reproducing a previous performance as closely as possible. They may create an entirely new interpretation, requiring an intense process of co-performer empathy: SIF. They may choose to use a combination of these two extremes, in places adhering to a pre-planned interpretation, and in other places creating moments of SIF. In all cases, the process of co-performer empathy is essential and must be present throughout.

Study 3: further exploration of co-performer empathy and SIF with a violin duo

A further video-recall study involving an expert violin duo, both players drawn from a professional string quartet, examined more closely the cyclical processes of co-performer empathy and of SIF, the special type of intense co-performer empathy. Rather than coding moments of intentional awareness, special connection and SIF, as in the string quartet study, the duo were asked to code for moments of intentional awareness, special connection and two types of response: expected response and novel response. These codes were drawn from the initial model of co-performer empathy/SIF in Figure 10.4. As in Study 2, the two players were interviewed separately to discuss their accounts in more detail with reference to some of the coded video moments they had logged, and to reflect on the processes of co-performer empathy and SIF in their experiences of ensemble playing. As part of this study, the violinists performed the B minor Double from J. S. Bach's Partita No. 1.

Familiarity and trust

Thematic analysis of the recall interviews revealed two main themes in addition to the recall codes: familiarity and trust. There were three different aspects to familiarity: musical tendencies, gestural idiosyncrasies and mechanics of the instrument.

Familiarity: musical tendencies

Violinist B explained that he was very familiar with Violinist A's musical tendencies because they had spent significant amounts of time rehearsing and performing together as members of the same quartet. He commented that this helped him to anticipate how she might approach or respond to particular moments in a piece of music. He felt that his familiarity with Violinist A's musical tendencies allowed him to accurately identify her musical intentions in each phrase in time to be able to respond flexibly when he was following, and to be able to gauge her likely response to his musical and expressive intentions in good time when he was leading. Violinist A commented that their shared history of quartet playing allowed them to draw on ideas developed in quartet rehearsals, sometimes a particular sound or colour, or, in one example, a type of musical moment:

> I kind of drew on our experiences to predict what was going to happen and sensed him doing the same thing. The 'Kung Fu Panda' thing, for example, that's a gesture we've talked about and I just could sense it. It came up, and we both applied it.
>
> (Violinist A from Violin Duo)

She went on to explain that a 'Kung Fu Panda moment' had once been described to them in a quartet coaching session by an eminent cellist as a way of building up and subsequently releasing energy in a passage as an ensemble. She had coded a moment of this in her recall log and, while watching the same excerpt during her interview, explained how she had felt a special connection with Violinist B at that particular moment. They had both simultaneously decided to create that particular musical moment during a certain passage of the duo without prior agreement. Their familiarity with one another's musical tendencies and shared history of working together allowed them, in that moment, to create something spontaneously and simultaneously without discussion.

Familiarity: gestural repertoire

Another aspect of the theme of familiarity concerned each player's knowledge of the other's individual repertoire of gestures. Violinist B commented that this was the thing that struck him most about his experience of completing the recall log. This shared understanding of one another's gestural repertoire was a result of familiarity with one another's use of gesture from all the time spent playing together in their quartet. Both players also agreed that their use of particular gestures to communicate different expressive or ensemble ideas was automatic rather than intentional. Since they have both worked together regularly as part of the same string quartet for a number of years, both players have developed gestures for leading and following in that ensemble's context that have become automatic, and that they were able to apply during the performances here without discussion or extra attention.

Familiarity: the instrument itself

Familiarity with the instrument itself was also suggested as an important indicator of the other player's musical or expressive intentions. During his recall interview, Violinist B described being able to navigate through the score and know that there were certain junctures within the music where different expressive decisions would be made. He explained that in addition to gesture, posture and familiarity with one another's musical tendencies, a shared familiarity with the mechanics of the instrument itself was useful in anticipating what the other player was likely to do at these moments:

> For example, if I play a passage and then reach a point at which we could do the second time *forte* or the second time 'echo', to take a really basic example, you're informed by where are they on the bow. How much tilt do they have? I mean, you don't register these things consciously of course. But if they're at the heel of the bow, odds are they're going to do something *forte*, versus something 'echo', because why would you prepare yourself to be at the heel otherwise?
>
> (Violinist B from Violin Duo)

Both players were able to draw on their expert knowledge of the violin itself, their understanding of its mechanics and use in ensemble settings through their experiences of quartet, chamber and orchestral playing. This allowed them to more accurately convey or anticipate one another's intentions at certain points within the music.

Trust

Several examples of trust and its importance to moments of empathy or SIF were given by both participants. Violinist B described at length the role of trust in successfully negotiating a moment of SIF in quartet performance.

> We just challenge each other to do these things in performance. Trusting that the work's been done, that all the specifics have been worked out. And say something happens that never happened before in performance: you trust each other that you've explored down all of these pathways, that if one comes up that you've never seen before, then you know how other ones work so you

can probably figure it out, and you trust that the others can figure it out and they trust you. There's this backwards and forth, so if something new comes up you trust that you can deal with it, and that is being flexible.

(Violinist B from Violin Duo)

His point was that SIF was rooted in trust that was built through rehearsing repertoire together over a period of time. The importance of trust between co-performers to the long-term success of a chamber ensemble has also been outlined by Gritten (2013; see also this volume), and was emphasised by several players in the focus group study.

The violinists' views on co-performer empathy

First, as expressed by Violinist B during his recall interview when considering the process of SIF, the initial stage in this cyclical process is perhaps better described as an 'expressive intention' rather than an 'expressive stimulus'. The word 'intention' suggests the deliberate formation of a certain musical, interpretative or expressive idea by one of the players at a given moment. An expressive stimulus, on the other hand, suggests that the idea or approach comes into being without the active input of one of the performers. Violinist B explained that the expressive intention was sometimes communicated very deliberately to co-performers, usually when the intention was to create a moment of SIF, or to negotiate a difficult musical moment in performance. He described the way in which he gathers his co-performers' attention in such moments through a gesture he called a 'butler sweep', in order to alert them that he is about to do something unexpected. By gathering their attention in this manner, he is warning or

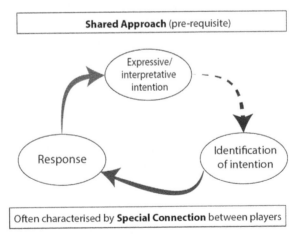

Figure 10.5 Final model of the cyclical process of co-performer empathy and SIF in expert ensemble playing.

encouraging them to be intentionally aware of his actions in that moment, so that they can identify his expressive intention and then respond appropriately.

He also explained the active role performed by the player(s) following, who must be alert and intentionally aware, in order to be able to identify the expressive intention of their colleague, and then respond appropriately. They cannot sit passively and wait to follow or there will be a delay and the process will be less successful. In her recall interview, Violinist A explained:

> [An eminent violinist] always says, you've got to be like a cat when it sits upright but at any moment it could just pounce. So you're kind of just sitting there and you're ready, but every single muscle in your body is ready to go in any direction. You're super alert.
>
> (Violinist A from Violin Duo)

In this way, the response could be regarded as always being flexible, to a degree. The player is prepared to move in any direction depending on the leader's expressive intention, how well it is identified by the other players, and how quickly, effectively and to what extreme the other players are able to respond. Violinist B suggested in his recall interview that perhaps it is better to think of response in terms of degree of flexibility, rather than simply 'flexible' or 'not flexible'. The latter view is perhaps too simplistic in the complex context of ensemble performance.

When asked about the process of musical interaction during ensemble performance, Violinist B articulated a process for SIF:

> There's ultimately an infinite loop going on … You gather whomever you want to play with and then you show them it's about to happen, and then while you're about to do it, and even while you're starting doing it, you're judging 'are they with me? Is this actually happening?' and if you get a re-doubled response, then you might do it more than you originally intended. If you know that they're with you then you'll just do as you wanted, and if they're not paying attention, if their heads are in the part or if you just don't feel their presence, then you're going to scale back. So … even when you're trying to lay it down, you're ultimately being flexible. In a way, the person who ends up leading is the one who is the least skilled … because the one who's the least skilled at having a clue what's going on is the one who's going to limit the possibility of what could happen. The reason I say it's an infinite loop, is because then from the person-who's-following's perspective, they're going 'Yeah OK I'm with you, but I'm giving you this. Are you with me?' So then I have to go, 'OK, yeah, I do recognise this, and I'm doing this in response to your doing that, in response to me doing my thing.' This all happens in the moment, several layers deep.
>
> (Violinist B from Violin Duo)

The continuous process of identification and response between leader and follower described by Violinist B as they negotiate a given moment within the music reflects the process of co-performer empathy presented above (Figure 10.5). His description of an 'infinite loop' concerns the cyclical nature of the process, with the players involved continuously identifying and responding to one another's musical intentions.

The point he raises about the least skilled member of an ensemble being the one who 'ends up leading' suggests that the success of the empathic process is limited by the ability of the ensemble's weakest member. Here, 'weakest' indicates the member of the ensemble who is least skilled in being able to transmit, identify, or respond to the other players' intentions. This could be a result of lesser technical skill, as suggested in Jane Davidson and James Good's (2002) student quartet case study, where the observations suggested that the members of the quartet were too focused on their own parts and the technical challenges contained therein, and as a result could not spare attention to work on expressive ideas. In a similar way, ensemble players' technical expertise might also influence their ability to divide their attention, looking up from their parts to direct their attention outwards and onto the intentions of their co-performers. It is possible that it may not only be technical expertise but also development of the skills involved in the process of co-performer empathy. After all, many concert soloists are highly skilled, technically proficient musicians, and yet some of these gifted solo performers are insensitive ensemble musicians. This suggests that an ensemble's success in producing expressive, novel performances could be limited not only by the individual technical expertise of the players, but also by how well each player within the ensemble is able to participate in the ongoing, cyclical process of co-performer empathy during performance.

If it is the case that an ensemble's success in producing expressive, novel performances depends on each player's ability to participate in a cyclical process of co-performer empathy throughout a performance, this presents important practical applications for chamber music pedagogy. While trust and familiarity both play critical roles in the development of a successful chamber ensemble, these are developed gradually over time spent rehearsing and performing together. However, it may be possible for techniques for the strengthening of the gathering of co-performers and the identification of expressive intentions to be developed and taught.

Conclusion

The results of the studies reported here have permitted the construction of a model (Figure 10.5) as well as a narrow definition of co-performer empathy in expert ensemble playing. Co-performer empathy is a cyclical process during expert ensemble playing that is based on a pre-requisite condition of a shared approach to musical interpretation and to working together. It is often characterised by a special connection between players and involves a process of empathic responding where players are aware of the expressive intentions of their colleagues and respond with some degree of flexibility. Parallels have also been drawn here between the process of co-performer empathy and the process of empathy more broadly.

SIF in ensemble playing was considered to involve an intense process of co-performer empathy, since it involves a similar process of identifying and responding, but a greater intentional awareness in order to respond with a greater degree of flexibility to a co-performer's expressive intention. Both the process of co-performer empathy and that of SIF were found to be characterised in some instances by a special connection between players. It is not yet clear what might influence the presence of a special connection, although one of the string quartet players suggested that it was sometimes based on the external circumstances of a particular performance, such as the importance of the occasion, the size and type of audience, or performer nerves.

The video-recall studies outlined here have involved only a string quartet and a violin duo. Further work should be undertaken to test the model of the process of co-performer empathy in ensemble playing using ensembles of different instrumental combinations, genres and levels of expertise. Another direction for future research may be to examine other indicators of co-performer empathy. The studies outlined here have incorporated only self-report measures of co-performer empathy. Empathy research in other fields has shown that physiological measures have had some success in indicating when an individual is experiencing empathy (for example, Hooker *et al.*, 2010; Krebs, 1975; Levenson & Reuf, 1992; Shamay-Tsoory *et al.*, 2005; Sonby-Borgstrom, 2002; Sterzer *et al.*, 2007; Westbury & Neumann, 2008). In the field of music, physiological measures have begun to be used to investigate empathy in various contexts (for example, Babiloni *et al.*, 2012; Miu & Balteş, 2012). An exploratory case study measuring the heart-rates of a violin duo in relation to self-reported moments of empathy has already been undertaken (Waddington, 2015), and further work in this direction may yield some interesting results.

Since co-performer empathy seems to be a vital process for expert ensemble performance, future work should also address techniques for facilitating co-performer empathy. This work could then have much-needed pedagogical applications for chamber music tuition. One possibility is an exploration of techniques for developing or improving ensemble musicians' capacity for the kind of musical perspective-taking described by the ensemble musicians in this chapter.

References

Babiloni, C., Buffo, P., Vecchio, F., Marzano, N., Del Percio, C., Spada, D., Rossi, S., Bruni, I., Rossini, P., & Perani, D. (2012). Brains 'in concert': Frontal oscillatory alpha rhythms and empathy in professional musicians. *Neuroimage*, *60*(1), 105–116.

Baron-Cohen, S. (2011). *Zero degrees of empathy*. London: Penguin.

Berliner, P. F. (1994). *Thinking in jazz*. Chicago, IL: University of Chicago Press.

Blum, D. (1986). *The art of quartet playing: The Guarneri Quartet in conversation with David Blum*. London: Victor Gollancz Ltd.

Coplan, A. (2011). Understanding empathy: Its features and effects. In A. Coplan & P. Goldie (Eds.), *Empathy: Philosophical and psychological perspectives* (pp. 3–18). Oxford: Oxford University Press.

Davidson, J. W. (1997). The social psychology of performance. In D. J. Hargreaves & A. C. North (Eds.), *The social psychology of music* (pp. 209–226). Oxford: Oxford University Press.

Davidson, J. W., & Good, J. M. M. (2002). Social and musical communication between members of a string quartet: An exploratory study. *Psychology of Music, 30*(2), 186–201.

Gabrielsson, A. (2001). Emotions in strong experiences with music. In P. N. Juslin & J. A. Sloboda (Eds.), *Music and emotion: Theory and research* (pp. 431–449). Oxford: Oxford University Press.

Gritten, A. (2013, 21–22 June). *Trust in collaboration: From policy to practice.* Paper presented at Creative Arts and Creative Industries: Collaboration in Practice Conference, Manchester Metropolitan University.

Haddon, E., & Hutchinson, M. (2015). Empathy in piano duet rehearsal. *Empirical Musicology Review, 10*(2), 140–153.

Hooker, C. I., Verosky, S. C., Germine, L. T., Knight, R. T., & Esposito, M. D. (2010). Neural activity during social signal perception correlates with self-reported empathy. *Brain Research, 1308*, 100–113.

Keller, P. E. (2008). Joint action in music performance. In F. Morganti, A. Carassa & G. Riva (Eds.), *Enacting intersubjectivity: A cognitive and social perspective to the study of interactions* (pp. 205–221). Amsterdam: IOS Press.

Keller, P. E. (2014). Ensemble performance: Interpersonal alignment of musical expression. In D. Fabian, R. Timmers & E. Schubert (Eds.), *Expressiveness in music performance: Empirical approaches across styles and cultures* (pp. 260–282). Oxford: Oxford University Press.

King, E. C. (2006). The roles of student musicians in quartet rehearsals. *Psychology of Music, 34*(2), 263–283.

Krebs, D. (1975). Empathy and altruism. *Journal of Personality and Social Psychology, 32*(6), 1134–1146.

Lipps, T. (1903). *Aesthetik: Psychologie des Schönen und der Kunst.* Hamburg: Voss.

Levenson, R. W., & Ruef, A. M. (1992). Empathy: A physiological substrate. *Journal of Personality and Social Psychology, 63*, 234–246.

Miu, A. C., & Balteş, F. R. (2012). Empathy manipulation impacts music-induced emotions: A psychophysiological study on opera. *PLoS ONE 7*(1), e30618.

Myers, S. A., & White, C. M. (2012). 'Listening with the third ear': An exploration of empathy in musical performance. *Journal of Humanistic Psychology, 52*(3), 254–278.

Privette, G. (1981). Dynamics of peak performance. *Journal of Humanistic Psychology, 21*(1), 57–67.

Sawyer, R. K. (2006). Group creativity: Musical performance and collaboration. *Psychology of Music, 34*(2), 148–165.

Seddon, F. A. (2005). Modes of communication during jazz improvisation. *British Journal of Music Education, 22*(1), 47–61.

Shamay-Tsoory, S. G., Lester, H., Chisin, R., Israel, O., Bar-Shalom, R., Peretz, A., Tomer, R., Tsitrinbaum, Z., & Aharon-Peretz, J. (2005). The neural correlates of understanding other's distress: A positron emotion tomography investigation of accurate empathy. *NeuroImage, 27*(2), 468–472.

Sloboda, J. (1985). *The musical mind: The cognitive psychology of music.* Oxford: Clarendon Press.

Sonnby-Borgström, M. (2002). Automatic mimicry reactions as related to differences in emotional empathy. *Scandinavian Journal of Psychology, 43*(5), 433–443.

Sterzer, P., Stadler, C., Poustka, F., & Kleinschmidt, A. (2007). A structural neural deficit in adolescents with conduct disorder and its association with lack of empathy. *Neuro-Image, 37*(1), 335–342.

Vischer, R. (1873/1994). Uber das Optische Formgefuhl. In H. Mallgrave & E. Ikonomou (Eds. and Trans.), *Empathy, form and space: Problems in German aesthetics, 1873–1893* (pp. 89–124). Santa Monica, CA: Getty Centre for the History of Art and the Humanities.

Waddington, C. E. (2013). Co-performer empathy and peak performance in expert ensemble playing. In A. Williamon & W. Goebl (Eds.), *Proceedings of the International Symposium on Performance Science 2013* (pp. 331–336). Brussels, Belgium: European Association of Conservatoires.

Waddington, C. E. (2015). *Co-performer empathy in expert ensemble playing* (Unpublished doctoral dissertation). University of Hull, UK.

Westbury, H. R., & Neumann, D. L. (2008). Empathy-related responses to moving film stimuli depicting human and non-human animal targets in negative circumstances. *Biological Psychology, 78*(1), 66–74.

Williamon A., & Davidson, J. W. (2002). Exploring co-performer communication. *Musicae Scientiae, 6*(1), 53–72.

11 Developing trust in others

Or, how to empathise like a performer

Anthony Gritten

1. Introduction: interaction rules

This chapter is about the relationship between empathy and trust in ensemble performing. My initial entry point to the subject is through the discourse of interaction, which is the public face that trust reveals to the world – its practical conduit. My argument is that trust is the ground upon which musical empathy is supervenient, that trust is the basis for empathy's emergence as a force relating ensemble co-performers and their live decisions, and that empathy can only be understood fully as a function of trust and trustworthiness. A fair amount has been written recently about empathy in music and in performing. There has, however, been far less discussion of how trust figures in performing, for probably all sorts of reasons from the trivial to the important.

The chapter is structured in five sections. This introductory section poses key questions and caveats. Section 2 outlines the key features of empathy and makes a brief comparison with trust. Section 3 considers the social value of ensemble interaction with respect to the concept of trust, positioning it alongside the related concept of social capital and noting the structural analogy between musical interaction and social interaction. Section 4 unpacks the basic phenomenology of ensemble interaction via reports in the literature of Music Performance Studies, noting along the way a strange characteristic of this literature. Section 5 returns to the comparison between trust and empathy, noting two areas that empathy alone is unable to explain and one area that trust is unable to explain, and aiming to synthesise the two concepts in the direction of a full explanation of interaction's social value. Section 6 concludes with a proposal for the direction of instrumental performance pedagogy.

Two caveats. First, my focus is on the performing of Western Classical ensemble music. Second, I ignore the logistics and legalities of interaction: funding, timetables, responsibilities, contracts and outputs. I simply note that they are neither trivial nor merely preliminary matters, but are central to the construction of a space within which performers can feel free enough to be creative and 'use symbolic resources intrinsic to their particular system of knowledge and, through communication, generate new and useful artifacts (the creative outcome) within a representational space of the group' (Glăveneau, 2011, p. 483).

An initial positioning of the value of ensemble interaction is appropriate in order to set the scene. Why interact with other performers? Why go to the undoubted effort of playing string quartets together, beyond the luxury of making wonderful music at one extreme, and at the other extreme the need to obtain gainful employment? In our everyday lives it is frequently assumed that interaction of the sort that we think we hear and see in a string quartet is a good thing, and of course the cultural industries are hugely dependent on it both financially and epistemologically. Indeed, interaction is a theme familiar to practitioners, theorists and policy makers alike. Given that interaction – usually under the name of collaboration (which is different, but often used as a convenient proxy, though not in this chapter) – is frequently positioned as an important kind of musical activity on the grounds of its wider social value both inside and outside music, it is worth asking what sorts of value ensemble interaction embodies. What lies behind the common assumption that interaction and/or collaboration is (always) a good thing, and what does musical ensemble performing contribute to the much wider Big Society-style debate on the merits of collaboration (which I ignore)?

2. Empathy and the decentering of the Cartesian subject

A summary of empathy's main characteristics is useful at the outset. This will help to clarify its relationship to trust, which is considered in more detail below in direct relation to the phenomenology of musical interaction.

Empathy has a diverse history within a number of disciplines – histories, more properly speaking. These include aesthetics (especially fiction), medicine, politics, psychiatry and psychoanalysis. Like trust, empathy can make a 'potential contribution to human capital' (Hodges & Klein, 2001, p. 439) based on its deep roots in human neurobiology. The term itself does not have an ancient etymology (Shakespeare does not use it, for example) (Valentino, 2005), but there are extensive cross-references with cognate concepts like attunement, care, compassion, contagion, entrainment, fellow-feeling, love, respect, sensitivity and (most obviously) sympathy (which Shakespeare did use) (Darwall, 1998). The most fundamental movement in empathy is a division of the subject's attention. The subject becomes aware simultaneously of herself and of the other, and directs her energy and attention inwards and outwards towards both subjects, viewing the world from both perspectives. She finds that she experiences similarity between her feelings and the other's feelings, and yet she can differentiate between experiencing (affectively) and recognising (cognitively) the dynamics of the other's experience. Different theories of empathy talk about 'projecting', 'simulating' and other ways of apprehending the other's experience *qua* other experience (Zahavi, 2008). For some, empathy is a fundamental moment of consciousness and an essential component of intentionality (Thompson, 2001). There is debate over the extent to which empathy is an automatic process managed by the 'shared manifold' (a mental mirror system affording the subject fast apprehension and sharing of intentions) (Gallese, 2001), and whether or not empathy is a simple matter of ever greater entrainment and 'adjustment' in the service of ever greater 'synchrony' between subjects (Rabinowitch, 2012).

Altogether, empathy effectively involves a decentering of the Cartesian subject, perhaps even a destabilising of it, a distracting passage in the direction of a more flexible and socially aware subject position. Hence empathy is frequently espoused as a tool for social negotiation, and sometimes characterised as a 'repair concept' (Depew, 2005, p. 105), by which is meant that empathy draws together subjects under the same experiential affect, and that it often involves 'the intention to respond compassionately to another person's distress' (Decety & Jackson, 2004, p. 73). In the musical world empathy is congruent with the discourse of 'musicking' (Small, 1988), in which musical processes and social protocols take precedence over objects and ontology.

Given that, at a broad evolutionary level (more detail is provided in the following section), trust is often defined as 'a confident expectation regarding another's behavior' (Barbalet, 2006, p. 5), and that trust is embodied in the subject's belief that the consequences of actions by another subject will prove conducive to the subject's own projects (Misztal, 1996), the relationship between trust and empathy can be understood in terms of the musical activities of which they can be configured as the theories. Thus, trust is a theory of what performance 'is', while empathy is a theory of what performing 'does'.

As a theory of 'performance', trust describes what performance 'is'. It emphasises the roles of concepts such as representation, expression, emotion, subjectivity, *werktreue*, interpretation, analysis, embodiment and consciousness, and defines the manner in which performances are prepared, given, interpreted, revised, recorded and forgotten. Trust is central to the systemic set up in which the performer operates. One of the central components of this set up is the technical apparatus of performance: the accuracy of the work and its editions, the entry-level threshold technical competency of the performers (trustworthiness: can they play the notes? Have they prepared? Do they understand and accept the interpretation?), the preliminary logistical stage management underpinning the event, and so on. Trust can often be dispensed with, fixed and put to one side prior to leaving the green room (albeit that the performer's judgements of trustworthiness remain subject to revision if, for example, it transpires during the course of live performance that one of her co-performers turns out to have not prepared their part as fully as had been assumed or hoped). It may be for a reason as simple as this, that trust and trustworthiness have been ignored hitherto in the scholarly literature.

As a theory of 'performing', empathy describes what performing 'does' as a process, event and affect, and it effectively tells the performer how to get from performance to performing, comprising a pragmatics. Empathy is about relating to other performers here and now, and it is what turns a performer into a co-performer, a technician into a musician. It is a performative quality that must arise in real time if it is to stand any chance of sustainable success. It is also something that is open-ended while the performing is going on ('you are the music/While the music lasts', to use T. S. Eliot's poetic words; Eliot, 1943); it only stops when the performer renters the green room afterwards.

3. Trust, social capital and the sound of community

Having outlined the essential features of empathy and a brief comparison with trust, a more formal description of trust and trustworthiness (and the related concept of social capital) will be useful at this point. This will help to contextualise the subsequent description of the phenomenology of ensemble interaction.

Trust is an ancient concept currently enjoying a renaissance in the public domain with respect to the behaviours of public figures and the management of public institutions. At a basic level, trust has been hailed as the 'basis of all human systems of morality' (Nowak & Sigmund, 2000, pp. 819–820). Hyperbole aside, there is certainly evidence that

> Without trust only very simple forms of human cooperation which can be transacted on the spot are possible, and [that] even individual action is much too sensitive to disruption to be capable of being planned, without trust, beyond the immediately assured moment.
>
> (Luhmann, 1979, p. 88)

Indeed, 'very few relationships would endure if trust were not as strong as, or stronger than, rational proof or personal observation' (Simmel, 1978, pp. 178–179).

Trust works across all domains of activity, from the relationships between infants and mothers (Glăveneau, 2011) to the economic stability of nations (Alan Greenspan's Harvard commencement address cited in Buchan, Croson, & Dawes, 2002). And it helps us to manage various important elements of social life: uncertainty (Barbalet, 2006; Luhmann, 1979); risk (Barbalet 2006); accountability (O'Neill, 2002); distributed labour; creative community; and so on – in general, all those situations that are resistant to normative subject-centered expectations (Misztal, 1996). At root, trust is an adaptive mechanism for two activities: first, it helps citizens to manage their future relationships with each other; second, it increases the willingness of citizens to cooperate with each other (an index of social capital). Trust is related to reliance, confidence, faith and familiarity, and its etymology encompasses the notion of 'leaning on others'. For this reason, the companion term to trust is trustworthiness, and it is this with which individual perceptions and judgements are concerned. Trust emerges between performers, while individual performers themselves become trustworthy to varying degrees through the perceptions and judgements of other performers. Individual perceptions and judgements are made on the basis of expectations of others' actions that are based on heuristic interpretations of the information at hand, which, given that it is always partial, also requires the suspension of the subject's normative desire for complete knowledge of others' actions (Möllering, 2001).

Theories of trust subdivide and categorise it variously, drawing it close to other concepts (among them empathy). One theory discerns two types of trust: strategic and moralistic (Uslaner, 2002). Strategic trust presupposes risk (Misztal, 1996) and aids the business of problem solving, while moralistic trust emerges when people are treated as if they are trustworthy, and changes more slowly than strategic risk. Another theory defines three dimensions to trust: personal, communal and systemic (Sztompka, 1999). An alternative theory defines three types of trust and associates them with three kinds of social order: trust as habitus is associated with stable order; trust as passion is associated with cohesive order; and trust as policy is associated with collaborative order (Misztal, 1996). These range, respectively, from trust acting as a routine background to everyday interactions, through trust based on familiarity and social bonds, through to trust as the means of fostering cooperation with others. The last is of most interest to me in this chapter.

Social capital is a concept that is familiar from the (separate) work of Pierre Bourdieu and Robert Putnam. It is often mentioned in the same breath as trust:

> Humans are social beings, and trust is widely seen as an essential element in any social setting. Without trust, people are loath to reach out, and to make the social connections that underpin any collaborative action. For sustainable success, trust needs to be matched by trustworthiness. ... trust has been seen sometimes as a proxy measure of social capital, or alternatively as a consequence or correlate of high levels of social capital. Like social capital, trust can be narrow or encompassing, identified by type and purpose, be affected by geographic, social and cultural distance, and take more time to build than to destroy.
>
> (Helliwell & Wang, 2010)

Social capital represents 'features of social organisations, such as trust, norms and networks that can improve the efficiency of society by facilitating coordinated actions' (Putnam, 1993, p. 167). It is often measured with questions about the level of trust, and it is usually described as an attribute of a community rather than of individuals (Glaeser, Laibson, Scheinkman, & Soutter, 1999). In this chapter, it is a fitting explanatory tool for what happens over time in string quartet performing.

With this formal description of trust in mind, the social context of ensemble interaction comes into focus with respect to its social value and where this value arises. The sociality of performing together and the phenomenology of distributed labour in ensemble interaction are central to Nicholas Cook's article, 'Making music together, or improvisation and its Others' (2004). This article, building on the work of Alfred Schütz though staking out a more sociological claim, focuses more on 'why' performing together is important than on 'how' it actually happens; more on what interaction reflects than on its sustaining mechanism. Cook explores the relationships between performing together and improvising together, and explores aspects of their cultural dynamics. His argument charts a trajectory from the idea of 'Music as Performance' (p. 5) to the idea of 'Performance as Improvisation' (p. 10) and from there to the idea that music is 'The Sound of Community' (p. 18). The move from 'Music as Performance' to 'Performance as Improvisation' is straightforwardly transitive. The first idea is relatively widely accepted now in Musicology (hence there is a sub-discipline called Music Performance Studies), and the second idea is easy enough to argue in at least its weak version, according to which it is improvisatory action rather than improvisation *per se* that is at issue (Cook, 2004, p. 18, n. 17). However, the third idea, namely that music, not merely represents, or embodies, but indeed may ultimately simply *be* 'The Sound of Community', involves a bigger leap. Notwithstanding his desire to annex new territories for Musicology and thus a programmatic element to his approach, Cook does not really explain what this leap entails in order that the claim might be plausible. What he correctly assumes but does not have time to unpack is the dynamic nature of the labour in a functioning first-world community. If, as he says, the act of listening 'to [Mozart's String Quartet] K. 387 is precisely [the act of listening to] the sound of social interaction, the sound of community' (Cook, 2004, p. 21), then this is because what subtends both the performance of Mozart and the social performance of community cannot be simply improvisation, however broadly the term is defined – and Cook finds it in Mozart and Sonny Rollins. What these multifarious practices share is the force that binds not just group improvisation but interactive performance per se. This binding force is the mutual 'trust network' (Tilly, 2005) that maintains the momentum of interaction into the future. Just as the social network that Facebook taps into and creates is sustained less by the labour of its contributors than by the various types, degrees and nuances of trust that resonate between them, so ensemble interaction is precisely interactive to the extent that its performers trust each other, independently of the degree to which each one contributes to the performance or the degree to which each contribution can be empirically measured. This claim, which buttresses Cook's argument in order to give teeth to his conclusions, involves two assumptions: first, that the smooth management of society and the accumulation of social capital require a type of labour called social interaction; second, that if this very social interaction is to be culturally meaningful, genuinely transformative, and sustainable, then it requires trust between citizens.

With this position regarding the sociology of trust in mind, and having acknowledged that the interaction within ensemble performing may not just represent but actually be 'The Sound of Community', it begins to become clear how successful interaction emerges and develops on the back of trust (or, in reverse, how interaction functions as the conduit for trust). Indeed, it could be claimed that interaction without trust is stillborn. Trust is certainly found in all kinds of interactions between performers, and underpins their activities as both an assumption and a goal. Trust enables and facilitates interaction, collaboration, risk taking, experimentation, interpretative leaps and all kinds of phenomena that are frequently associated with 'wonderful' performance. As such, trust should be incorporated more explicitly into performance curricula (as I propose at the end), because being good at trusting is a widely transferable skill with a variety of benefits.

Acknowledging that trusting is a transferable skill involves certain corollaries: first, that trust generates a lasting affective resonance in performers' lives after the performance; second, that performers learn from, as well as during, interaction; and third, that, however trust is configured (whether as an attitude, a trait, a temperament, a frame of mind, an ideology, a mind-set, an outlook, a style, a disposition, a habitus or a virtue), it affords the performer the potential for creative transformations of matter, mind, music and perhaps even morality as a result of ensemble interaction. In short, put schematically: interaction is a conduit for trust, and trust is a conduit for social capital. Thus the best answer to the question in Section 1, 'Why interact with other performers?' is as follows: on the back of trust, ensemble interaction generates social capital, albeit in ways that often seem indirect, and it behoves us to remain cognisant of this underlying rationale, for it makes us better citizens and improves the quality of life in the *polis*.

Without wishing to expand this answer further into the theory of social capital, what is of interest in the next section are the pragmatic implications of this answer for music performing, for these seem to coalesce around a second question. To wit: if it is true that, on the back of trust and trustworthiness, the performer interacts with co-performers not only in order to create wonderful music but also in order through trust to generate social capital, then what characterises successful interaction and makes it both such a sought-after commodity in the Western Classical music business and such a slippery matter for practical pedagogy? Exploring this second question, the following section looks under the bonnet of ensemble interaction and seeks to understand trust as the engine of successful ensemble performing, its basic phenomenological *qualia*. Investigating aspects of how the psychology of performance is reported, it becomes clear that theories of interaction premised on assumptions about the kinds of distributed labour emerging from the music's stylistic identity (performance initiatives on the back of assumptions about the musical style of, for example, Mozart's String Quartet K. 387) are meaningless without an *a priori* theory of trust and trustworthiness, and that interaction without trust has no pragmatic means to get itself beyond microscopic, atomistic, local interactions and begin developing its own self-sustaining ecology – what is often called an expert performance practice. Of particular interest below is the way in which trust plays both a political *and* an existential role in the performer's actions. Without interaction, no social capital; without trust, nothing.

4. The phenomenology of ensemble interaction

In this section, I describe the basic phenomenology of ensemble interaction in relation to the trust that affords the performer a means of interacting productively. How does the performer become an effective co-performer in an ensemble? How does she deal with distributed labour? How does she develop interactive skills for navigating 'The Sound of Community'? What kinds of social skills might these be?

Consider the principles. Interaction is broader than the linguistic paradigm of communication. Whatever else interaction is, it involves certain basic principles: it is interpersonal, participative, distributed, shared and collaborative.

Its outputs are emergent, however well it is planned, and jointly owned. Two or more performers undertake the interactive task jointly with a collective goal in mind, in addition to whatever individual intentions each might bring to the task. The labour driving the interaction is distributed between them according to mutually agreed criteria that may include skill, aptitude, experience, preference, time available, financial support, physical location and institutional affiliation. Interaction is simultaneously the goal, the process and the result of such social, distributed, emergent labour. It is a good example – indeed, perhaps *the* paradigm – of social performing, of performing as a social activity with social value (as Cook, 2004 notes).

With these principles in mind, it is very strange that the scholarly literature on ensemble interaction tends to shy away from analysing the pragmatic 'how' of ensemble interaction, concentrating instead on the descriptive 'what' of ensemble interaction. Besides largely technical matters such as how cues and signals are shared between performers (Ginsborg, Chaffin, & Nicholson, 2004), joint action and synchronisation (Goebl & Palmer, 2009; Keller, 2008), the meanings of body language (Ginsborg & King, 2009), and technical matters (Ginsborg & King, 2007a; Davidson & King, 2004; McCaleb, 2011), the most common theme in the literature on ensemble interaction is leadership, followed closely by expertise (Ginsborg, 2009; Ginsborg, Chaffin, & Nicholson, 2006; Ginsborg & King, 2007b), the two often in fact being construed as a symbiotic pair. This is perhaps because leadership is more easily measurable than trust. For example, Elaine King (née Goodman) writes in a textbook chapter on ensemble performance that 'Ensemble performance is about teamwork: half the battle of making music together (and ultimately staying together as an ensemble) is fought on social grounds. The most important issue to consider is leadership, for every group needs at least one leader' (Goodman, 2002, pp. 163–164). And at the end of another article, she concludes that

> To return to the issue of leadership, the interview data revealed that the establishment of a leader within a student ensemble is perhaps the most difficult, yet crucial part of building up an ensemble. Arguably, a leader can only fulfil his or her role effectively if the remaining members of a group oblige, allowing that person to take control. ... It is probably through respect of her musicianship, above all, that the rest of the group felt that they could, and wanted to, "follow" her.
>
> (King, 2006, p. 280)

In neither of these texts is trust mentioned, nor is the possibility entertained that, if 'the battle of making music together ... is fought on social grounds' (Goodman, 2002, p. 163), then trust might well require acknowledgement as an equally fundamental component of ensemble interaction. After all, the possibility that 'the members of a string quartet might endeavour to work together democratically, [or that ...] the orchestral conductor might strive towards a less dictatorial approach by gradually relinquishing control' (Goodman, 2002,

p. 164) are decisions that can only happen if the interaction is already grounded in trust. Schematically put: Leadership requires trust, trust does not require leadership.

On a wider level, in fact, not only does the literature on ensemble interaction generally stick with the 'why' and 'what' of performing at the expense of descriptions of 'how' it happens pragmatically, but also the discourse of trust tends to be absent (despite trust being a large part of precisely 'how' ensemble performing happens). I write 'discourse of trust' rather than 'concept of trust' to emphasise that trust is absent from the vocabulary and rhetoric of ensemble interaction, although it may be present elsewhere, as I argue below. It is discussed in the literature on collaborative learning (Gaunt & Westerlund, 2013), but not in the literature that claims to address the mechanics of ensemble interaction. It is the missing link in Murphy McCaleb's *Embodied knowledge in ensemble performance*, being mentioned only in the meta-observations on his own practice in the final chapter (McCaleb, 2014), and it seems to be strangely absent from the interview subjects' responses in Susan Hallam's '21st century conceptions of musical ability' – or at least, it needs careful unpicking and extrapolation from the idea of 'being able to successfully engage musically with others' (Hallam, 2010, p. 308). To go a little further afield, trust is also absent from – or only implicit in – Michael Hooper's article on Christopher Redgate's completely redesigned oboe, even though the subject matter is the early stages of interaction between Redgate and the composers commissioned to work with him on the generation of new repertoire (Hooper, 2012). And it is also absent from Sam Hayden and Luke Windsor's article on 'Collaboration and the composer', which focuses on assessing when and whether 'collaborations' are merely 'interactive' or 'directed', although there is one allusion to a trust network in the remark that 'professions ... tend to build a repertoire of technical procedures which are only questionable by individuals within that profession' (Hayden & Windsor, 2007, p. 30). A rare acknowledgement, albeit in passing, of trust's key role in ensemble interaction comes in Mine Doğantan-Dack's article 'The art of research in live performance'. She writes that:

> For any collaborating group of people to work well, there needs to be a sense of trust and support between them, as well as a sense of belonging in the group ... The chemistry of an ensemble in live performance is the site where the trust and support between the performers get tested, confirmed and re-confirmed, and acquire their true practical meaning; the willingness and ability to create an emotional comfort zone during the live event when performers need it is crucial for the success of the performance.
>
> (Doğantan-Dack, 2012, p. 43)

Another isolated acknowledgement of trust can be found in the theoretical model of performance constructed by Dimitra Kokotsaki (2007). Other than that, mention of trust is limited to such places as the conclusion of Caroline Waddington's conference paper, 'Creativity in ensemble performance: A case of intense co-performer empathy', where the opportunity to investigate the phenomenological details of how 'trust and familiarity both play critical roles in the development of a successful chamber ensemble' (2014, p. 9) is not taken up, despite the obvious overlap between trust and the way that Waddington uses empathy within her own argument.

In general, the absence – or at least down-playing – of trust from the scholarly literature on ensemble interaction is strange, given its regular presence in more naturalistic musical situations, such as Amanda Bayley's interviews with Michael Finnissy and the members of the Kreutzer Quartet about the composers' Second Quartet (Bayley, 2013), not to mention its almost ubiquitous presence in the literatures on collaboration and creativity in other disciplines (not just the Arts and Humanities). It is more than a matter of the word itself simply not being used in Music Performance Studies. In contrast, the huge literatures in Management Studies on leadership, innovation and creativity, all three of which are invoked as explanatory tools in the literature on ensemble interaction, make repeated references to the importance of trust in the effective operation of creative groups.

Nevertheless, despite the apparent absence of trust from the (written) discourse of ensemble interaction, much can be gleaned – sometimes by reading between the lines – about how trust functions in performing situations, about the phenomenology of trust in ensemble interaction. A good place to start is King's (née Goodman) textbook chapter discussed above. She writes:

> The coordination of sound can be assisted by the planning of visual signals – for instance, by determining who gives the lead at the beginning of the piece, or who makes eye contact with whom following a large pause. As suggested above, however, such choreography might be detrimental to the spontaneity of the performance. Interestingly, the members of the Guarneri String Quartet state that their physical movements are mutually absorbed at an unconscious level over a period of time, so they are hardly aware of visual signals relayed in performance: 'There's a certain body language that each of us has when he plays. You get to know that about your colleagues and react accordingly. Over the years a great deal of it becomes intuitive'.
>
> (Goodman, 2002, p. 158)

This is a staple position in the literature on ensemble interaction. It is all true and sensible advice, particularly about the importance of understanding the development of ensemble skills longitudinally and in terms of absorption and assimilation. But this is only because of what the long duration affords, namely the nurturing of a trust network between performers – here overwritten as intuition. Indeed, there is a whole discourse of trust and a set of protocols for trustworthiness operating within this paragraph, subsuming all of the interactions between agents described, from the 'planning of signals' through to the 'determining' of leads and of 'making' eye contact. More generally, trust functions as a way of linking microscopic and macroscopic levels of interaction. Although it is overwritten here by the technical discourses of signaling and coordination, the point is that:

> Trust is a functional alternative to rational prediction for the reduction of complexity. Indeed, trust succeeds where rational prediction alone would fail, because to trust is to live *as if* certain rationally possible futures will not occur. Thus, trust reduces complexity far more quickly, economically, and thoroughly than does prediction. Trust allows social interactions to proceed on a simple and confident basis, where, in the absence of trust, the monstrous complexity posed by contingent futures would again return to paralyse action.
>
> (Lewis & Weigert, 1985, p. 969)

Even at localised, microscopic levels, the goal of ensemble interaction, both in rehearsal and in live performance, is not just interaction per se but what it affords the performer. Here are five representative comments about a rehearsal: 'There was a *sense of determination* from each of the students because of *the desire to* work through the whole movement in one rehearsal'; '*quietly absorbing* the advice'; 'her *reliability* in executing a number of functional roles'; 'her position *was perceived* in different ways, including "supportive" and "happy-go-lucky"'; 'the remaining two players *are considered* to be supportive' (King, 2006, pp. 272, 272, 274, 275, 276 respectively; italics mine). Each of these comments should be understood in terms of the way it represents – indeed, performs – a commitment to trust other performers, and that the performer's perceptions in ensemble interactions are first and foremost perceptions about the trustworthiness of her individual fellow performers and her perception of the reliability of their individual actions (trust is non-transitive) (Barbalet, 2006).

The perceptions and actions reported in King's article show how the performer needs to find reliable ways of articulating and maintaining her trust, and this means finding workable ways of perceiving and judging the trustworthiness of information and of co-performers. In the way that they 'carry out complex predictions that are intimately bound to reactions gained through feedback: [for example] on the basis of the previous note, when is the next note of a fellow performer going to sound?' (Goodman, 2002, p. 154), it is trust that affords such prediction, given the necessarily incomplete information available. For trust is more than 'a sense of personal reliance and security between persons' (Barbalet, 2006, p. 8), and it is different to confidence: the performer needs to be able to rely on the music, but place trust in the other performers (Barbalet, 2006, p. 13).

This is one of the primary ways in which labour is exhibited in musical interaction: as value judgement. Indexes of trustworthiness chart how performers 'communicate with one another, don't withhold information, and allow the free flow of ideas' (Glăveneau, 2011, p. 483) and try to avoid 'impatience, ownership, conflict, and unfriendliness and the ever-present possibility of not being able to unify dichotomies' (Glăveneau, 2011, p. 482). Here Cook's list of performative qualities begins to make sense both with reference to historical issues of musical style (Hunter, 2012) and as a way of mapping out how trust might be played out in musical interaction: 'statements, assertions, allegations, questions, requestings, implications, mockings, and occurrences' (Cook, 2004, p. 22). Such qualities map loosely onto the fragmentary vocabulary used by performers to describe what 'clicking together' empathically feels like and what its mechanisms are: 'gelling', 'exactly synchronised', 'an intimate connection', 'in harmony', 'eyes', 'ears', 'radar', 'instinctively aware', 'sympathy', 'clicking', 'locking in', 'getting into each other's heads', 'being able to read the other person's mind' (Waddington, 2014, p. 2; see also Waddington, this volume). Cook's list of qualities is also related to the nine team roles categorised by the management guru Meredith Belbin, who is often cited in the literature on ensemble interaction: plant, resource, investigator, coordinator, shaper, monitor, evaluator, teamworker, implementer, completer and specialist (Belbin, 1993). They are also congruent with the seven Nolan principles of public life: selflessness, integrity, objectivity, accountability, openness, honesty and leadership. This is to be expected, given trust's role in the accumulation of social capital. Placing Cook's list alongside these wider world frameworks for public action, it is clear that string quartet performing – and ensemble interaction in general – maps directly onto what is happening beyond the footlights, and this (as I argue at the end) places performing in a key pedagogical position with respect to the education of a more socially able and responsible *polis*.

Such indexes of trustworthiness as Cook lists are consolidated in the various ways in which performers form working relationships with each other within the overarching pattern of distribution of labour. These relationships are played out variously over the duration of an interaction:

> We can use the word 'relationship' in two ways: to stand for the bond which links two or more people, or to stand for the attitudes which bonded people have to each other. As examples of the first kind of relationship we might mention kinship, marriage, business association, or teacher–pupil. As examples of the second kind we might mention fear, pride, respect, envy, contempt, etcetera.
>
> (Downie & Jodalen, 1997, p. 129)

Trust figures within and between these roles in various ways, as the texts discussed above make clear, and there is 'a fine line between flexibility and stability: successful teams will sometimes thrive on "simple" and "uncomplicated" actions as individuals maintain distinctive team roles; at other times, they will rely on the flexibility of their members' (King, 2006, p. 265). The key point, of course, is that such a withdrawal from complexification towards simplicity of intention requires a certain kind of assumption of trust between co-performers.

Many of the elements of interaction that I have described as being central to productive ensemble interaction are also present in solitary individual creative acts. They are also often presented by those in power as ideals that govern citizens' everyday transactions – and presumably theirs, too. This is exactly as it should be, if we desire musicking in general and interactive musicking in particular to enjoy a healthy relationship with and within society, if we desire our ensemble interactions to feed (back) into the broader development and accumulation of social capital that we need to pursue in the developed world. However, the special creativity governed by the interactive attitude provides a heightened and more socialised version of general creativity, and a useful complement to those still influential lone-ranger models of creativity. Even if we do not want to go as far as dialogic theorists and argue that 'Human thought becomes genuine thought, that is, an idea, only under conditions of living contact with another and alien thought, a thought embodied in someone else's voice' (Bakhtin, 1984, pp. 87–88), it is nevertheless clear that every action benefits from some kind of exposure to the responses of others, indeed, needs to be configured dialectically as such. Just as no man is an island, so no thought is an oasis. Hence my conclusion: if Cook is right, as indeed I think he is, to argue that music 'symbolises social interaction even when it doesn't actually present it' (Cook, 2004, p. 22), then it is the duty of *musical* interaction to ensure that *social* interaction happens, a duty that falls on the shoulders of the performer and her co-performers, and this will only happen if the concept of trust is incorporated more centrally into our models of performing. On which note, I return to the article by King discussed above. She concludes:

> Finally, it should be mentioned that this study exposed the difficulties faced by students in learning how to collaborate effectively in rehearsal, especially in dealing with the issue of leadership. The students sometimes faced the problem of 'what to do' to improve pieces besides running through them several times, and their relative lack of experience in working together in a small group context exposed issues of 'how to get on' effectively to enable goals to be achieved. These concerns highlight the need for students to obtain both further musical training and greater skills in social interaction. One way in which the latter might be addressed is by providing some kind of 'role learning' education to expose self-insight and group awareness of team-role actions along with an understanding of how particular roles blend to enable successful teamwork.
>
> (King, 2006, pp. 280–281)

Although this is all eminently sensible, it seems to me, given that 'The social dynamics among the performers in an ensemble are as important as the musical dynamics for a successful performance, and [that] each live performance is in fact an opportunity to further develop and strengthen the social bonds between the performers' (Doğantan-Dack, 2012, p. 43), that the pedagogical problems identified here would disappear or at least shrink in size if trust were acknowledged as playing a more prominent role within the discourse of ensemble interaction. For under the figure of trust:

> The acknowledgement of each person's role as [performer], and of the ultimate [performance] of the group is based on a recognition of the truth of human interaction; the curious bumping together of individuals, groups,

ideas and knowledge which becomes the engine of creativity. The energy of exchange, once set in motion, fuels a network which endures long after the project has passed, a testament to the vitality of the process and a reminder of the human at the centre of creative work.

(Boddington & Bannerman, 2004, p. 80)

5. Synthesising trust and empathy

In this section I return to the intimate relationship between trust and empathy as this is played out in ensemble performing, offering a simple and musically intuitive way of comparing the two concepts.

The two theories of 'performance' and 'performing' mentioned above – of trust and empathy – are dialectically related, and the passage between them needs to be worked through. There needs to be a movement from trust towards empathy in performing, and from empathy towards trust in analysis. Moralistic trust comes to sound rather like empathy. The point is that trust and empathy are needed together in order to provide a full explanation of ensemble interaction. With the synthesis between trust and empathy in mind, I now discuss two specific areas in which empathy on its own is an inadequate explanatory tool and where trust is a better explanatory tool, and one area where the reverse is the case – or, better: where their mutual synthesis affords a genuine understanding of ensemble interaction.

First, interaction is the business of trusting other performers. This is where much of the conscious energy is focused in practice and in performance: dealing with others. But obviously there is also the vital, more primary place towards which trust is directed, also during live performance: the self. Each performer in an ensemble must rely on herself: on her memory holding up, her fingering working and her articulation in the recapitulation coming off. This 'reliance' (trust may not be quite the right word), which is normally operative below the level of conscious thought and which is essential to the performer's sense of subjectivity, has to be implicit: she must be able to literally give no thought to it in order to focus instead on the ensemble interaction. Empathy cannot explain this relationship of the performer to herself, for its purpose is rather to explain how two different subjects relate non-verbally to each other and to account for those particular moments when contact happens (Goldie, 2000). To put the matter schematically: empathy accounts for what I try to do in the ensemble, while trust accounts for what we try to do together as an ensemble.

Second, in the above discussions I have said little about ensemble interactions that fail: when performers cannot resolve differences; cannot meet their end of the bargain; cannot complete their part of the labour; cannot bring themselves to trust other performers musically; when the artistic product is inadequate to one or more of the goals; and so on. And I have ignored situations where performers may continue to work together at the highest professional musical levels, but refuse to communicate with each other socially in everyday life (Doffman, 2012; see also Laurence, this volume; Waddington, this volume; King & Roussou, this volume) – where the balance between strategic and moralistic trust seems to have collapsed. In certain cases, similarly, an increased professionalism of subjects correlates with an increased depersonalisation of the trust network; in, for example, medical activity, this correlation is vital for the success of the labour. Empathy does not explain these situations, though it is certainly invoked often enough in musically successful situations in order to explain quickly how productive parallels have arisen between music and life, the assumption being that increasing empathy in one domain increases the productivity of the other domain. Trust, however, explains how, across stylistic divides, there are ensembles that embrace each other musically on stage but avoid each other socially in the green room (and why this is not actually a problem). This is because trust avoids the central step of empathy, namely 'feeling into' the other, preferring instead to afford performers the ability to make judgements about fellow co-performers' trustworthiness that do not have to assume an unbreakable positive link between music and life. Such judgements of trustworthiness leave a certain element of the ensemble interaction, not just under-determined, but un-determined, the point being that the relation between what Cook (2004) calls the 'sound of social interaction' and the 'The Sound of Community' is dynamic, not fixed. Trustworthiness involves fewer predictions and investments than empathy about the future, and is thus better placed to deal with it (Luhmann, 1979), and to assimilate the quite radical – but eminently pragmatic – idea put forward by Andrea Schiavio and Simon Høffding (2015) that ensemble performing is able to arise perfectly successfully 'without attention to either shared goals, or to the other ensemble musicians' – something which theories of empathy (and certain ideologies of listening) find it difficult to countenance.

Having just provided two examples where trust/trustworthiness provides a better explanation than empathy alone, I now describe a third example where the reverse is the case. The entire discussion above describing the role of trust and social capital in ensemble interaction needs to be underpinned with something ontologically prior to trust: love. A productive musical interaction is a labour of love. Trust and love are closely related in performing as they are in everyday life (Clarke, 2012), and their relationship needs to be unpacked so that love provides the underlying ground for the trust and trustworthiness present within ensemble interaction. This task, which requires a separate essay, configures cognate terms like 'respect for' and 'confidence in' others centrally in the constellation around trust (King, 2013), and it is a task in which, having a closer connection to love than trust (because empathy is often psychologised), empathy comes into its own as a means of explaining the intimate gestures that characterise the micro-level phenomenology of ensemble interaction.

6. Conclusion: enhancing practical pedagogy

I conclude with a proposal for the direction of performance pedagogy. Here I follow up, *inter alia*, the suggestive separate conclusions of King (2006, pp. 277–281) and Waddington (2014, p. 10).

A subsequent stage of research into musical empathy might take this chapter's ideas about interaction and the development of trust and social capital in ensemble performing and expand them into a manifesto on behalf of the important social value that musicking, the performing arts, and the creative industries more widely contribute to society. It is easy to imagine a manifesto arguing for maintaining the level of funding apportioned to the Arts and Humanities, and to the performing arts in particular. The manifesto would have a claim like the following at its heart: The creative industries, and ensemble performing as one such industry, provide a means of generating social capital that is vital for the long-term health of the *polis*, namely a common desire to work together and a shared understanding that doing so has individual *and* civic benefits for all.

The acceptance of such a manifesto would have many benefits. One benefit would be that it would afford practical performance pedagogy a space in which, while still firmly in the grip of trust and trustworthiness, it could nevertheless feel able to configure the role of trust more explicitly within its practice, in order that 'the social climate in the group will be conducive to enjoyable and effective playing' (Young & Colman, 1979, p. 15). After all, as I suggest above, notwithstanding its apparent absence, there is already a pedagogy of trust hidden within the scholarly literature on ensemble interaction. This pedagogy would offer a useful complementary way of teaching chamber music and of setting up the goals and values of such music making without having to resort to 'black box' approaches (you can either do it or you cannot). It would also offer the performer more privileged access to the inner workings of the culture of ensemble interaction earlier on in her education, as well as the opportunity to grasp more quickly empathy's potential, grounded by trust, to act as a 'facilitative tool' (Waddington 2014, p. 1) for peak performance. In due course, learning 'how to empathise like a performer' would involve, alongside developing basic technical skills at the instrument, spending time creating ways of behaving socially, intimately, responsibly and daringly alongside your co-performers – time developing trust in others.

References

Bakhtin, M. (1984). *Problems of Dostoevsky's poetics.* C. Emerson (C. Emerson, Trans.). Minneapolis, MT: University of Minnesota Press.

Barbalet, J. (2006). A characterisation of trust, and its consequences. *Social Contexts and Responses to Risk Network (SCARR) Working, 13,* 1–21.

Bayley, A. personal communication, 23 April 2013.

Belbin, R. M. (1993). *Team roles at work.* Oxford: Butterworth-Heinemann.

Boddington, G., & Bannerman, C. (2004). Sharing the process: A consideration of inter-authorship in the performing arts. *Digital Creativity, 15*(2), 76–80.

Buchan, N., Croson, R., & Dawes, R. (2002). Swift neighbours and persistent strangers: A cross-cultural investigation of trust and reciprocity in social exchange. *American Journal of Sociology, 108*(1), 168–206.

Clarke, E. Personal communication. 27 March 2012.

Cook, N. (2004). Making music together, or improvisation and its others. *The Source: Challenging Jazz Criticism, 1,* 5–25.

Darwall, S. (1998). Empathy, sympathy, care. *Philosophical Studies, 89*(2–3), 261–282.

Davidson, J. W., & King, E. C. (2004). Strategies for ensemble practice. In A. Williamon (Ed.), *Musical excellence: Strategies to enhance performance* (pp. 105–122). Oxford: Oxford University Press.

Decety, J., & Jackson, P. (2004). The functional architecture of human empathy. *Behavioral and Cognitive Neuroscience Review, 3*(2), 71–100.

Depew, D. (2005). Empathy, psychology, and aesthetics: Reflections on a repair concept. *Poroi, 4*(1), 99–107. http://dx.doi.org/10.13008/2151-2957.1033 (accessed 4 May 2015).

Doffman, M. Personal communication, 18 March 2012.

Doğantan-Dack, M. (2012). The art of research in live music performance. *Music Performance Research, 5,* 34–48.

Downie, R., & Jodalen, H. (1997). 'I-thou' and 'doctor-patient': A relationship examined. In H. Jodalen & A. J. Vetlesen (Eds.), *Closeness: An ethics* (pp. 129–141). Oslo: Scandinavian University Press.

Eliot, T. S. (1943). The dry salvages. In *Four quartets.* New York: Harcourt Brace.

Gallese, V. (2001). The shared manifold hypothesis: From mirror neurons to empathy. *Journal of Consciousness Studies, 8*(5–7), 33–50.

Gaunt, H., & Westerlund, H. (Eds.). (2013). *Collaborative learning in higher music education.* Farnham: Ashgate.

Ginsborg, J. (2009). Focus, effort, and enjoyment in chamber music: Rehearsal strategies of successful and 'failed' student ensembles. In A. Williamon, S. Pretty & R. Buck (Eds.), *Proceedings of International Symposium on Performance Science* (pp. 481–486). Auckland, New Zealand.

Ginsborg, J., Chaffin, R., & Nicholson, G. (2004). Sharing performance cues in collaborative performance: A case study. In S. Lipscomb, R. Ashley, R. Gjerdingen & P. Webster (Eds.), *Proceedings of the 8th International Conference on Music Perception and Cognition, Evanston, Illinois* (pp. 252–255). Adelaide, Australia: Causal Productions.

Ginsborg, J., Chaffin, R., & Nicholson, G. (2006). Shared performance cues: Predictors of expert individual practice and ensemble rehearsal. In M. Baroni, A. Addessi, R. Caterina & M. Costa (Eds.), *Proceedings of the 9th International Conference on Music Perception and Cognition* (pp. 913–919). Bologna, Italy.

Ginsborg, J., & King, E. (2007a). Collaborative rehearsal: Social interaction and musical dimensions in professional and student singer-piano duos. *Proceedings of the Inaugural Conference on Music Communication Science* (pp. 51–55). Sydney, Australia.

Ginsborg, J., & King, E. (2007b). Expertise versus partnership in collaborative rehearsal. In K. Maimets-Volt, R. Parncutt, M. Marin & J. Ross (Eds.), *Proceedings of the Third Conference on Interdisciplinary Musicology* (pp. 50–51). Tallinn, Estonia.

Ginsborg, J., & King, E. (2009). Gestures and glances: The effects of familiarity and expertise on singers' and pianists' bodily movements in ensemble rehearsals. In J. Louhivuori, T. Eerola, S. Saarikallio, T. Himberg & Eerola, P-S. (Eds.), *Proceedings of the 7th Triennial Conference of the European Society for the Cognitive Sciences of Music* (pp. 159–164). Jyväskylä, Finland.

Glaeser, E., Laibson, D., Scheinkman, J., & Soutter, C. (1999). What is social capital? The determinants of trust and trustworthiness. *National Bureau of Economic Research Working Paper, 7216*(2), www.nber.org/papers/w7216 (accessed 4 May 2015).

Glăveneau, V-P. (2011). How are we creative together? Comparing sociocognitive and sociocultural answers, *Theory and Psychology, 21*(4), 473–492.

Goebl, W., & Palmer, C. (2009). Synchronisation of timing and motion among performing musicians. *Music Perception, 26*(5), 427–438.

Goldie, P. (2000). *The emotions: A philosophical exploration.* Oxford: Clarendon Press.

Goodman, E. (2002). Ensemble performance. In J. Rink (Ed.), *Musical performance: A guide to understanding* (pp. 153–167). Cambridge: Cambridge University Press.

Hallam, S. (2010). 21st-century conceptions of musical ability. *Psychology of Music, 38*(3), 308–330.

Hayden, S., & Windsor, L. (2007). Collaboration and the composer: Case studies from the end of the 20th century. *Tempo, 61*(240), 28–39.

Helliwell, J., & Wang, S. (2010). Trust and well-being. *National Bureau of Economic Research Working Paper, 15911*(1), www.nber.org/papers/w15911 (accessed 4 May 2015).

Hodges, S., & Klein, K. (2001). Regulating the costs of empathy: The price of being human. *Journal of Socio-Economics, 30*(5), 437–452.

Hooper, M. (2012). The start of performance, or, does collaboration matter? *Tempo, 66*(261), 26–36.

Hunter, M. (2012). The most interesting genre of music: Performance, sociability and meaning in the classical string quartet, 1800–1830. *Nineteenth-Century Music Review, 9*(1), 53–74.

Keller, P. (2008). Joint action in music performance. In F. Morganti, A. Carassa & G. Riva (Eds.), *Enacting intersubjectivity: A cognitive and social perspective on the study of interactions* (pp. 205–221). Amsterdam: IOS Press.

King, E. C. (2006). The roles of student musicians in quartet rehearsals. *Psychology of Music, 34*(2), 262–282.

King, E. C. Personal communication, 16 May 2013.

Kokotsaki, D. (2007). Understanding the ensemble pianist: A theoretical framework. *Psychology of Music, 35*(4), 641–668.

Lewis, D., & Weigert, A. (1985). Trust as a social reality. *Social Forces, 63*(4), 967–985.

Luhmann, N. (1979). *Trust and power.* New York & Chichester: John Riley.

McCaleb, J. M. (2011, 14–17 July). Communication or interaction? Applied environmental knowledge in ensemble performance. Paper presented at the CMPCP Performance Studies Network 1st International Conference, Cambridge University.

McCaleb, J. M. (2014). *Embodied knowledge in ensemble performance.* Farnham: Ashgate.

Misztal, B. (1996). *Trust in modern societies: The search for the bases of social order.* Cambridge: Polity Press.

Möllering, G. (2001). The nature of trust: From Georg Simmel to a theory of expectation, interpretation and suspension. *Sociology, 35*(2), 403–420.

Nowak, M., & Sigmund, K. (2000). Shrewd investments, *Science, 288*(5467), 819–820.

O'Neill, O. (2002). *A question of trust.* Cambridge: Cambridge University Press.

Putnam, R. (1993). *Making democracy work: Civic tradition in modern Italy.* Princeton, NJ: Princeton University Press.

Rabinowitch, T-C. (2012). Musical games and empathy. *Education and Health, 30*(3), 80–84.

Schiavio, A., & Høffding, S. (2015). Playing together without communicating? A pre-reflective and enactive account of joint musical performance. *Musicae Scientiae, 19*(4), 366–388.

Simmel, G. (1978). *The philosophy of money* (T. Bottomore & D. Frisby, Trans.). London: Routledge & Kegan.

Small, C. (1998). *Musicking: The meanings of performing and listening.* Middletown, CT: Wesleyan University Press.

Sztompka, P. (1999). *Trust: A sociological theory.* Cambridge: Cambridge University Press.

Thompson, E. (2001). Empathy and consciousness. *Journal of Consciousness Studies,* *8*(5–7), 1–32.

Tilly, C. (2005). *Trust and rule.* Cambridge: Cambridge University Press.

Uslaner, E. (2002). *The moral foundations of trust.* New York: Cambridge University Press.

Valentino, R. S. (2005). The oxymoron of empathic criticism: Readerly empathy, critical explication, and the translator's creative understanding. *Poroi, 4*(1), 108–114. http://dx.doi.org/10.13008/2151-2957.1034 (accessed 4 May 2015).

Waddington, C. E. (2014, 17–20 July). Creativity in ensemble performance: A case of intense co-performer empathy. Paper presented at the CMPCP Performance Studies Network 3rd International Conference, Cambridge University.

Young, V., & Colman, A. (1979). Some psychological processes in string quartets. *Psychology of Music, 7*(1), 12–18.

Zahavi, D. (2008). Simulation, projection and empathy. *Consciousness and Cognition,* *17*(2), 514–522.

12 The empathic nature of the piano accompanist

Elaine King and Evgenia Roussou

The ways in which humans interact in any society or culture have occupied the attention of researchers from different disciplinary backgrounds over centuries, including philosophers, psychologists, historians, sociologists, anthropologists and musicologists. Indeed, relationships among people are a constant source of fascination, not least because they are unique (based upon time, place and circumstance) and dynamic (subject to change over time), but because they are open to interpretation (that is, they may be understood in different ways both within and outside the relationship according to the varying perspectives of individuals). Over the past several decades there has been a growing preoccupation with the notion of empathy in human relationships, or, broadly (and perhaps somewhat crudely) speaking, 'the ability to understand and share the feelings of another' (*Oxford English Dictionary*).[1] For the purposes of this chapter, empathy will be regarded as an 'intersubjectively motivated experience marked by affective, cognitive and motor attunement' (after Doğantan-Dack, 2015) that, in the context of music ensemble playing, is shaped primarily through 'interpersonal awareness', or acute listening and communication skills (after Myers & White, 2012). This definition makes three assumptions about empathy (Doğantan-Dack, 2015): first, empathy is biologically and culturally embedded as a fundamental response to human interaction; second, empathy is a dynamic and emerging phenomenon that underpins creative collaborative processes; and third, empathy is a crucial factor in group music-making.[2] Indeed, in their study of empathy in musical performance, Sharon Myers and Catherine White (2012) claim that 'being in a relationship where one is understood by another is something to which people respond and highly value'; moreover, in the case of music ensemble playing, they state that 'interpersonal awareness dictates success' (p. 255). This chapter will focus on further investigating empathic relationships in ensemble music performance by exploring the perspectives of professional performers working in the specialist context of the Western art solo–accompaniment duo chamber ensemble. The stereotypical myths of inferiority surrounding the pianist within this medium present a particularly interesting case for study, not least because the empathic nature of the piano accompanist might be seen to dictate the success of the soloist.

Existing research on ensemble music performance provides insight into the complex processes involved in group music-making that necessarily contribute towards an understanding of interpersonal awareness among co-performers. Peter Keller's (2008; Keller, Novembre, & Hove, 2014) theoretical framework highlights three core cognitive–motor skills that underpin joint action: anticipation (to plan the production of one's own sound and predict that of others); adaptation (to engage in mutual temporal adjustment; cf. the phenomenon of entrainment); and attention (prioritised towards one's own action over those of co-performers; see also Waterman, 1996). Keller posits that these core skills are influenced by four factors: knowledge (about the music and familiarity with co-performers; see also Davidson & Good, 2002; King & Ginsborg, 2011); goals (concerning the interaction); strategies (used to facilitate interaction); and social–psychological issues, including empathy. For instance, there is evidence to suggest that individuals with higher empathic predispositions (according to measurements on the 'perspective-taking' subscale of empathy questionnaires) are better able to anticipate micro-timings than those with lower empathic predispositions (Novembre, Ticini, Schütz-Bosbach, & Keller, 2012).

Whilst Keller's framework effectively explains the operational skills and contributory factors involved in group music-making, the ways in which chamber ensemble musicians experience their relationships with co-performers during performance is less well documented, although first-hand accounts by professional musicians provide valuable lenses into their work (for example, Blum, 1986). There are, however, three recent research projects that set out to expose systematically the views of musicians on their relationships with co-performers in small ensembles with an emphasis on exploring the notion of empathy that provide preliminary informed insight into this aspect of music-making: Myers and White's (2012) enquiry using self-reflective narratives by nine professional performers, including accompanists; Elizabeth Haddon and Mark Hutchinson's (2015) self-reflective diaries of working together in a piano duet; and Caroline Waddington's (2015) focus-group interview study with nineteen professional musicians from five established Western art chamber groups. The motivation for Myers and White's (2012) research was to seek parallels between empathy as experienced in musical relationships and those described in therapeutic encounters. They claim that empathy is 'mutually created in a relational context' (p. 255) and cite accounts by piano accompanists to contextualise their research, drawing upon Gerald Moore's books on piano accompaniment (1962, 1978) as well as a broadcast in 2008 with renowned accompanist Malcolm Martineau: they refer to Moore's belief about trying to be '*at one*' with a soloist, and Martineau's notion of the interaction between soloist and accompanist as a 'circle of energy'; that is, when one performer does something different, it brings about something different in the other (p. 259). They indicate (perhaps unintentionally) that the soloist–accompanist partnership specifically may resemble something of the client–therapist dyad.

Myers and White interpreted their data in three stages. The first, 'forming an empathic connection', reflected performers' views on the importance of experiencing a 'special connection' when engaging in professional relationships with other musicians, fostering 'interpersonal awareness' through having well-developed skills in listening and communication, and approaching music with 'respect and integrity'. In effect, the latter aspects reflect directly upon Keller's core cognitive–motor skills and the importance of having shared goals. The second, likened to the 'working relationship', depicted how the performers endeavoured to create synchrony in their playing, such as through staying tuned to one another by listening to themselves and the other player (or by 'attending', to use Keller's term), reported willingness to embark on emotional journeys together, displayed commitment and effort in their work, and acknowledged that there were sometimes 'detours' (problems and tensions in the process). The third, on 'making music', was likened to the therapeutic process and referred to ensemble playing as an 'intense and specialized enterprise' that might potentially lead to a 'transformative connection' among players. This was further depicted as a connection that was considered to be 'beyond words', 'all about the relationship', a 'spiritual experience' and a 'circle of energy'.

Empathic connections were thus described positively, even idealistically, across Myers and White's report, including 'special', 'transformative', 'beyond words', 'ephemeral', 'spiritual' and 'magical', with all of them based upon performers' recollections of sharing and understanding the feelings of another in a musical relationship. Haddon and Hutchinson (2015) also draw parallels with therapist/counsellor–client relationships in their self-reflective study of working together in a musical partnership. They describe the 'fluidity of roles' between co-pianists and the establishment of the rehearsal environment as a 'safe space' for delineating empathic processes in their ensemble (pp. 148–149). Furthermore, they report that empathy facilitates different aspects of their duet work, including easing practical difficulties which can arise with two players at a single instrument, aiding the construction of shared musical concerns, enabling creative 'flow' via socio-emotional bonding, and helping negotiate and resolve possible areas of conflict. Their study portrays empathy in a similarly idealistic way, through enabling, facilitating and easing aspects of group music-making. It is plausible to suggest that a cyclical relationship between musicking (Small, 1998) and empathising could potentially lead to less positive encounters (see Laurence, 2009; see also Doğantan-Dack, 2015).

As part of a wider study on empathy in expert ensemble performance, Waddington (2015; see also Waddington, this volume) explored musicians' optimal experiences of performance, their general experiences of working together and their views on co-performer empathy. She revealed that co-performer empathy was described by these performers as comprising three main components: 'a "shared approach" to interpretation and to working together; a "special connection" between players; and an "intentional awareness" of how colleagues are operating on both a musical and a practical level' (p. 64). Furthermore, she found that 'whilst in empathy, players felt able to vary aspects of musical expression spontaneously'. This 'spontaneous interpretative flexibility' was considered to be a central feature of optimal performance, perhaps something that might enable the 'transformative', 'spiritual' or 'magical' experiences alluded to by the performers in Myers and White's enquiry. And, likewise, Waddington uses the term 'special connection' to capture the varying comments from the performers about how they experienced empathy between themselves, even though the term was not used directly by the performers themselves.

These accounts draw upon the views of a range of professional musicians about experiencing empathy in ensemble performance, although to date less specific attention has been given to the empathic nature of the piano accompanist. Arguably, piano accompanists present a special case within ensemble playing, for they are not always considered to be part of a specific chamber group; rather, they may be expected to work with different soloists (instrumentalists or vocalists), in different scenarios (for example, in auditions, as répétiteurs, in rehearsals and performances), and sometimes with little or no prior rehearsal time. Unlike other chamber performers, pianists, including accompanists, traditionally perform with the full score (for example, solo and piano parts) and, while this may be seen as advantageous for the purpose of navigating the ensemble, this, in turn, may place specific demands on them, such as to accommodate co-performers. An existing interview study by Dimitra Kokotsaki (2007) with twenty professional pianists from a range of chamber ensembles, including duos, trios, quartets and quintets, provides detailed insight into pianists' perspectives on the achievement of high-quality ensemble playing and, of particular relevance to this research, uncovers critical points on piano accompanying and on empathy. References to empathy were made in the context of familiarity and time availability about performance preparation: '[pianists] expressed the desire to connect and empathize with one another for a musical performance of high quality. In turn, these feelings assisted them to perform at their best and achieve integration with the co-performers' (p. 656). In Kokotsaki's theoretical framework, empathy thus features as a contextual condition of time availability and is influenced by the partner's involvement in achieving integration. It is unclear, however, what these 'feelings' of connection and empathy might entail and how they are established within the ensemble.

Kokotsaki referred to the accompanist as a 'guide' or 'facilitator' when considering the pianist's regulating role in an ensemble. Various strategies were identified for 'bringing out potential' within a group, notably through offering moral support and musical support, being alert, showing musical adaptation and, when working with singers, providing 'vocal coaching' (p. 653). Similar points are made in earlier accounts of piano accompanists who have been under the scrutiny of musicians and audiences alike for decades (Adami, 1952; Brown, 1917; Lyle, 1923; Moore, 1943; Zeckendorf, 1953). Over the last century, the piano accompanist's role has been criticised and challenged (Butler, 1940; Cecil, 1907; Cranmer, 1970; Foss, 1924; Hoblit, 1963; Moore, 1962; Tomes, 2004). Recently, the term 'piano collaborator' (Katz, 2009) has been suggested as an alternative to the term 'piano accompanist', for it implies equality between two performers in a duo context, although there is still widespread usage of the term accompanist.

The word 'accompany' has its roots in the old French *compaignon*, meaning companion and, later, *accompagner*, to go along with or keep someone company. This might involve guiding, leading, following, helping or assisting a fellow individual. By definition, therefore, in keeping someone company, one may or may not be responsible for their actions. In the context of music-making, the accompanist is an individual who 'plays with' or 'plays for' another musician, hence keeping them company. Yet, the piano accompanist seems to have assumed the latter meaning of 'playing for' rather than 'with' another musician in certain areas of Western music culture through and beyond the twentieth century, implying that they occupy a supporting or following role within a partnership. The pianists in Kokotsaki's study alluded to the 'derogatory attitude' of some audience members regarding the subordinate and inferior role of the accompanist, or the 'derogatory behaviour and exaggerated expectations' of some singers evidenced by a 'lack of appreciation towards the accompanist' (p. 659). There are numerous explanations for these attitudes, including socio-cultural and musical pressures, such as the expectation upon solo musicians to take the so-called limelight on stage and to lead in the delivery of musical material.

To this end, it is plausible to suggest that in 'playing for' a soloist, the piano accompanist might be seen to act as an empathiser, while the soloist is an empathisee; in other words, the pianist is responsible for connecting with the soloist by understanding and sharing their feelings even if this connection is not reciprocated. Furthermore, as Felicity Laurence explains in phenomenological terms according to a Steinian perspective, 'the empathised experience "appears differently" for the person directly experiencing it from how it appears for the empathiser' … so they do not have the same quality of "givenness" or reality' (Laurence, this volume). The aim of this interview study was to probe the perspectives of professional piano accompanists and instrumental soloists about their understandings and experiences of empathy in the solo–accompaniment duo chamber context with a view to exploring more specifically the empathic nature of the piano accompanist.

Interview study with piano accompanists and instrumental soloists

Following ethical approval from the Faculty of Arts and Social Sciences Ethics Committee at the University of Hull, fourteen professional performers were interviewed about their views on empathy in the Western art solo–accompaniment duo chamber ensemble context. The sample included seven experienced piano accompanists (mean age 53.9 years) and seven instrumental soloists (mean age 35.7 years). The accompanists' experiences varied between working evenly across four instrumental categories, namely voice, strings, woodwind and brass, whilst at the same time specialising in one or two of them. The seven soloists represented the same four instrumental categories: voice (two singers), strings (one violinist and one cellist), wind (one flautist and one clarinettist) and brass (one French horn player). All of the accompanists regularly worked

with instrumentalists of different levels and abilities, from beginner, interme-
diate and advanced students, to amateur, semi-professional and professional
musicians. All participants were European with the majority being British, and
others recruited from Bulgaria, Cyprus, Greece, France and Poland. All participants were known personally to either both researchers or the second researcher
only and were approached independently. Discriminate sampling (Strauss &
Corbin, 1990) was used as the primary selection criterion to ensure that participants displayed individuality in the specialised field of solo–accompaniment
duo ensemble performance and could offer a wealth of experiences in order to
contribute to the research. The participants signed consent forms prior to interview. In order to preserve anonymity, pianists and soloists will be identified
with letters and numbers in this chapter: pianists as P1, P2 and so on; soloists
as S1, S2 and so on.

Interviews were carried out as part of a larger-scale study to explore the attributes of experienced piano accompanists. All interviews were undertaken by
the second researcher and audio-recorded, transcribed and coded into themes
(Arksey & Knight, 1999; Tracy, 2013). The interview questions were devised
specifically to explore how empathy is perceived and experienced between
pianist and soloist within the solo–accompaniment duo ensemble, ultimately to
expose and subsequently understand the empathic nature of a piano accompanist
within this context. There were four key areas of discussion: (a) defining empathy: to explore participants' understandings of the term empathy and how they
would define it within the solo–accompaniment duo context; (b) presence of empathy: to ascertain their views on whether or not empathy should exist between
soloist and accompanist; (c) functions of empathy: to find out whether or not
the participants personally experienced empathy in this context and, if so, how;
and (d) alternatives to empathy: to explore which other words might be used to
describe the relationship between soloist and piano accompanist.

Defining empathy

To start with, the participants were asked to explain their understanding of the
word empathy and how they would define it in the solo–accompaniment duo
chamber ensemble context. The data revealed general, rather than specific, understandings of the term that could be applied within and beyond the duo medium. Empathy was defined in four ways. First, it was regarded in terms of the
relationship with a co-performer, such as when an accompanist was being understanding, instinctively aware and sensitive towards a partner's feelings, both
musically and emotionally. It was described as the ability 'to sense the soloist's
intentions' (P4), as an 'unspoken kind of awareness and understanding of what
someone else is feeling or thinking' (P5), or, similarly, 'picking up what the person's sensitivities might be at the particular point' (P7). Second, it was perceived
according to *actions towards co-performers*, notably as being flexible and prepared to compromise. Indeed, according to some of the pianists, empathy was
about 'being open for other people's feelings or emotions or reactions to certain

things' (P6) or 'being prepared to compromise' (P1). One of the soloists commented that empathy is about

> flexibility, sensitivity, listening, sharing; just being at one ... Sometimes it's just something you both express while playing, sometimes you have to discuss it, sometimes you've got to talk it through to come to an agreement, just like friendship or a relationship (S3).

Third, empathy was defined according to *character traits*, such as being supportive, friendly, kind and easy going. One of the soloists remarked that one had to be 'emotionally compatible with the feelings of the other musician' (S7). Finally, empathy was seen to be related to the *working ethos* of the performers, that is being able to work together towards a common goal: 'two people having an equal goal in mind' (S3); or 'having the same understanding of the music' (S6); or 'being mentally, psychologically and emotionally on the same road' (S4). One of the soloists described this ethos more carefully as being able 'to work together in a way that you are kinder to them, you are sensitive to their needs, you are ready to help them if needed at any point, not to make them feel at any point unsupported' (S2). The distinctive empathic nature of a piano accompanist is not immediately clear from these data. What is apparent is that all of the participants provided general ideas of what empathy might (or might not) be in the context of ensemble playing more broadly, and that these chimed with previous accounts discussed above (Myers & White, 2012; Waddington, 2015).

Presence of empathy

The majority of participants indicated that empathy should be present between a soloist and a pianist: eight of the fourteen performers (four pianists and four soloists) responded that it existed, whilst five performers (three pianists and two soloists) were indifferent and one soloist remarked that it was not needed. Positive responses sometimes left no room for dispute, such as 'definitely' (S2), 'absolutely' (S3), 'there has to be empathy' (P2) and 'of course it is always present' (P6), whilst others offered explanations, including that it is required 'so as to perform a piece of music as the composer wanted' (P2) and 'without it, it is impossible to do anything' (P3). Some of the performers' responses promoted empathy as a prerequisite for success: 'it benefits the music and the performance' (S6) and '[it has to be present] so the work would not fall apart' (P6). Saying this, one of the soloists made the point that the existence of empathy between soloist and accompanist 'depends on how you cultivate it' (S1). Another commented that it can exist 'only up to a certain point' (S4) and that it 'depends on the person you are working with' (P5). One of the pianists offered that 'sometimes musical material sets up a competition between soloist and accompanist ... there are some contemporary works where the two musicians are set up to be at odds with one another' (P1). Interestingly, a similar viewpoint was shared by another pianist who remarked that 'being empathic will not necessarily be reciprocated or bring about the desirable results' (P5), and another who claimed that 'it could be boring to be completely empathic all the time as sometimes you need to spar against each other' (P7). This point was also reinforced by the pianist who commented that 'great performances can be achieved by having two contrasting minds at work which are not necessarily in empathy' (P4). The one participant who indicated that empathy should not be present between soloist and accompanist made the point that it was not necessary if the musicians 'already accepted each other' (S5).

The presence of empathy therefore reflects something about the nature of the relationship between soloist and accompanist. The participants' responses determined that empathy is present, must be present, may be present, is not present, or that empathy can be cultivated, depending on the specific relationship between the two performers as well as the kind of musical repertoire being performed. To this end, performers might consider themselves to be 'in empathy' or 'out of empathy' during performance activity, although there could be times when they are working towards achieving these experiences. The specific empathic nature of the piano accompanist is, once again, blurred in these data with the potential experiences of ensemble players in general, although contrary to previous studies (Haddon & Hutchinson, 2015; Myers & White, 2012), these participants do not assume that empathy is always a positive phenomenon (cf. Laurence, 2009; see also Laurence, this volume). Furthermore, while it was assumed at the outset that empathy is both dynamic and emergent, and that it underpins collaborative creative music-making, these participants suggested that it is not always desirable or indeed necessary in the achievement of ensemble playing. Rather, empathy may be perceived to be a divergent and unwanted phenomenon in group music-making.

Functions of empathy

Most of the participants reported that they had experienced empathy with their duo partners and could identify specific scenarios based upon either personal incidents or hypothetical situations whereby an accompanist might demonstrate empathy towards a soloist. Three functions of empathy were described, reflecting both musical and socio-emotional aspects of the relationship between co-performers: dealing with interpersonal dynamics; offering support and reassurance; and experiencing a connection. With regard to *dealing with interpersonal dynamics*, performers commented on the communication between soloist and accompanist as empathic when one is on the same wavelength, whether this involves agreeing or being in conflict with one other. On the one hand, this communication might be essentially non-verbal: it is 'when you share an almost telepathic communication' (P3); 'when you communicate musically without words' (S7). On the other, verbal communication might underpin the interpersonal dynamic: it is 'when you arrive at an accumulative decision about the interpretation' (P1); or 'when you have different opinions about interpretation and discuss alternatives' (P6).

In the second function, *offering support and reassurance*, performers expressed understanding and discretion towards their partner, such as through knowing when to keep a distance ('when you are aware of the soloists' behaviour pattern before a performance and letting them be, allowing them to deal with it as they feel, rather than well-intentionally interfering which could result in making matters worse' (P3)) and when to offer direct support ('when your partner takes on board your technical difficulties adjusting their performance in order to accommodate you' (P1); or 'when you or your partner make a mistake and they feel really bad about it, and the other reassures them that it is okay' (S3)). Similarly, performers described situations of this kind which involved coping with nerves and diffusing tense situations: 'when the accompanist takes the upper hand to help with the soloist's tempo fluctuations due to stress during a performance' (S4); 'when the pianist is not affected by the soloist's nervousness, and manages to calm them down by being supportive and solid' (S6); 'when the accompanist has been very calm and relaxing during a soloist's stressful situation, such as an audition' (S3); 'when the accompanist helps in regaining the performance flow after a soloist's memory lapse' (S2), or 'when the soloist is made to feel comfortable during a very important performance in their life' (S3). Crucially, in the majority of these examples given, emphasis was largely placed upon the accompanist to morally and musically support and reassure the soloist rather than vice versa.

The third function, *experiencing a connection*, included incidents whereby the two performers experienced a notable bond, whether musically, emotionally and/or socially. Examples included moments when a pianist was described as 'knowing and anticipating correctly what your soloist is going to do' (P7), or 'when you enjoy performing with your partner' (P2), or 'when both experience a difficult situation during a performance where they are both affected, ultimately resulting in increasing the bond between them' (S3). Outside of the rehearsal and performance arena, one soloist remarked that an empathic connection could be made 'when the two performers make time to socialise and become friends' (S4).

As distinct from other ensemble players, then, the piano accompanist was described as offering high levels of moral and musical support and reassurance. The examples provided by these participants reflected the specific actions of accompanists towards soloists in accommodating partnerships, indicating that the empathic nature of the piano accompanist is more one-sided than that of soloists (and potentially other ensemble players). Even though empathy may still be regarded as intersubjectively motivated and shaped by interpersonal awareness, that motivation and awareness may be fundamentally skewed towards the piano accompanist in this context.

Influences on empathy

Other issues arose through discussion of certain scenarios that highlighted a range of influences on empathy in the solo–accompaniment context: liking, familiarity, friendship and experience. In one scenario, empathy was related to either liking or disliking a co-performer. Interestingly, this issue was raised by pianists only. P2 and P6 underlined the importance of liking a partner whereas P3 emphasised that it may be necessary to empathise with a co-performer that one dislikes but has to work with, thus retaining a professional stance by overriding personal feelings (see also Gritten, this volume). Another scenario raised the question of whether differences in personal opinion and musical backgrounds could lead to a breakdown of empathy (P1 and S1). To avoid this breakdown, P1 expressed the view that empathy should be more like a 'compromise than a dictatorship' with 'overtones of kindness' and consideration towards a partner. S2 believed that empathy is about having a good working relationship and musical chemistry with a partner, whereas S4 considered that two people should be able to create musical synergy despite differences in character. Negativity through disliking, therefore, was put across as something to be dealt with so as to be avoided.

Issues of liking were often related to the notion of familiarity in developing empathy (see King & Prior, 2013; Waddington, 2015). Specifically, S1 commented that the presence of empathy depends on how one cultivates it. P1 suggested that it is possible that empathy has a timescale, nurturing an empathic relationship with someone over a period of time. Further, this relationship could be long term or short term depending on the nature of the partnership, the empathy present over one single performance being different to the empathy blossoming over a longer collaboration. P2 claimed that 'empathy can grow the more you perform together' (P2), thus allowing a piano accompanist to get to know their soloist's musical and technical trends. P3 emphasised the importance of being able to be completely open with their partner to the extent that it feels like 'going to a psychiatrist'; the reason behind this view was that soloists and accompanists should be able to talk about absolutely anything within the boundaries of the rehearsal room, provided that it would help the music. The importance of trust is implicit in these remarks (see also Gritten, this volume).

Friendship was also associated with familiarity. Participants separated friendship from empathy, one not necessarily being the prerequisite of the other. For example, P5 and S3 reported that developing empathy with an individual that one is regularly working with and building a long-term relationship with them does not necessarily lead to friendship; instead, they implied that it could lead to an empathic understanding shared on professional grounds for the sake of the music. This point resonates with aspects of Laurence's (2009; see also Laurence, this volume) work on musical empathy and, in particular, the relationship between musicking (Small, 1998) and empathising. Laurence finds that empathy does not always transcend shared musical experiences. On the other hand, according to S4, becoming friends with your partner has other advantages to the music as 'the closer you become to your partner the more comfortable you feel during a performance'.

Finally, the pianists talked about demonstrating empathy towards their soloist through offering practical help as if assuming the role of a coach. In such cases, experience in working with soloists as well as with different repertoire was considered to be fundamental. P1 suggested that 'empathy can have a technical dimension' where, for instance, the pianist could offer technical solutions to issues raised during the rehearsals, such as repeatedly rehearsing a passage where the breathing is difficult for the soloist (P1), or offering advice on alternative fingering to a wind player for a note which is not quite in tune with the piano (P7). Knowledge of repertoire could also assist accompanists in recognising potential danger areas within certain pieces. P5 commented that they would normally like to establish what the soloists' difficulties are so they can adjust their playing to accommodate them, such as by playing a chordal passage in a way that allows the soloist more space to breath. Moreover, analytical expertise could be applied in helping a soloist to understand why a breathing issue arises and guidance could be offered in assisting the soloist to analyse the situation in order to discover what they need to do to make sure they do not run out of breath.

To this end, all of the pianists were asked whether or not they can detect and consequently attempt to prevent technical, musical or other issues that may arise either in rehearsal or in performance. P1 mentioned that there are certain clues concerning imminent mishaps, such as the soloist altering their articulation in order to compensate for running out of breath, while P5 stated that the pianist instinctively senses the soloist's intentions by being 'attuned' to what is happening. There was a common belief amongst the pianists that the rehearsals are about minimising such risks (P1), by setting the expectations and the boundaries of flexibility (P1), and being prepared about what could happen in the real performance (P2). The actual performance is less predictable as there are many factors which could derail the preparation (P1), therefore the pianists indicated that they would apply techniques which would help in rectifying a possible error, such as skipping a passage or shaping a phrase in a different way (P2). P3 insisted that 'in performance, you simply cover, always cover, you must never ever allow an audience to feel that the other person has gone wrong, ever'. If part of the empathic process involves identifying and responding to the intentions of co-performers (see Waddington, 2015; see also Waddington, this volume), this further implies that for piano accompanists, the empathic process is rather one-sided as levels of identification and response may be greater than for soloists.

Alternatives to empathy

The final part of the interview provided performers with the opportunity to identify other words or terms that might be used to describe the relationship between soloists and accompanists in the duo ensemble. Table 12.1 summarises the data. Some of the participants' responses overlapped with elements of their definitions of empathy that emerged earlier on in their interviews, notably through describing the relationship itself (marriage, collaboration, interaction, friendship, equality), actions towards their co-performers (support, flexibility, sensitivity, responsiveness) and character traits (open, honest, reliable, sympathetic, trusting). It is interesting to note that one pianist used the word 'sympathetic' having spoken previously about empathic aspects of accompanying. These two terms, as discussed elsewhere in this volume, have a shared history (for example, see

Table 12.1 Alternative words used by participants to describe the relationship between soloists and accompanists.

Pianists' Responses	Common Responses	Soloists' Responses
Dynamism	Collaboration	Bonding
Exploration	Connection	Familiarity
Marriage	Creativity	Friendship
Open	Equality	Honesty
Partner	Flexibility	Other-half
Respect	Interaction	Reliability
Responsiveness	Sensitivity	Support
Sympathetic	Understanding	Trust

Laurence, this volume). Indeed, it was noted by these participants that some of their suggested terms could be used interchangeably to describe similar aspects of relationships among co-performers in ensemble playing, both within and beyond the solo–accompaniment duo context, indicating that empathy is one of many facets of group activity, all of which are potentially interlinked.

Conclusions

To summarise, the data acquired from current professional practitioners indicate that empathy is likely to be present among soloists and accompanists working together in the Western art duo chamber context. Even though there are differing opinions about the sustainability and even desirability of its presence – one may be 'in' or 'out' of empathy at any one time during rehearsal and/or performance subject to the nature of the repertoire and individual performers – there was a sense that empathy could and should be cultivated. Nevertheless, at times, empathy could be regarded as a divergent, rather than emergent, phenomenon. According to these performers, empathy is defined by the character traits and working ethos of the performers in a partnership, similar to the 'shared approach' identified by the participants in Waddington's (2015) research. Moreover, these performers considered empathy to be portrayed through the relationship between co-performers and one's actions towards co-performers, hence it is dependent upon the 'partner's involvement' (Kokotsaki, 2007) and is shaped by 'interpersonal awareness' (Myers & White, 2012) as well as 'intentional awareness' (Waddington, 2015). The functions of empathy described by these performers further reflect upon the nature of this interpersonal awareness: empathy exists when performers deal with interpersonal dynamics, offer moral and/or musical support and reassurance to one another, and experience a particular bond, or, to use Waddington's term, a 'special connection'. Factors influencing the experience of empathy – including degrees of liking and familiarity among players as well as levels of friendship and performance experience – were considered to impact upon the nature of that empathic interpersonal awareness and connection. Kokotsaki's (2007) pianists referred to familiarity in the context of time availability in performance preparation and these pianists similarly explained that empathy might grow across short- and long-term collaborations. Likewise, there are allusions to the importance of trust in group music-making, which resonate with ideas put forward by Anthony Gritten (see Gritten, this volume)

Similar perspectives, therefore, were ascertained from these performers compared with those in previous studies exploring the notion of empathy in ensemble playing. What is interesting, however, is that in the context of the solo–accompanist partnership, empathic interpersonal awareness involving support and reassurance among players was only described from the direction of accompanists towards soloists, whilst other scenarios referred to mutual experiences. This suggests that there could be a prevalent expectation for this particular kind of empathy to be more one-sided than evident in other Western art chamber music ensembles: the accompanist, rather than the soloist, is normally expected to cushion the partnership through offering support and reassurance to the soloist, thus acting in the majority of instances as the assumed empathiser (or even therapist). It is perhaps mostly in this regard then – through offering levels of (moral and musical) support and reassurance – that an accompanist may be seen to determine or at least strongly contribute towards the success of a soloist, for this kind of empathic interpersonal awareness may distinguish one accompanist from another and from other co-performers working in chamber groups. If socio-cultural and musical expectations of Western art performers have contributed towards determining the empathic nature of the piano accompanist, one must also consider whether or not the conditions of the partnership are influenced in any way by related circumstantial factors, such as the physical presence or absence of scores during performances. For instance, if the soloist performs from memory, or if the pianist works from a piano part only (without sight of the full score), the empathic relationship between the performers may be affected. Further research is necessary to fully investigate these claims.

The alternative words used to describe the relationship between soloists and accompanists reflected similar attitudes among the performers about the nature of the duo partnership as well as the possibility that empathy could be explained in other terms. The performers' perspectives pointed towards the fact that the general opinion about the piano accompanist is changing among contemporary practitioners: the stereotypical and mythical perception of the pianist as inferior to the soloist was not reinforced. These soloists regarded the accompanist as 'playing with' rather than 'playing for' them, or, in the words of one soloist, as their 'other half'. A sense of equality was expressed via references to collaboration, connection, interaction, flexibility, trust and understanding. Even though, as Katz (2009) and others imply, there is still a need to increase awareness about the contribution of piano accompanists in duo chamber ensemble performance, these performers underlined their significance within this context through discussion of empathy. And, while the data indicated that there may be unevenness in the empathic relationship in terms of the levels of support and reassurance operating between soloist and accompanist, this was not portrayed via allusions to musical or social supremacy within partnerships. Evidently, empathy in this context and other ensemble music domains needs to be explored further so that the experiential aspects of co-performer relationships continue to be scrutinised and more fully understood.

Notes

1 Other definitions and conceptualisations of empathy are presented throughout this volume: for a preliminary account, see the Introduction (King & Waddington, this volume); for an extended critique, see the Prologue (Laurence, this volume).
2 There is sometimes an assumed innateness about empathy as well as in related discussions about theory of mind and the mirror neuron system. According to Cecilia Heyes (2010), it is plausible that such skills are learned rather than innate (as explained according to the 'associative' and 'adaptation' hypotheses respectively).

References

Adami, G. (1952). Accompanying: An art. *Music Journal, 10*(6), 27–40.

Arksey, H., & Knight, P. (1999). *Interviewing for social scientists: An introductory resource with examples.* London: SAGE Publications.

Blum, D. (1986). *The art of quartet playing: The Guarneri Quartet in conversation with David Blum.* New York: Cornell University Press.

Brown, A. (1917). Hints on the art of accompanying. *Musical Herald, 830,* 138–139.

Butler, H. L. (1940). The accompanist. *The National Association for Music Education, 27*(1), 42.

Cecil, G. (1907). The art of accompanying. *English Illustrated Magazine, 54,* 596–598.

Cranmer, P. (1970). *The technique of accompaniment.* London: Books Ltd.

Davidson, J. W., & Good, J. M. M. (2002). Social and musical co-ordination between members of a string quartet: An exploratory study. *Psychology of Music, 30*(2), 186–201.

Doğantan-Dack, M. (2015). Response to Haddon and Hutchinson: Empathy in ensemble performance. *Empirical Musicology Review, 10*(2), 154–156.

Foss, H. J. (1924). The art of accompanying songs. *Musical Times, 65*(981), 979–984.

Haddon, E., & Hutchinson, M. (2015). Empathy in piano duet rehearsal and performance. *Empirical Musicology Review, 10*(2), 140–153.

Heyes, C. (2010). Where do mirror neurons come from? *Neuroscience and Biobehavioural Reviews, 34,* 575–83.

Hoblit, H. A. (1963). The art of accompanying. *Music Educators Journal, 50*(1), 139.

Katz, M. (2009). *The complete collaborator. The pianist as a partner.* Oxford: Oxford University Press.

Keller, P. E. (2008). Joint action in music performance. In F. Morganti, A. Carassa & G. Riva (Eds.), *Enacting intersubjectivity: A cognitive and social perspective to the study of interactions* (pp. 205–221). Amsterdam: IOS Press.

Keller, P. E., Novembre, G., & Hove, M. J. (2014). Rhythm in joint action: Psychological and neurophysiological mechanisms for real-time interpersonal coordination. *Philosophical Transactions of the Royal Society B, 369*: 20130394.

King, E. C., & Ginsborg, J. (2011). Gestures and glances: Interactions in ensemble rehearsal. In A. Gritten & E. King (Eds.), *New perspectives on music and gesture* (pp. 177–202). Farnham: Ashgate.

King, E., & Prior, H. M. (Eds) (2013). *Music and familiarity: Listening, musicology and performance.* Farnham: Ashgate.

Kokotsaki, D. (2007). Understanding the ensemble pianist: A theoretical framework. *Psychology of Music, 35*(4), 641–668.

Laurence, F. (2009). Music, empathy and intercultural understanding. Retrieved from http://www.slideshare.net/WAAE/music-empathy-and-intercultural-understanding-felicity-laurence.

Lyle, W. (1923). Accompanying and accompanists. *Sackbut, 4,* 6–8.

Martineau, M. (2008). Radio broadcast on piano accompaniment (15 April). In W. Robbins (Executive Producer), *Studio Sparks with Eric Friesen.* Ottawa: Canadian Broadcasting Corporation.

Moore, G. (1943). *The unashamed accompanist.* London: Hamish Hamilton.

Moore, G. (1962). *Am I too loud? Memoirs of an accompanist.* London: Macmillan.

Moore, G. (1978). *Farewell recital: Further memoirs.* London: Taplinger.

Myers, S. A., & White, C. M. (2012). 'Listening with the third ear': An exploration of empathy in musical performance. *Journal of Humanistic Psychology, 52*(3), 254–278.

Novembre, G. Ticini, L. F., Schütz-Bosbach, S., & Keller, P. E. (2012). Distinguishing self and other in joint action: Evidence from a musical paradigm. *Cerebral Cortex, 22,* 2894–2903.

Small, C. (1998). *Musicking: The meanings of performing and listening.* Hanover, NH: Wesleyan University Press.

Strauss, A., & Corbin, J. (1990). *Basics of qualitative research: Grounded theory procedures and techniques.* Newbury Park, CA: Sage.

Tomes, S. (2004). *Beyond the notes: Journeys with chamber music.* Woodbridge: The Boydell Press.

Tracy, S. J. (2013). *Qualitative research methods: Collecting evidence, crafting analysis, communicating impact.* Oxford: Wiley-Blackwell.

Waddington, C. E. (2015). *Co-performer empathy in expert ensemble playing* (Unpublished doctoral dissertation). University of Hull, UK.

Waterman, M. (1996). Emotional responses to music: Implicit and explicit effects in listeners and performers. *Psychology of Music, 24,* 53–67.

Zeckendorf, S. (1953). Accompanying is a partnership. *Music Journal, 11*(6), 28–29.

Index

Interpersonal Reactivity Index (IRI) 13, 141
intra-parietal area 210

Jackson, Vivian 'Yabby You' 203–4
Jamaican popular music 6, 194–206; dub mixing in 6, 194, 201–5; *see also* groove; reggae
jazz performance 5–6, 146–7; empathy in 2, 148–9, 157–69; improvisation 158, 159, 211; performance of spontaneity in 168; viewing 161–9
Jodalen, H. 259
Juslin, P. N. 130
Juslin, Patrik 42

Kalliopuska, M. 2, 151
Katz, M. 279
Keller, Peter 268, 269; Distinguishing self and other in joint action 147; Ensemble performance 230; Perceiving bodies in motion 151; Perceiving performer identity and intended expression intensity in point-light displays of dance 151
Kenneth M. Bilby oral history collection on foundations of Jamaican popular music 194, 195, 196, 197, 198, 199–200
Kiel, Charles: Grooving on participation 189; Participatory discrepancies and the power of music 175, 176, 177; theory of participatory discrepancies, The 176–7, 188, 189
Kimura, D. 105
King, Elaine 1, 7, 255–6, 267; roles of student musicians in quartet rehearsals, The 255, 258, 259, 260, 262; *see also* Goodman, Elaine
Kirschener, S. 2
Koelsch, S.: Investigating emotion with music 104; Processing of hierarchical syntactic structure in music 106–7
Kohler, E. 99
Kokotsaki, Dimitra 256, 270, 271, 278
Krebs, Angelika: Phenomenology of shared feeling 24; *Zwischen Ich und Du, Eine dialogische Philosophie der Liebe* 19
Kreutz, Gunter 149

Lahav, A. 104
Laurence, Felicity 3, 11, 158, 271; Empathic creativity in musical group practices 42, 59; Music, empathy and

intercultural understanding 276; Music and empathy 26, 33n38, 157, 159
Lavy, M. M. 130
League, Michael 161, 162, 165, 167, 168, 170n8
learning disabilities, music development with 39, 53–5, 57–74
Lee, Vernon 18
Leman, M. 141
Levinas, Emmanuel 6, 178, 179, 191n7; *Time and the other* 178, 189; *Totality and infinity* 178, 180, 181, 182, 183, 184, 187–8, 189, 191n5
Levinson, J. 140, 141
Levitin, D. J. 107
Levy-Bruhl, Lucien 176, 189
Lewis, D. 258
Lewis, Larnell 162, 163, 164, 165, 166, 167, 168, 170n6
limbic system 109, 210
Lipps, Theodor 19, 142; *Aesthetik* 1; Einfühlung, inner Nachahmung, und Organ-empfindungen 101–2, 125; *Foundations of aesthetics* 142–4, 145, 148, 153; *Foundations of psychology* 142
Litweiler, John 158
Locke, David 199
Luchin, Adam 18
Luhmann, N. 251
Lyn, Robert 'Robbie' 196, 200

McAdams, S. 131, 132
McCalem, Murphy: *Embodied knowledge in ensemble performance* 256
McDaniel, Kris: *Ten Neglected Classics of Philosophy* 20
magnetoencephalography (MEG) 107, 209, 210, 212
Martin, Shaun 164
Martineau, Malcolm 268
Martins, M. D. 107
master-student relationship 185–7
medial frontal (premotor) cortex 211
MEG *see* magnetoencephalography (MEG)
Meltzoff, Andrew 40, 59, 64
Menon, V. 107
merged subjectivity 93
mesolimbic dopaminergic system 98
Meyer, Leonard 47
middle cingulate gyrus 101
mimicry 12; automatic 127, 133, 134; emotional 126–7; reflex 126